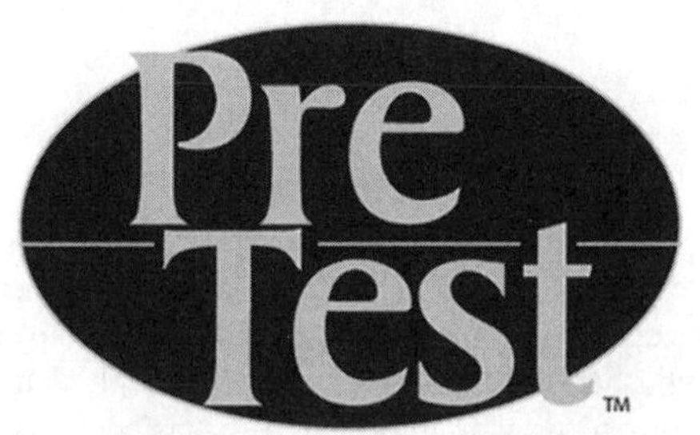

Pharmacology

PreTest™ Self-Assessment and Review

Notice

Medicine is an ever-changing science. As new research and clinical experience broaden our knowledge, changes in treatment and drug therapy are required. The authors and the publisher of this work have checked with sources believed to be reliable in their efforts to provide information that is complete and generally in accord with the standards accepted at the time of publication. However, in view of the possibility of human error or changes in medical sciences, neither the authors nor the publisher nor any other party who has been involved in the preparation or publication of this work warrants that the information contained herein is in every respect accurate or complete, and they disclaim all responsibility for any errors or omissions or for the results obtained from use of the information contained in this work. Readers are encouraged to confirm the information contained herein with other sources. For example and in particular, readers are advised to check the product information sheet included in the package of each drug they plan to administer to be certain that the information contained in this work is accurate and that changes have not been made in the recommended dose or in the contraindications for administration. This recommendation is of particular importance in connection with new or infrequently used drugs.

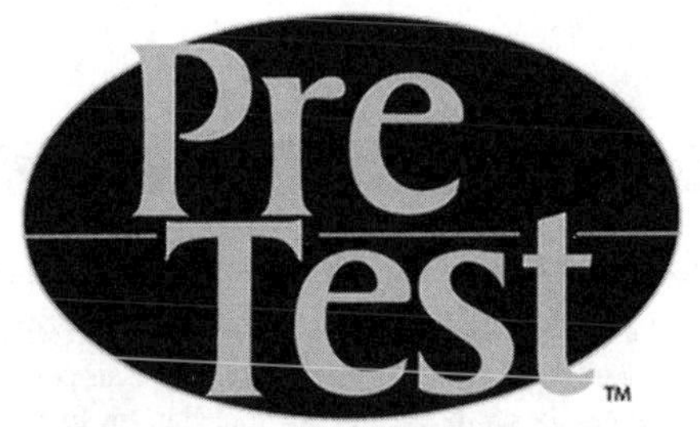

Pharmacology

PreTest™ Self-Assessment and Review
Thirteenth Edition

Marshal Shlafer, PhD
Professor of Pharmacology
Director of Undergraduate Medical Pharmacology Education
Department of Pharmacology
University of Michigan Medical School
Ann Arbor, Michigan

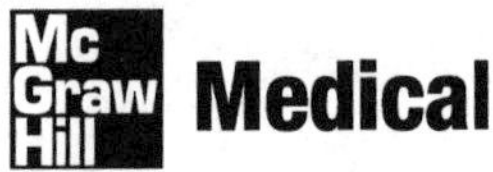

New York Chicago San Francisco Lisbon London Madrid Mexico City
Milan New Delhi San Juan Seoul Singapore Sydney Toronto

The McGraw·Hill Companies

Pharmacology: PreTest™ Self-Assessment and Review, Thirteenth Edition

1 2 3 4 5 6 7 8 9 0 DOC/DOC 14 13 12 11 10

ISBN 978-0-07-162342-1
MHID 0-07-162342-6

This book was set in Berkeley by Glyph International.
The editors were Kirsten Funk and Cindy Yoo.
The production supervisor was Sherri Souffrance.
Project management was provided by Somya Rustagi, Glyph International.
The cover designer was Maria Scharf.
RR Donnelley was printer and binder.

This book is printed on acid-free paper.

Library of Congress Cataloging-in-Publication Data

Shlafer, Marshal.
Pharmacology : PreTest self-assessment and review.—13th ed. /Marshal Shlafer.
p. ; cm.
Rev. ed. of: Pharmacology. 12th ed. / [edited by] Marshal Shlafer.
c2007.
Includes bibliographical references and index.
ISBN-13: 978-0-07-162342-1 (pbk. : alk. paper)
ISBN-10: 0-07-162342-6 (pbk. : alk. paper) 1.
Pharmacology—Examinations, questions, etc. I. Pharmacology. II. Title.
[DNLM: 1. Pharmaceutical Preparations—Examination Questions. 2. Drug Therapy—Examination Questions. QV 18.2 S558p 2010]
RM301.13.P475 2010
615′.1076—dc22

2009054285

Student Reviewers

Joseph Bart
Lake Erie College of Osteopathic Medicine
Class of 2008

Scott J. Cameron, MD, PhD
NYU Presbyterian Hospital
Weill Cornell Medical College PGY-1

Jessica Gleason
SUNY Stony Brook
School of Medicine
Class of 2010

Melisa Nika
University of Michigan Medical School
Class of 2011

Daniel Scoville
University of Kansas
School of Medicine
Class of 2011

Contents

Preface

Welcome to this, the thirteenth edition, of *Pharmacology: PreTest™ Self-Assessment and Review.* I'm pleased to have been invited back to write this edition after doing the previous two. Whether you're studying for Step 1 of the USMLE, or for a course exam that includes pharmacology content, I think you'll find this helpful to assess and strengthen your intensive and extensive knowledge of pharmacology and therapeutics—your knowledge of basic facts and principles, and your ability to apply that knowledge to some basic clinical situations.

Among the changes here you'll find in this edition are

- Many new or extensively revised questions, most based on clinical vignettes or scenarios, most pretested on hundreds of first- and second-year medical students, and all but a select few in a format you'll likely see on Step 1.
- More integration of content between the various areas of pharmacology and therapeutics, with many questions that encourage you to connect new material with content presented earlier.
- A better blend of questions that integrate basic pharmacology content with basic information from other preclinical disciplines.
- More complete explanations for why correct answers are correct and the others aren't.
- Updated cross-references to two widely used pharmacology texts in the answers so you can find additional information or explanations if you wish.
- An updated list of abbreviations of terms you will find in this text or elsewhere as they apply to drugs and drug therapy.
- A new resource that lets you look at suffixes of many generic drug names and deduce the chemical or pharmacologic group or class to which the drug belongs.

Introduction

"Even though your profs may tell you otherwise, pharmacology is pure memorization . . . the ultimate challenge in medical memorization . . . some remedy to dull the pain of the subject is needed."

That was the admonition to students in a popular exam study aid written, of course, by students.

"*Baloney*," I say.

My Perspectives on and Approaches to Learning "Pharm"

Before you get on with your studying, I'd like to give you a little insight into who another otherwise faceless author might be, because it might explain where I'm "coming from" when I prepared this book.

Having taught many areas of pharm over the last 25 years, to more University of Michigan Medical School students than I can count, I know that things pertaining to pharmacology and therapeutics are overwhelming in terms of breadth, detail, number, and consequences. A generation or so ago the pharmacologic armamentarium (and what you ostensibly needed to know) was a small fraction of what it is now. Now the number of drugs is in the thousands, and new drugs are coming at a mind-boggling frequency. Do you need to know about them all? Can you possibly be taught about, or be expected to learn, everything? In my opinion, no.

There's simply too much information, and too much presented to you in the preclinical years. Even though a host of drugs "exist" there's little point in knowing about them all explicitly. Trying to do so would be a futile and needless task, and truth be told many of the new drugs are not-so-creative spin offs of what I refer to as the "oldies but goodies." No matter how well you think you know your information (pharmacology or otherwise), no matter how completely or comprehensively you've been taught, all the content tends to become jumbled and incomprehensible when you're faced with the task of "knowing it all" all at once. You lose sight of the proverbial forest. Knowing too much about trees and too little about the forest they're in may not be sufficient once you get into a clinical situation. You can't put yourself in the position of knowing so much about the details that you can't think in broader terms.

Borrowing from literature, you are expected to be like the cheerful Major General in Gilbert and Sullivan's *Pirates of Penzance*. You seemingly need to know "all the facts" and be able to spit them back almost without having to strain to think. Sure, it's rewarding and often important to answer an ostensibly complicated or detailed question correctly (you possess the main positive attributes of Gilbert and Sullivan's Major General). But you don't want to find yourself so bogged down in knowing the details that you miss seeing the more important big picture, or how the facts apply or relate to one another (the Major General's main flaw). The simplest or most basic concepts can be overlooked with teaching or learning that is too detailed in terms of fact and focus. (I'll also go out on a limb and state that you've also been taught, and expected to learn, a ton of information that is trivial or, at best, not necessary for your understanding and ultimate application of basic pharmacology to clinical reality.)

One example of what I'll call the Major General's syndrome involves a fairly common clinical problem, hyperuricemia and gout. A doc in the ER where I showed up one hot summer day, with a horrific gout attack (big, red, hot metatarsophalangeal joint, nothing more) asked me about my medical history (it included years of asymptomatic hyperuricemia) and what I had been doing during the prior 24 hours (drinking adult beverages while searching for ground squirrels for some lab experiments—honest!). Then he asked what I did "for a living." After hearing I taught pharm, he proceeded to cite every metabolic intermediate and enzyme in the biosynthesis of uric acid by the so-called purine degradation pathway. This is, of course, the metabolic crux of the problems in hyperuricemia and gout. He also correctly stated that xanthine oxidase generates oxygen free radicals and H_2O_2, which contribute to the pathophysiology. Inhibit xanthine oxidase with allopurinol and none of those nasty oxidants or the poorly soluble xanthine and uric acid are produced, he said. That's great. I gave him an A for his intensive knowledge.

Unfortunately, that young physician then dogmatically stated what seemed so mechanistically rational but in actuality was wrong: Given the role of uric acid in the pathophysiology of gout, and the ability to inhibit urate synthesis with allopurinol, his first choice therapy for my acute gout would be that xanthine oxidase inhibitor if his hunch about my problem was correct. (Of course it was gout!) Oops. "And what about the pain and inflammation I have now, dear doctor?" Acetaminophen or aspirin, he said. Oops times two. He flunked my critical test. I knew he made incorrect drug choices and I quickly checked myself out of the ER as soon as he said he was leaving to find a polarizing microscope. (I knew what was coming next!)

But what if I didn't know anything about gout, or pharmacology? I'd be getting an inappropriate treatment from a decidedly smart physician, but after days on his selected drugs I'd probably be hurting just as bad as when I came to the ER. (After starting an OTC NSAID—not aspirin, of course—I was quite comfortable the next morning.) So there you go: knowing a lot doesn't mean knowing the right stuff.

And So, a Disclaimer of Sorts

Your experiences from the courses and exams you've taken may be quite different from those of students in other medical schools, the medical students I've taught, or the very same students here or elsewhere taught by different profs. Therefore, the focus of questions you'll see here, and the way they're stated, may be different from those you've encountered on your exams. The explanations may differ too.

There's no one "standard" pharmacology curriculum for all medical schools. Some have separate preclinical courses for the basic sciences (anatomy, physiology, pharm, and so on). Others, such as ours, have a discipline-based curriculum in which, for example, the basic sciences applicable to cardiovascular diseases are all in one section (we call them "sequences"). And when we think about individual faculty it's obvious that points emphasized by a particular instructor may differ (sometimes markedly) in scope and orientation from those made by others.

Some faculty place considerable emphasis on detailed or complex mechanisms of drug action; detailed pathways of drug metabolism; chemical structures and perhaps structure-activity relationships; mathematical approaches to pharmacokinetics; and so on. Students leave lecture wondering what the clinical implications are. Conversely, other faculty address the clinical "relevance" of certain drugs, but do little more than say "Your 50-year-old male patient has recently been diagnosed with Type 2 diabetes mellitus. Prescribe metformin." (As Homer Simpson might say, "duh—oh, ok." But why? Always start with metformin?)

How do I know? The students are quite comfortable just chatting with me, and they tell me about it all the time.

For better or worse, I try to balance the basic science and the clinical relevance in teaching and testing. My focus usually is on the "whys" of things probably more than the "whats," and I try to reduce the number of what you'd call rat facts to a minimum. I don't spend time teaching about all the angiotensin converting enzyme inhibitors when I can teach the essentials by focusing on captopril. I prune the teaching of β-blockers by focusing on propranolol as the prototype (most representative drug), then spend some time talking about the so-called cardioselective β-blockers (atenolol, metoprolol), those that have vasodilator activity (whether by virtue of α-blockade or nitric oxide generation), trying to show how or why those drugs are different and important clinically. No discussion or testing on the two dozen or so other β-blockers.

Since there is no universally adopted or "official" medical pharmacology course or course content (and even though the National Board of Medical Examiners, who prepare your Step exams, have relatively focused learning and testing objectives), I choose material I think is important, exclude what I deem unnecessary, simplify that which can be unnecessarily complicated, try to bridge learning of basic facts and concepts and apply them clinically, and largely ignore content I think is irrelevant. For lack of a better phrase, I skip things that are just something else to learn. That's what I do in class and on exams, and that's my main approach to writing questions and explaining the answers in this book.

Suggestions on How to Use This Book

Prepare yourself to answer the questions in each chapter by studying first the corresponding material from your lecture notes and favorite (or, at least, assigned) text. This book that you hold in your hands is, after all, a review and self-assessment tool, not an original source of learning information.

Before you work on the questions and your studying overall, try to do the following:

Be able to identify main drug classes, recognizing that sometimes we use more than one classification scheme (eg, chemical; by main mechanism(s) or site(s) of action; by clinical use); and be able to cite a prototype drug for each. Conversely, given a named prototype or otherwise representative drug, be able to work backward and know the rest of the most relevant information, including the class(es) to which it belongs.

For example, you should be able to identify a group of drugs that are called dihydropyridines as a main chemical class of calcium channel blockers (CCB) that are mainly vasodilators and are used for such indications as hypertension or other conditions in which vasodilation is desired. You should know that nifedipine can be considered a prototype of the large and growing class.

You should be able to take the reverse approach by identifying nifedipine as the prototype dihydropyridine CCB; identifying the main actions of the drug and its overall class; and recognizing the main uses and adverse effects. Then you need to be able to do the same with the "other" CCBs-the nondihydropyridies-picking, say, verapamil as the best example. And once you're familiar with the basics of verapamil, you should have no problem comparing and contrasting it with a dihydropyridine. It's also important to know about what might be described as "subprototypes"—for example, what's special about atenolol or metoprolol, or labetalol, compared with the overall and prototypic β-adrenergic blocker, propranolol?

Be able to identify the class to which a drug belongs by looking at its generic name or other name.

You should have some knowledge of a drug's class by looking at it's generic name—for example, a drug that ends in the suffix "-stigmine" is a reversible acetylcholinesterase inhibitor; one that ends in "-pril" is an angiotensin converting enzyme inhibitor; and so on. Although this "look at the generic name and you'll know the drug group" technique doesn't apply to all drugs, it does apply to dozens. (To that end, I've included a table, new for this edition of PreTest™, to help you do just that.) You also need to be able to give a reasonable working definition for certain drug classification terms, such as catecholamine, SSRI, reverse transcriptase inhibitor. You get the point, I hope.

Be able to state the main expected effects or side effects of major drugs or drug classes. This should give you a good idea of what the relevant precautions or contraindications are, even if you haven't been taught about the latter, even if your learning focus hasn't been too clinical.

For example, you know that β-adrenergic blockers can reduce cardiac rate, contractility, and electrical impulse conduction velocity (especially through the AV node), and sometimes these drugs are used specifically to cause one or more of those effects. You should then realize that excessive doses may cause unwanted degrees of suppression of those cardiac parameters. And you should realize that the effects of these drugs warrant extra caution or contraindicate altogether the use of a β-blocker in patients who already have bradycardia, significantly reduced ventricular contractility, or some degree of heart block. Making these associations or extrapolations is not rocket science that you must have been taught about explicitly. You should be able to use your basic knowledge of pharmacology and drug action and of physiology and pathophysiology, to piece things together and get the correct (or most logical or likely) answer. But then again, you need to think deeper. You know that (low output) heart failure is a reduction of cardiac output, and that cardiac output is the product of heart rate and stroke volume. But do you understand why and when β-adrenergic blockers, which lower both heart rate and stroke volume, are beneficial for many patients with heart failure?

Be able to state the most important (eg, serious or life-threatening) unwanted side effects, adverse responses, and clinically relevant drug interactions for the main drugs or drug classes.

Such "must know" adverse responses to certain drugs aren't necessarily common ones, but you need to know about them anyway. For example, myopathy and rhabdomyolysis from statins are relatively rare, but you certainly need to know about them and their clinical consequences. The same applies to gingival hyperplasia from phenytoin when administered to (mainly) children; paradoxical thrombocytopenia from unfractionated heparin; coagulopathies (including paradoxical thrombosis) from loading doses of warfarin—and embryopathy when administered during the first 12 weeks of pregnancy; and so on.

Each question is written to elicit the one "best" or "most likely" correct response. Mark your answer by each question, or download, print, and use the "answer sheets" I've posted on my personal teaching web site. (The URL is www.umich.edu/~mshlafer/pharm.html. When you get there, click the PreTest™ button at the top of the page.) Don't rush. There are no penalties for going through this review and answering incorrectly, and no rewards for speed. This isn't a timed exam.

After you finish all the questions in a chapter, spend as much time as you need verifying your answers and carefully reading all the explanations. This is particularly important if you chose a wrong answer, didn't have a clue about what the right answer might be, or just made a lucky guess, perhaps because of your test-savvy skills. I wrote most of the explanations to reinforce and supplement the information sought by the questions, and sometimes to gently encourage you to look at (usually earlier) parts of this review book. Do revisit your class notes for further clarification too.

I urge you not to do one rather tempting thing: read, or even peek, at the answers to individual questions in a chapter before you've answered all the questions. I know this may be painful in a variety of ways ("no pain, no gain" as they say). Nonetheless, explanations for the answer to one question may give you a tip-off (if not the outright correct answer) to another question that might address the same drug or drug class, but from a different perspective. There is "planned redundancy" in some of the questions and the answers I've written for you, and I hope that helps.

Addendum

In 1964 Bob Dylan said it better than anyone before or since: "The times they are a-changin." I've never been a fan of change when the only apparent reason is simply to do something different. (It took years for me to forgive Dylan's switch from acoustic guitar solos to the electric guitar and a band.) If it ain't broke, don't fix, is good advice to follow in life.

Throughout my 30 plus years of professional life I've learned and taught about diseases, signs, symptoms, syndromes, and the like, called Addison's, Cushing's, Parkinson's, Prinzmetal's, and the like. I'd guess 99% of the faculty who teach here still use those possessive forms with which we Neanderthals are so familiar.

But the American Medical Association's latest "style" mandates apparently include "no possessives" as we've been using them for decades when referring to things named for their founders. (Being a cynic, or more likely a realist, I think someone equated the word possessive with oppressive, and more than a wee bit of political correctness, once again, led to . . . *change*!) At any rate, McGraw-Hill Medical subsequently adopted the new AMA style for the entire pre-test series. I'd write the possessives, the editors crossed 'em out; I'd put them back in, and you can guess the rest.

So, you'll find no attributions written in this book as a possessive applied to a specific person. Apologies, then, to Drs. Thomas Addison, Alois Alzheimer, Harvey Cushing, James Parkinson, Myron Prinzmetal, Carl Wernicke (and Sergei Korsakoff too), and many others, who earned and I think deserve some recognition of "ownership" to their seminal findings. Those ostensibly damnable and offensive apostrophes and s's are gone! It looks funny to me without them, but I invoke another adage: It is what it is.

Acknowledgments

Quick but sincere thanks to my McGraw-Hill Medical editors, Kirsten and Cindy; and to Somya Rustagi at Glyph International, who engaged in the back-and-forth insertions and deletions of apostrophes, s's, and all other sorts of stuff.

Finally, from "S" to all the first and second year students at the University of Michigan Medical School: You rock! It's been not only a privilege being part of your education, but also a ton of fun for me. And always remember: Don't be the first kid on the block to prescribe a drug just because it's new—at least, don't prescribe it for me.

And so now, as you turn the pages for your review and self-assessment, do as one of my favorite comics would encourage you to do: "Git er done!"

Good luck.

Marshal Shlafer, PhD
Department of Pharmacology
University of Michigan Medical School
Ann Arbor, MI 48109
mshlafer@umich.edu

Cross-References (for Answers) to Selected Pharmacology Texts

Brunton L, Lazo J, Parker K, eds. *Goodman & Gilman's The Pharmacological Basis of Therapeutics,* 11th ed. McGraw-Hill; 2006.

Katzung BG, Masters SB, Trevor AJ, eds. *Basic and Clinical Pharmacology,* 11th ed. McGraw-Hill; 2009.

Explanations for the answers provided in this edition of *Pharmacology: PreTest™* are cross-referenced to one or both of the above pharmacology texts.

Each text excels in certain respects, yet they differ in terms of content (what's included or not) and how it is presented. Look at the text cross-references in each of my answers and you'll see the differing focus. One text may be more mechanistic or more detailed; another may be more clinical; one may paint a discussion about certain drugs or drug groups, or a particular medical condition, with broader brush strokes than another. One text may address a particular point on several pages, the other on one or two, or may have no specific coverage at all. This is not surprising, and it parallels the way you were probably taught pharmacology: no one standard preclinical pharmacology curriculum for all medical schools nor any standard or consistency in how the content may be presented at a particular school, or by a particular prof, compared with another.

Generic Drug Name Recognition Guide

I've compiled this list with the hope that it may help you look at a drug's generic name and figure out the group or class to which it belongs. I am sure there are some omissions, but the list is nonetheless quite complete. Most of the entries are arranged alphabetically by suffixes, but in a couple of instances the listing is for a prefix (eg, *ceph-* for cephalosporins) or some sequence of letters consistently found in the drugs' names (eg, *quin* in quinidine, quinine, chloroquine). **Drug names in bold** are ones I consider to be a prototype or most important example(s).

Where and how do generic drugs get their "official" names, at least in the United States? They are assigned by the United States Adopted Names Council (USANC). The USANC states that their purpose is to provide "simple, informative, and unique nonproprietary names for drugs"—the USAN. They do this by "establishing logical nomenclature classifications" based on drugs' pharmacologic relationship with others (of the same or similar type) or based on chemical similarities (eg, the core chemical structure of drugs). The USANC is sponsored by three organizations: the AMA, the U.S. Pharmacopoeia Convention (the "USP"), and the American Pharmacists Association (APhA; not to be confused with APHA, the American Public Health Association). USANC also works with the U.S. FDA and the World Health Organization's International Nonproprietary (ie, generic) Name program. Nonetheless, in the United States the FDA, not some international body, has the final say on whether a drug name is acceptable and, therefore, "official."

A side note: although many generic names are identical worldwide, there are also some glaring inconsistencies, some of which you're apt to encounter. For example, the British (and others) call acetaminophen paracetamol and meperidine is pethidine.

Where can you get more information about drug names? Point your browser to:

http://www.ama-assn.org/ama/pub/about-ama/our-people/coalitions-consortiums/united-states-adopted-names-council.shtml

Generic Drug Name Suffix	Selected Examples	What the Drug Usually Is—Drug Class	Some Noteworthy Exceptions (Drugs that Don't Fit Naming Convention) or Comments
-abine	**Cytrarabine**, gemcitabine	Pyrimidine analog antimetabolite anticancer drug, phase nonspecific	**Fluorouracil**, floxuridine
-abinol	**Tetrahydrocannabinol, dronabinol**	Cannabinoid, mainly used therapeutically for emesis control	—
-actant	Beractant, calfactant, poractant alfa	Surfactant for prevention or treatment of (mainly premature) neonatal respiratory distress syndrome	—
-afil	**Sildenafil**, tadalafil, vardenafil	Drug used for male erectile dysfunction, inhibits cGMP breakdown by inhibiting phosphodiesterase (PDE 5)	—
-al (also see -barbital, later)	**Thiopental**, thiamylal, methohexital	Ultrashort-acting thiobarbiturate given IV for anesthesia induction (methohexital is an ultrashort-acting oxybarbiturate)	Thiopental, thiamylal, and a few others are thiobarbiturates; methohexital is the noteworthy example of an oxybarbiturate
-amivir	**Oseltamivir**, zanamivir	Antivirals, neuraminidase inhibitors (largely equieffective for Influenza A and B)	Also see -avir and -mivir below

-ane (also see -flurane, later)	**Enflurane**, desflurane, **halothane**	Usually a halogenated hydrocarbon inhaled volatile liquid anesthetic	—
-avir	**Ritonavir**, **saquinivir**, lopinavir, many others	Protease inhibitor antiretroviral drugs	Also see -amivir above and -mivir below
-azepam (also see -azolam, later)	**Diazepam, lorazepam**, flurazepam, many others	Usually a benzodiazepine-type anxiolytic, hypnotic, or related CNS depressant	not all benzodiazepines end in –azepam (eg, **midazolam**, chlordiazepoxide)
-azide	**Hydrochlorothiazide**, chlorothiazide, others	Thiazide (benzothiadiazide) diuretic	note that some important thiazide-like diuretics (chemical structures not truly like those of benzo-thiadiazides), have uses and most other properties very similar, eg, **chlorthalidone, metolazone**
-azine	**Chlorpromazine**, fluphenazine, thioridazine	Phenothiazine antipsychotics/ neuroleptics	—
-azolam (see also -azepam, earlier)	**Midazolam**, alprazolam	Certain benzodiazepines	**Diazepam, lorazepam**, flurazepam, others
-barbital (see also -al, earlier)	**Phenobarbital**, secobarbital, pentobarbital, metharbital	Mainly oxybarbiturates indicated for insomnia, anxiety, but all except for phenobarbital now seldom used; phenobarbital still used for certain epilepsies	**Thiopental**, thiamylal

(*Continued*)

Generic Drug Name Suffix	Selected Examples	What the Drug Usually Is—Drug Class	Some Noteworthy Exceptions or Comments
-bendazole	**Thiabendazole**, mebendazole, albendazole	Anthelminthic for systemic/intestinal roundworms, pinworms, etc	—
-caine	**Lidocaine, procaine, benzocaine, cocaine**, others	Local anesthetic	If drug's generic name contains only one letter "i" it is an ester (procaine, tetracaine); if the letter "i" appears twice, it is an amide (lidocaine, mepivicaine)
cef- (or ceph-) prefix	**Cefaclor, cefazolin, cephalexin**, many others	Cephalosporin antibiotic (but gives no information about generation, antibiotic spectrum, etc)	Note: you will see some listings where ceph- is replaced with cef-, or vice versa
-choline	**Acetylcholine, succinylcholine**, methacholine, others	Cholinergic receptor agonist; may be an agonist for both muscarinic and nicotinic receptors (eg, acetylcholine), or more selective for one type of cholinergic receptor over the other (eg, succinylcholine and its selective effects on skeletal muscle nicotinic receptors)	**Bethanechol, pilocarpine**

-ciclovyr (or -cyclovir)	**Acyclovir**, ganciclovir	Antiviral agents (inhibit DNA polymerase, cause premature DNA chain termination) mainly for CMV	**Foscarnet**, fomivirsen
-cillin	**Penicillin, amoxicillin**, ticarcillin	β-Lactamase inhibitor antibiotic	Note that suffix does not tell whether the drug has narrow-, broad- or extended-spectrum activity or whether it is penicillinase (β-lactamase) resistant
-codone	**Oxycodone**, hydrocodone	Synthetic or semisynthetic and relatively weak opioid (codeine-like) analgesic	—
-conazole	**Ketoconazole**, fluconazole, itraconazole	Azole antifungal drug for systemic or cutaneous mycoses	**Amphotericin B**
-coxib	**Celecoxib**	"Selective" cyclooxygenase-2 (COX2) inhibitor NSAID	—
-curine (or -curonium)	**Pancuronium**, vecuronium, metocurine	Nondepolarizing and competitive skeletal neuromuscular blocker (N_M antagonist)	Note that the prototype/oldest agent, **(*d*-)tubocurarine,** and **mivacurium,** do not fit this nomenclature
-cycline	Tetracycline, doxycycline	Macrolide antibiotic	—
-dipine (see also -ine, above)	**Nifedipine**, amlodipine, felodipine	Dihydropyridine calcium channel blocker, used mainly as antihypertensive drug	—

(*Continued*)

Generic Drug Name Suffix	Selected Examples	What the Drug Usually Is—Drug Class	Some Noteworthy Exceptions or Comments
-dronate	**Etidronate**, pamidronate	Bisphosphonate, used mainly for management of osteoporosis, sometimes used to manage hypercalcemia	—
-emide	**Furosemide**, torsemide	Loop diuretic (Na-Cl symport inhibitor; also called high-ceiling diuretic)	Bumetanide, ethacrynic acid
-ephrine	**Epinephrine, norepinephrine, phenylephrine**	Usually a direct-acting α-adrenergic receptor agonist	Of course EPI and NE also activate β-adrenergic receptors
fab	**Digoxin immune fab**	Antibody fragment	Mere presence of "fab" does not indicate antigen against which antibody or fragment is directed
-fentanyl	**Fentanyl**, alfentanyl, sufentanyl	Strong opioid (μ and κ) agonist approximately 50-100x as potent as morphine, usually given IV for severe acute pain and/or as anesthetic adjunct	Note that fentanyl is also used as a topical (transdermal) and oral analgesic (lozenge or "lollipop") for chronic pain management or as a preoperative adjunct
-floxacin	**Ciprofloxacin**, norfloxacin	Second-generation or newer fluoroquinolone antibiotic	—

-flurane	**Enflurane**, desflurane, isoflurane, sevoflurane	Volatile liquid halogenated hydrocarbon general anesthetic	**Halothane**
-gatran	Dabigatran	Anticoagulant, direct thrombin inhibitor	Slated for U.S. approval in 2010; some other direct thrombin inhibitors are not -gatrans
-glitazone	**Pioglitazone, rosiglitazone**	Oral hypoglycemic (for Type 2 diabetes mellitus) drug, more properly classified as thiazolidinediones	—
-grel	**Clopidogrel, prasugrel**	Antiplatelet drugs that work by blocking ADP receptors on platelets, eg, clopidogrel;	Ticlopidine, also an ADP blocker; seldom used because of greater risk of adverse hematologic responses (neutropenia, TTP)
-idone	**Risperidone**	Certain atypical antipsychotics, mainly used as adjunctive therapy of bipolar disorder	Aripiprazole, olanzapine

(*Continued*)

Generic Drug Name Suffix	Selected Examples	What the Drug Usually Is—Drug Class	Some Noteworthy Exceptions or Comments
-[i]mab	**Abciximab, omalizumab**	Monoclonal antibody; note that although the suffix indicates drug is an antibody, it gives no information about the antigen/ligand against which it is directed.	—
-ine	**Atropine, codeine, morphine, theophylline**	Alkaloid (nitrogen-based chemical, usually but not necessarily obtained originally from a botanical source). Note that many drugs in radically different pharmacologic classes are alkaloids, and so the suffix alone is not helpful in telling you more about the drug; however, there are some tip-offs, eg, dihydropyridine calcium channel blockers (nifedipine, amlodipine, felodipine, etc) all end in "-dipine"	—

-leukin	**Interleukin 1, etc**	Cytokine, primarily target function of B or T cells or enhance actions of another interleukin	—
-lukast	**Montelukast, zafirlukast**	Leukotriene (B) receptor used as control medication for asthma	—
-mantadine	**Amantadine**, rimantadine	Antiviral agents (mainly effective against Influenza A vs B)	—
-mivir (see also –avir, above)	**Oseltamivir**, zanamivir	Antiretroviral agents, now widely used for "swine flu" (influenza A virus subtype H1N1) prophylaxis	—
-mustine	**Carmustine**, lomustine	Nitrosourea anticancer drug, alkylating agent, phase nonspecific	Streptozocin
-mycin (see also -omycin, above)	**Tobramycin**, others	Aminoglycoside antibiotic	**Gentamicin** (with this drug an "i" replaces the usual "y"), amikacin
-novine	**Ergonovine**, methylergonovine	Ergot alkaloids used as postpartum uterine stimulants	—

(Continued)

Generic Drug Name Suffix	Selected Examples	What the Drug Usually Is—Drug Class	Some Noteworthy Exceptions or Comments
-olol	**Propranolol, atenolol**, many others	β-Blocker; name does not indicate whether nonselective $\beta_{1/2}$, "cardioselective (atenolol, metoprolol), or has other properties (eg, vasodilator)	—
-olone	**Prednisolone, methylprednisolone**	Certain glucocorticoids	—
-omycin	(1) **Bleomycin**, mitomycin, dactinomycin (2) **Erythromycin, azithromycin**	(1) Nonanthracycline antitumor antibiotics, phase-nonspecific, G_1 and S phase most sensitive (2) Certain macrolides used as typical antibiotics, not anticancer drugs	**Vancomycin** (fits neither 1 nor 2)
-osin (see also -zosin below)	**Prazosin**, doxazosin, **tamsulosin**	Selective α_1-adrenergic blocker for hypertension or (some drugs in class) for benign prostatic hypertrophy	—
-oxifen (or -oxifene)	**Tamoxifen**, raloxifene	Antiestrogen for estrogen-responsive breast cancer	**Fulvestrant**, toremifene
-oxynol	Nonoxynol, cocoxynol	Spermicide	—
-peridol	**Haloperidol, droperidol**	Butyrophenone-class antipsychotic	—

-penem	**Imipenem**, meropenem	β-Lactamase antibiotics, very broad spectrum	—
-phenidate	**Methylphenidate**, dexmethylphenidate	Amphetamine-like drugs used mainly for ADHD	—
-phetamine	**Amphetamine, dextroamphetamine, methamphetamine**	Indirect-acting (norepinephrine-releasing) sympathomimetic in the amphetamine class	—
-phylline	Theophylline, aminophylline	Methylxanthine bronchodilator	Caffeine
-plase	**Alteplase**, tenecteplase, reteplase	Thrombolytic (fibrinolytic) drug pharmacologically related to tissue plasminogen activator (tPA)	**Streptokinase** and lesser-used urokinase are thrombolytics that do not follow this nomenclature, are not tissue plasminogen activators
-platin	**Cisplatin**, carboplatin, oxiliplatin	Platinum-based anticancer drugs, phase nonspecific	—
-poside	**Etoposide**, teniposide	Topoisomerase inhibitor anticancer drug, G_2 most sensitive	—
-pramine	**Imipramine**, desimipramine	Tricyclic antidepressants	Amitriptyline, nortriptyline, maprotiline
-prazole	**Esomeprazole**, lansoprazole, omeprazole, pantoprazole	Proton pump inhibitor (inhibitor of parietal cell H^+-K^+-ATPase)	—
-pressin	**Vasopressin**, desmopressin	ADH-like, renal water-conserving drug, including vasopressin itself	—

(*Continued*)

Generic Drug Name Suffix	Selected Examples	What the Drug Usually Is—Drug Class	Some Noteworthy Exceptions or Comments
-pril	**Captopril**, enalapril, others	angiotensin converting enzyme (ACE) inhibitor	—
-profen	**Ibuprofen**, ketoprofen, flurbiprofen	NSAID, propionic acid derivative	Naproxen
-prost	**Carboprost**, latanoprost	Prostaglandin analog for open-angle glaucoma, control of postpartum labor (depending on drug)	Dino*prost*one (for cervical ripening before inducing labor), miso*prost*ol (prophylaxis of NSAID-induced ulcers) don't use this suffix, have "prost" in the generic name.
-quine	**Chloroquine**, primaquine, mefloquine	Antimalarials	Quinine is used as antimalarial (and off-label for other uses), does not use this suffix, but has "quine" in the name
-rubicin	**Doxorubicin**, daunorubicin, idarubicin	Anthracycline antibiotic/ antitumor drug, phase-nonspecific	**Mitoxantrone**
-sartan	**Losartan**, valsartan	Angiotensin II receptor blocker	—

-setron	**Ondansetron**	5-HT_3-receptor antagonist such as and others, mainly used to suppress nausea and vomiting associated with emetogenic cancer chemotherapy, radiation therapy, or several other causes	—
-sone (see also -olone above)	**Beclomethasone, cortisone, dexamethasone, prednisone,** many others	Synthetic corticosteroid with variable and drug-dependent glucocorticoid-to-mineralocorticoid activity	—
-statin	**Atorvastatin**, rosuvastatin, simvastatin, several others	HMG-CoA reductase inhibitor-type antihyperlipidemic (antihypercholesterolemic) drugs	—
-stigmine	**Neostigmine, physostigmine**, pyridostigmine, others	Acetylcholinesterase inhibitor (AChEIs), most	All "stigmines" are AChEIs, but not all AChEIs are "stigmines" (eg, **edrophonium** and the **organophosphate insecticides and nerve gases**, eg, SOMAN, SARIN)
-stim	**Filgrastim**, pegfilgrastim, sargramostim	Leukopoietic growth factor, granulocyte or granulocyte/ macrophage colony stimulating factor	—
-taxel	**Paclitaxel**, docetaxel	Taxane-type mitotic inhibitor anticancer agent, G_2 specific	—

(Continued)

Generic Drug Name Suffix	Selected Examples	What the Drug Usually Is—Drug Class	Some Noteworthy Exceptions or Comments
-tecan	Topotecan, irinotecan	Topoisomerase inhibitor, S-phase specific	—
-terol	**Albuterol**, formoterol, **salmeterol**, others	Relatively selective (and orally inhaled) β-2-adrenergic agonist such as, used for maintenance control or rescue therapy of asthma (whether for rescue or control depends on pharmacokinetic properties of individual drug, eg, albuterol for rescue or control, salmeterol for control only)	**Terbutaline** (bronchodilator and uterine relaxant [tocolytic])
-terone	**Testosterone**, fluoxymesterone, methyltestosterone	Androgens used for male hypogonadism, delayed puberty, certain breast cancers	Oxandrolone, testolactone
-tidine	**Cimetidine**, **famotidine**, nizatidine, ranitidine	Selective histamine H-2 receptor blocker	—
-triptan	**Sumatriptan**, almotriptan, zolmitriptan	Selective serotonin receptor ($5\text{-HT}_{1B/1D}$) agonist, used mainly to abort migraine headaches	—

-tropin	**Corticotropin**, somatropin, cosyntropin, thyrotropin	Modifier of anterior pituitary-hypothalamic-endocrine axis	—
-tropine	**Atropine**, homatropine, **benztropine**	Antimuscarinic (muscarinic receptor-blocking) drug	Glycopyrrolate; note that other drugs with strong antimuscarinic activity (eg, diphenhydramine, imipramine, chlorpromazine), but with other pharmacologic properties too, do not have this suffix
-tropium	**Ipratropium**, tiotropium	Orally inhaled antimuscarinic bronchodilator for COPD	—
-trozole	**Anastrozole**, letrozole	Aromatase/estrogen synthesis inhibitors	—
-triptyline (see also -ipramine, above)	**Amitriptyline**, nortriptyline	Certain tricyclic antidepressants	—
-xone	**Naloxone, naltrexone**	Opioid receptor (μ, κ) "pure" antagonist	**Nalmephene** (long-acting naltrexone analog)
-zepam	**Diazepam, lorazepam**, oxazepam	Benzodiazepine	Alprazolam, chlordiazepoxide, clorazepate
-zolamide	**Acetazolamide**, dorzolamide, methazolamide	Carbonic anhydrase inhibitor (diuretics or anti-glaucoma agents)	—

(*Continued*)

Generic Drug Name Suffix	Selected Examples	What the Drug Usually Is—Drug Class	Some Noteworthy Exceptions or Comments
-zosin (see also -osin, above)	**Prazosin**, doxazosin, terazosin	Selective, competitive α-1 adrenergic (postsynaptic) blocking drug, eg,, used as antihypertensives	**Tamsulosin**, which is used for benign prostatic hypertrophy because of its relative selectivity for α-receptors on prostate smooth muscle vs those on vascular smooth muscle cells

List of Abbreviations

Here are some common abbreviations you are likely to encounter in this edition of *Pharmacology: PreTest™ Self-Assessment and Review* or many other places where abbreviations related to pharmacology and therapeutics are found. I've tried to spell out the full word(s), and give the abbreviation parenthetically, at the first occurrence in each question or answer in this book.

Nonetheless, there are other common abbreviations that don't appear in the following pages. I've omitted symbols for chemical elements or their cationic or anionic forms (eg, Ca^{2+}, Cl^{-}), chemical formulae (eg, NaCl), abbreviations of common biochemicals (ATP, ADP, DNA, etc), Greek letters, most units of measure (volume, weight, time), and abbreviations for some common lab tests (but there are some exceptions).

I want to note that by listing abbreviations here I'm not condoning or encouraging their use when, for example, entering information into a patient's chart or medication order or record. Indeed, some of these abbreviations in patient-related documents (prescriptions and medication orders in particular) should be avoided, in large part to help avoid errors in interpreting them or their meanings or intent.

$[X]_i$—intracellular concentration, where *X* is an anion or cation
$[X]_O$—extracellular ("outside") concentration, where *X* is an anion or cation
1°—first degree (eg, 1° heart block)
2°—second degree (eg, 2° heart block)
3°—third degree (eg, 3° heart block, also called complete heart block)
5-FU—5-fluorouracil
5-HT—5-hydroxytryptamine; serotonin
6-MP—6-mercaptopurine (active metabolite of azathioprine)
A
A-II—angiotensin II
AA—arachidonic acid; amino acid
AAPMC—antibiotic-associated pseudomembranous colitis
Ab—antibody
a.c.—before meal(s) or, simply, before eating
AC—adenylyl cyclase
ACE—angiotensin converting enzyme (also known as bradykininase, kininase II)
ACh—acetylcholine
AChE—acetylcholinesterase
AChEI—acetylcholinesterase inhibitor
ACS—acute coronary syndrome
ACTH—adrenocorticotropic hormone; corticotropin
ADD/ADHD—attention-deficit (/hyperactivity) disorder
ADH—antidiuretic hormone (vasopressin [VP])
ad lib—(take) freely as desired, as much as needed, as much as you'd like
ADR—adverse drug reaction(s)
AED—antiepileptic (anticonvulsant) drug
AF (or AFIB)—atrial fibrillation
AFL—atrial flutter

Ag—antigen
AIDS—acquired immunodeficiency syndrome
ALL—acute lymphocytic leukemia
ALT—alanine aminotransferase
AMI—acute myocardial infarction
AML—acute myelogenous leukemia
ANA—antinuclear antibody
ANS—autonomic nervous system
AP—action potential
APAP—*N*-acetyl para-amino phenol (acetaminophen; known as paracetamol in the United Kingdom and elsewhere)
APD—action potential duration
APTT—activated partial thromboplastin time (eg, a measurement of anticoagulation, eg, as caused by unfractionated heparin)
ARB—angiotensin receptor blocker
ARC—AIDS-related complex
ASA—acetyl salicylic acid (aspirin); Anesthesiology Society of America
AST—aspartate aminotransferase
AUC—area under the (blood) concentration versus time "curve" (of a drug)
AV(N)—atrioventricular (node)
A-V—arteriovenous (as in A-V shunt; or differences in concentrations of a substance in arterial vs venous blood, as used to calculate clearance of a drug)
AZT—azidothymidine (zidovudine)

B

BAL—British Anti-Lewisite (dimercaprol; chelator, antidote for arsenic poisoning)
BBB—bundle branch block
bid—twice daily; spelling out twice daily is preferred
BMI—body mass index (body weight/body surface area in m^2)
BMR—basal metabolic rate
BP—blood pressure (= cardiac output × total peripheral resistance)
BPH—benign prostatic hypertrophy
BPM—beats per minute
BUN—blood urea nitrogen
BZD—benzodiazepine

C

C_{av}—average (mean) plasma concentration of a drug
C_{max}—maximum plasma concentration
C_{min}—minimum plasma concentration
C_{ss}—steady-state plasma (or drug) concentration
CABG—coronary artery bypass graft(ing)
CAI—carbonic anhydrase inhibitor
CAD—coronary artery disease; coronary heart disease (CHD)
CBC—complete blood count
CCB—calcium channel blocker
CDC—(U.S.) Centers for Disease Control and Prevention

CF—cystic fibrosis
CGL—chronic granulocytic leukemia
CHD—coronary heart disease; coronary artery disease (CAD)
CHF—congestive heart failure
CHI—closed-head injury
CI—cardiac index (cardiac output normalized to body surface area)
CK—creatine kinase
Cl—clearance (of drug); chloride
CML—chronic myelogenous leukemia
CMV—cytomegalovirus
CNS—central nervous system
CO—cardiac output (heart rate × stroke volume)
COLD—chronic obstructive lung disease
COMT—catechol *O*-methyltransferase (catecholamine-degrading enzyme)
COPD—chronic obstructive pulmonary disease (eg, emphysema, chronic bronchitis)
COX—cyclooxygenase(s); COX-1 and/or COX-2
CPZ—chlorpromazine; also used as abbreviation of a brand name product of prochlorperazine; avoid use of this abbreviation to avoid improper substitution of one drug for another
CRF—corticotropin-releasing factor
CRP—c-reactive protein
CSF—cerebrospinal fluid
CTZ—chemoreceptor trigger zone (vomiting center) in the brain stem
CVA—cerebrovascular accident (stroke)
CVP—central venous pressure
CYP—cytochrome P450 (system or member of it)

D

D_1 (D_2)—dopamine D_1 (or D_2) receptor
DA—dopamine
DBH—dopamine β-hydroxylase (enzyme involved in catecholamine synthesis)
DBP—diastolic blood pressure
DC—discontinue (also D/C)
DDI—drug-drug interaction
DFX—deferoxamine (chelator used mainly for iron poisoning)
DHT—dihydrotestosterone
DIG (or dig)—digoxin
Disp—dispense
DKA—diabetic ketoacidosis
DM—diabetes mellitus
DMARD—disease-modifying antirheumatic drug (eg, etanercept, methotrexate, many others); sometimes referred to as SAARD (slow-acting antirheumatic drug)
DOPA—dihydroxyphenylalanine
DPH—diphenylhydantoin (phenytoin)
DPI—dry powder inhaler (administration system for certain drugs, usually pulmonary drugs)
dP/dt—rate of pressure change (eg, left ventricular pressure) versus time
DU—duodenal ulcer

DVT—deep venous thrombosis
Dx—diagnosis
E
eAG—estimated average plasma glucose, calculated by a formula that converts HbA_{1C} units (expressed as a %) into more familiar units (mg/dL, mmol/L)
ECG—electrocardiogram; EKG
ED—effective dose; emergency department
ED_{50}—median effective dose
EDRF—endothelium-derived relaxing factor (nitric oxide)
EEG—electroencephalogram
EKG—electrocardiogram; ECG
EPI—epinephrine
ERP—effective refractory period (eg, of a nerve); see also RP, RRP
EtOH—ethanol (also ETOH)
F
FAB—antibody fragment
FDA—(U.S.) Food and Drug Administration
FdUMP—5-fluoro-2′-dexoyuridine-5′-monophosphate, active anticancer (anti)metabolite of fluorouracil
FEV—forced expiratory volume; FEV1, forced expiratory volume in 1 second
FFA—free fatty acids
FH_2—7,8-dihydrofolic acid
FH_4—5,6,7,8-tetrahydrofolic acid
FSH—follicle-stimulating hormone
Fx—function
G
G6PD—glucose-6-phosphate dehydrogenase
GABA—γ-aminobutyric acid
GAD—generalized anxiety disorder
GCSF—granulocyte colony–stimulating factor
GERD—gastroesophageal reflux disease
GFR—glomerular filtration rate
GH—growth hormone
GHB—γ-hydroxybutyrate (mainly a "date-rape" drug)
GI—gastrointestinal
GLP—glucagon-like peptide (eg, GLP-1)
GM-CSF—granulocyte macrophage colony–stimulating factor
G protein—guanine nucleotide–binding protein
Gp IIb/IIIa—platelet membrane glycoprotein receptor responsible for linking (via fibrinogen) activated platelets
GSH, GSSG—glutathione (reduced, oxidized)
GTT—glucose tolerance test (involving either oral [OGTT] or parenteral glucose administration); drop(s) (as in amount or dose of liquid drug; largely archaic term)
g*X*—membrane conductance of an ion, where *X* is potassium, calcium, etc (eg, gK)
GU—genitourinary

H

H_1—histamine H_1 receptor
H_2—histamine H_2 receptor
HAART—highly active antiretroviral therapy
Hb—hemoglobin (also HGB)
HbA_{1c}—glycosylated (or glycated or glyco-) hemoglobin, used to monitor glycemic control long-term
hCG—human chorionic gonadotropin
Hct—hematocrit
HCTZ—hydrochlorothiazide
HDL—high density lipoprotein(s)
HEENT—head, eyes, ears, nose, and throat (eg, as parts of a physical examination)
HF—heart failure (or CHF, heart failure with signs and symptoms of venous congestion)
HDL—high density lipoprotein (cholesterol)
HGB—hemoglobin (also Hb)
HHNKS—hyperosmolar hyperglycemic nonketotic syndrome; also abbreviated HHNS
HIT—heparin-induced thrombocytopenia
HIV—human immunodeficiency virus
H^+,K^+,ATPase—proton (hydrogen)–potassium ATPase (eg, the gastric parietal cell "proton pump")
HLBI—Heart, Lung and Blood Institute (of the National Institutes of Health)
HMG—CoA-β-hydroxy-β-methylglutaryl-coenzyme A
HPA—hypothalamic-pituitary axis
h.s.—at bedtime
HSV—herpes simplex virus
HTN—hypertension
Hx—history

I

I&O—intake and output (eg, of foods, fluids)
IBD—inflammatory bowel disease
ICP—intracranial pressure
IDDM—insulin-dependent diabetes mellitus; usually means Type 1 diabetes mellitus, however many patients with Type 2 diabetes need (are "dependent" on) insulin, so IDDM is not a suitable term nor one that automatically implies Type 1
IgE, G (etc)—immunoglobulin E, G, etc
IGF—insulin-like growth factor
IHSS—idiopathic hypertrophic subaortic stenosis
IL (-1, -2, etc)—interleukin(s)
IM—intramuscular(ly)
INH—isoniazid
INR—International Normalized Ratio, derived from and used to standardize results of prothrombin time (PT) measurements (eg, when monitoring warfarin therapy)
IOP—intraocular pressure
IP_3—inositol trisphosphate
ISA—intrinsic sympathomimetic activity; subclass of β-adrenergic blockers that also have weak agonist activity, for example, pindolol

ISMP—Institute for Safe Medical Practice (health care/safety and monitoring organization)
IT—intrathecal (administration route)
ITP—idiopathic thrombocytopenic purpura
IV—intravenous(ly)
IVP—intravenous pyelogram; IV push (rapid, bolus injection of a drug)

J

JCAHO—Joint Commission on Accreditation of Healthcare Organizations (now known as The Joint Commission)
JNC—Joint National Committee (of the National Institutes of Health), as in JNC-7—more properly known as the Seventh Report of the Joint National Committee on Prevention, Detection, Evaluation, and Treatment of High Blood Pressure

K

k_e—elimination rate constant

L

L&R—norepinephrine + phentolamine (occasionally used as IV alternative to dobutamine for short term cardiac inotropic support, enables norepinephrine to stimulate heart without causing vasoconstriction)
LA—local anesthetic
L-DOPA—levodopa
LD—lethal dose
LD_{50}—median lethal dose
LDL—low density lipoprotein(s)
LE—lupus erythematosis (see also SLE)
LH—luteinizing hormone
LHRH—luteinizing hormone–releasing hormone (hypothalamic)
LMWH—low molecular weight heparin (enoxaparin)
LR—lactated Ringer solution
LSD—lysergic acid diethylamide
LT—leukotriene
LV—left ventricle/ventricular
LVEDP—left ventricular end-diastolic pressure
LVH—left ventricular hypertrophy

M

MAC—minimum alveolar concentration (eg, of inhalation anesthetic/analgesic) expressed percent of agent in total gas mixture needed to abolish response to certain painful stimuli in 50% of patients
MAP—mean arterial pressure
MAR—medication administration record
MBC—minimum bactericidal concentration
MAO—monoamine oxidase
MAO-A, -B—monoamine oxidase type A, type B
MAOI—monoamine oxidase inhibitor
mcg—microgram; noted here because it is preferred abbreviation, instead of μg (which might be misinterpreted as mg), when writing prescriptions, making notes in the medication administration or patient chart, etc

MDI—metered dose inhaler (delivery system for some liquid orally-inhaled drugs, usually targeted to the respiratory tract)
MEC—minimum effective concentration
MH—malignant hyperthermia
MI—myocardial infarction
MIC—minimum inhibitory concentration (usually applied to antimicrobials)
mmol—millimole
MMR—measles, mumps, rubella
MOPP—chemotherapy combination used to treat Hodgkin disease, derived from generic or trade names of four drugs: **m**echlorethamine, **O**ncovin® (vincristine), **p**rednisone, and **p**rocarbazine
mOsmol—milliosmole
MP—(6-)mercaptopurine
MRSA—methicillin-resistant *S aureus*
MS—morphine sulfate; multiple sclerosis
MTX—methotrexate
N
Na-K ATPase—the sodium pump (eg, on nerve, muscle cells and some other excitable cells)
NBME—National Board of Medical Examiners (the folks who write and score your thoroughly enjoyable step and shelf exams)
NE—norepinephrine
NADH—nicotinamide adenine dinucleotide
NADPH—nicotinamide adenine dinucleotide phosphate
Na^+,K^+,ATPase—sodium–potassium–adenosine triphosphatase ("sodium pump")
NAPA—*N*-acetylprocainamide, metabolite of procainamide; type of cabbage that is the main ingredient in kim chee
NE—norepinephrine
NET—norepinephrine transporter
NIDDM—noninsulin-dependent diabetes mellitus; more properly called Type 2 diabetes mellitus, although some patients with Type 2 diabetes may require (depend on) supplemental insulin (see IDDM)
N_M—nicotinic-skeletal muscle receptors (ie, those postsynaptically at the skeletal-somatic neuromuscular junction)
N_N—nicotinic-neural receptors (those found postsynaptically in autonomic ganglia and on cells of the adrenal [suprarenal] medulla)
NMDA—*N*-methyl-D-aspartate (glutamate channel)
NMS—neuroleptic malignant syndrome
NNRTI—nonnucleoside reverse transcriptase inhibitor
NO—nitric oxide
NOS—nitric oxidase synthase
NPH—neutral protamine Hagedorn (type of intermediate-acting insulin); isophane insulin suspension
NPO—nothing by mouth (nil per os)
NRTI—nucleotide reverse transcriptase inhibitor
NS—normal saline (ie, 0.9% NaCl in sterile water)

NSAID—nonsteroidal anti-inflammatory drug; see also tNSAID
NSTMI—non-ST (elevation) myocardial infarction
NTG—nitroglycerin (glyceryl trinitrate)

O

O_2 SAT—oxygen saturation (eg, of blood sample)
OA—osteoarthritis
OC—oral contraceptive
OCD—obsessive-compulsive disorder
OD—overdose; right eye
OS—left eye
OTC—over-the-counter (nonprescription), eg, OTC drug
OU—both eyes

P

P450—cytochrome P450 mixed-function oxidase system
PA—pulmonary artery; physician-assistant
PAO_2—arterial partial pressure of oxygen
PABA—*p*-aminobenzoic acid (ingredient in some sunscreens, common preservative in some multiuse parenteral medication containers)
PAC—premature atrial contraction
PAD—peripheral arterial disease
PAF—platelet aggregating factor(s)
PAM (2-PAM)—pralidoxime (cholinesterase reactivator)
PAS—para-aminosalicylic acid
PAT—paroxysmal atrial tachycardia (see also PSVT)
PBP—penicillin-binding protein(s)
p.c.—after meal(s)
PCA—percutaneous angioplasty
PCO_2_partial pressure of CO_2
PCN—penicillin
PCOS—polycystic ovarian syndrome
PCP—*Pneumocystis* pneumonia; phencyclidine ("angel dust")
PCWP—pulmonary capillary wedge pressure
PDGF—platelet-derived growth factor
PFT—pulmonary function test(s)
PG—prostaglandin
PGE_1—prostaglandin E_1 (alprostadil)
PGE_2—prostaglandin E_2 (dinoprostone)
PGI_2—prostaglandin I_2 (prostacyclin)
P-gp—P-glycoprotein(s); permeability glycoprotein(s)
PI—protease inhibitor
PICC—peripherally inserted central (venous) catheter (eg, used for drug delivery, often referred to as a "PICC line")
PID—pelvic inflammatory disease
PKC—protein kinase c
PKU—phenylketonuria
PLC—phospholipase C

PMS—premenstrual syndrome
PNS—parasympathetic nervous system (not to be confused with peripheral nervous system)
PO—(administration route) by mouth (per os)
Po_2—partial pressure (tension) of oxygen
PPAR—peroxisome proliferator-activated receptor(s), eg, PPAR-γ, the cellular target (in nuclei) of insulin-sensitizing effects of thiazolidinediones ("glitazones," ie, pioglitazone, rosiglitazone)
PPI—proton pump inhibitor (gastric acid-antisecretory drug, esomeprazole etc)
PR—(administer) via the rectum (per rectum)
PRN—as needed (pro re nata)
PRP—pressure (eg, peak LV systolic)—(heart) rate product; platelet-rich plasma
PSVT—paroxysmal supraventricular tachycardia
PT—prothrombin time
PUD—peptic ulcer disease
Pt—patient
PT—prothrombin time (also see INR); physical therapy
PTH—parathyroid hormone
PUD—peptic ulcer disease
PVB or PVC—premature ventricular beat, premature ventricular contraction
Q
q4h—every 4 hours (or other number inserted)
qd—each day; best to spell out "daily" than use abbreviation
qid—4 times daily, spelling out 4 times a day is preferred
QTc—corrected QT interval (on electrocardiogram)
R
RA—rheumatoid arthritis; right atrium
RBC—red blood cell; erythrocytes
RBF—renal blood flow
RDA—recommended daily allowance (eg, of a nutrient)
rDNA—recombinant DNA, for example, molecular biologic technology used to synthesize or modify protein drugs such as many insulins
RP—refractory period, for example, of a nerve (also see ERP, RRP)
RRP—relative refractory period
RR—respiratory rate
Rx—prescription; abbreviation for Latin word meaning take or take thou
S
SAARD—slow-acting antirheumatic drug; also see DMARD
S-A(N)—sinoatrial (node)
SBP—systolic blood pressure
SC—see subQ
SERM—selective estrogen receptor modifier
SERT—serotonin transporter
SH—sulfhydryl
SIADH—syndrome of inappropriate ADH (arginine vasopressin) secretion, manifest as hypervolemia, hyponatremia, and reduced blood osmolality
sig—write on prescription label
SK—streptokinase

SL—sublingual (administration route)
SLE—systemic lupus erythematosus
SMBG—self-monitoring (by the patient) of blood glucose
SR—sarcoplasmic reticulum (in myocytes)
SRS-A—slow-reacting substance of anaphylaxis
SSRI—selective serotonin reuptake inhibitor
STAT—immediately
STD—sexually transmitted disease
STE—ST elevation (as in STE myocardial infarction)
SubQ—subcutaneous (eg, injection type), preferred to the abbreviation SC
SuCh—succinylcholine
SVR—systemic vascular resistance; total peripheral resistance (TPR)
SVT—supraventricular tachycardia, or sustained ventricular tachycardia
Sx—symptom(s)

T

$T_{1/2}$—half-life (of a drug)
T_3—triiodothyronine
T_4—thyroxine, levothyroxine, tetraiodothyronine
TB—tuberculosis
TCA—tricyclic antidepressant
TDP—torsades de pointes (from French, "twisting of the points")
TG—triglyceride(s)
TI—therapeutic index (LD_{50}/ED_{50})
TIA—transient ischemic attack
tid—3 times daily, spelling out 3 times a day is preferred
TKO—to keep open (as an IV infusion at a rate just sufficient to keep venous access open)
TNF—tumor necrosis factor
tNSAID—traditional nonsteroidal antiinflammatory drug, eg, aspirin, ibuprofen, many others, but not including selective COX-2 inhibitors
tPA—tissue plasminogen activator
TPR—total peripheral resistance (systemic vascular resistance)
TRH—thyrotropin-releasing hormone
TSH—thyroid stimulating hormone
TTP—thrombotic thrombocytopenic purpura (and ITTP: idiopathic TTP)
TXA_2—thromboxane A_2
TZD—thiazolidinedione (class of oral antidiabetic drugs, ie, pioglitazone, rosiglitazone)

U

UFH—unfractionated heparin (see also LMWH)
USAN—United States Adopted Name (official naming council and system for generic drugs)
UTI—urinary tract infection

V

V_d—volume of distribution (eg, of a drug)
VIP—vasoactive intestinal peptide
VLDL—very low density lipoprotein
VP—vasopressin (antidiuretic hormone [ADH])

V/Q—ventilation/perfusion (as used in pulmonary function tests)
VRE—vancomycin-resistant enterococcus
VT (VTACH)—ventricular tachycardia

W

WBC—white blood cell
WITDOOMS?INSH—Who is the dean of our medical school? I've never seen him (her).
WPW—Wolff-Parkinson-White (cardiac electrophysiologic anomaly)

X

XD—xanthine dehydrogenase
XO—xanthine oxidase

Z

ZES—Zollinger-Ellison syndrome

General Principles of Pharmacology

Dosage regimens and their consequences
Dose-response relationships
Drug-receptor interactions, signal transduction
Factors affecting drug dosage
Metabolism of drugs
Pharmacodynamics (mechanisms of drug action)
Pharmacokinetics (time-, dose-, and concentration-related phenomena)
Regulation of drug approval and use

Questions

1. Such substances as inositol trisphosphate (IP_3), diacetyl glycerol (DAG), cyclic AMP (cAMP), cAMP-dependent protein kinases, and changes in such functions as membrane ion conductance (eg, of gK^+ and gCa^{2+}) are important with respect to the effects of ligands on cell responses. Which best summarizes where they are found or what they do?

a. Are present in nerve cells, but not the various types of muscles or glands
b. Are the receptors for various agonists and antagonist drugs
c. Interact with neurotransmitters or hormones (endogenous ligands), but not to chemicals that are not found naturally in the body
d. Mediate excitatory, but not inhibitory, responses in various target structures
e. Transduce a chemical "signal" from a ligand into the final cell response(s)

2. Azithromycin, an antibiotic, has an apparent volume of distribution (V_d) of approximately 30 L/kg. What is the main interpretation of this information?

a. Effective only when given intravenously
b. Eliminated mainly by renal excretion, without prior metabolism
c. Extensively distributed to sites outside the vascular and interstitial spaces
d. Not extensively bound to plasma proteins
e. Unable to cross the blood-brain or placental "barriers"

3. A cardiovascular pharmacologist is assessing the inotropic (contractile) responses of cardiac muscle to a variety of drugs. She uses a small animal (eg, rabbit or rat)–isolated papillary muscle preparation to gain her data. The experimental setup is shown here:

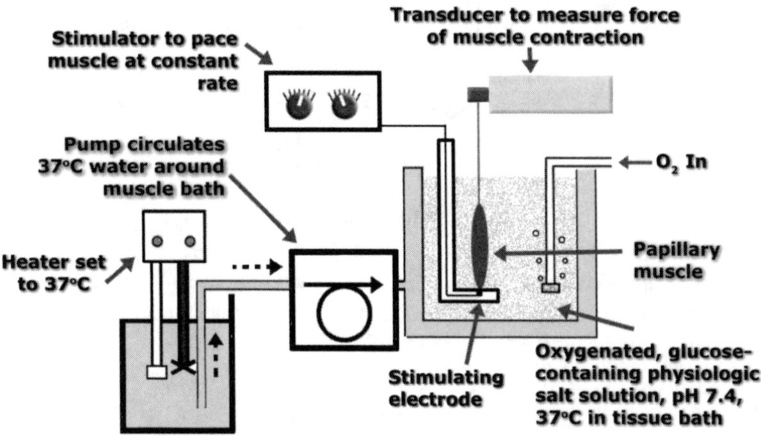

The diagram shows a papillary muscle that has been excised from the animal's heart and put into a physiologic salt solution that contains glucose, electrolytes at usual extracellular concentrations, and pH and oxygen tensions that will keep the muscle alive and functional for several hours. The papillary muscle is electrically stimulated at a constant rate so there are no rate-dependent effects on contractile force development, and all neural influences on papillary muscle function or drug responses are absent because the muscle is not innervated.

A reference standard positive inotropic drug is administered, in varying concentrations, to determine the maximum increase of contractile force (the inotropic response; maximum increase of force caused by the reference is set at 100%). Thereafter, three other drugs—X, Y, and Z—are tested, and their ability to increase contractile force development (compared with the standard or reference drug) is measured. A comparison of the positive inotropic effects of X, Y, and Z is then plotted. The dose-response curves are shown here:

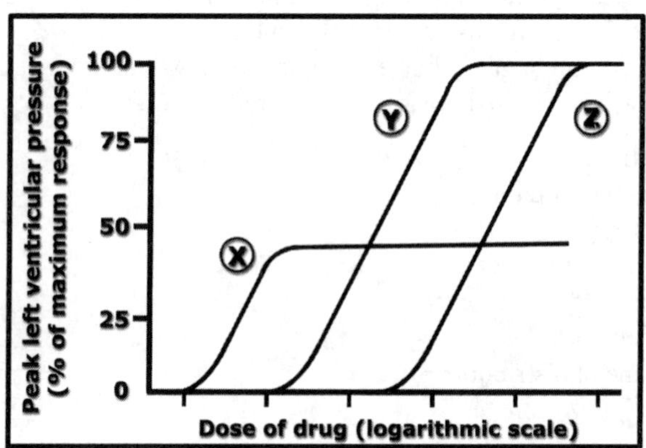

Which statement describes the findings of this experimental study involving drugs X, Y, and Z?

a. Drug X is most efficacious because its ED50 is lowest
b. Drug Y is the least potent drug among the three drugs shown
c. Drug Z is the most potent cardiac inotrope
d. Drug Y is more potent than drug Z, and more efficacious than drug X
e. Drug X is more potent than drug Y, and more efficacious than drug Z

4. We are repeatedly administering a drug orally. Every dose is 50 mg; the interval between doses is 8 hours, which is identical to the drug's plasma (overall elimination) half-life. The bioavailability is 0.5. For as long as the drug is administered no interacting drugs are added or stopped, and there are no applicable factors affecting such things as absorption or elimination that might change the drug's pharmacokinetics.

Which formula gives the best estimate of how long it will take for the drug to reach steady-state plasma concentrations (C_{SS})?

Abbreviations:
Cl = clearance (mL/min)
D = dose (mg)
F = bioavailability
k_e = elimination rate constant
$t_{1/2}$ = half-life (h)
V_d = volume of distribution

a. $(0.693 \times V_d)/\mathrm{Cl}$
b. $1/k_e$
c. $4.5 \times t_{1/2}$
d. $(t_{1/2}) \times (k_e)$
e. $D/(F \times t_{1/2})$

5. We want to estimate, following drug administration, some measure that most reliably reflects the total amount of drug reaching target tissue(s) over time. We're giving the drug orally. Which of the following would you assess to get the desired information?

a. Area under the blood concentration-time curve (AUC)
b. Peak (maximum) blood concentration
c. Product of the volume of distribution and the first-order rate constant
d. Time to peak blood concentration
e. Volume of distribution

6. Experiments show that 95% of an oral 80-mg dose of verapamil is absorbed in a 70-kg test subject. However, because of extensive metabolism during its first pass through the liver the bioavailability was only 0.25 (25%). Assuming a liver blood flow of 1500 mL/min, what is the hepatic clearance of the verapamil in this situation?

a. 60 mL/min
b. 375 mL/min
c. 740 mL/min
d. 1110 mL/min
e. 1425 mL/min

7. A classmate is doing summer research in your school's clinical pharmacology division between her first and second years of medical school. Her topic involves new investigations into the roles of P-glycoprotein. Which statement accurately summarizes the biologic role of P-glycoproteins, particularly as it affects drugs and their actions?

a. Conjugates a variety of drugs, or their metabolites, to facilitate their ultimate renal elimination from the body
b. Maintains structural integrity of cell membranes and the surface receptors found on them
c. Phosphorylates certain substances, such as in the conversion of adenosine monophosphate (AMP) into the diphosphate and triphosphate forms (ADP, ATP)
d. Transports certain drugs and xenobiotics across cell membranes
e. Works, in conjunction with various G proteins, to transduce (convert) interactions between drugs and their receptors into biologic responses

8. We are conducting pharmacokinetic studies on a new drug that we hope will be approved for clinical use. We insert a venous catheter to sample blood immediately before and at various times after drug administration. After assaying the blood samples for the drug we make a graph that plots plasma drug concentrations over time, continuing until tests reveal undetectable blood levels. What can you calculate or estimate based on the ratio of the area under the curve (AUC) obtained with oral administration versus the AUC for intravenous administration of the same drug?

a. Absorption
b. Bioavailability
c. Clearance
d. Elimination rate constant
e. Extraction ratio
f. Volume of distribution

9. We orally administer a weak acid drug (A) with a pK_a of 3.4. Gut pH is 1.4, and blood pH is 7.4. Assume the drug crosses membranes by simple passive diffusion. Which of the following observations would be true?

a. Only the ionized form of drug, will be absorbed from the gut
b. The concentration ratio of total drug ($A + HA^-$) would be 10,000:1 (gut:plasma)
c. The drug will be hydrolyzed by reaction with HCl and so cannot be absorbed
d. The drug will not be absorbed unless we raise gastric pH to equal pK_a, as might be done with an antacid
e. The drug would be absorbed, and at equilibrium the plasma concentration of the nonionized moiety (HA) would be 10,000 times higher than the plasma concentration of A^-

10. Identical doses of a drug are given orally and intravenously, we sample blood at various times, measure blood concentrations of the drug, and plot the data shown here:

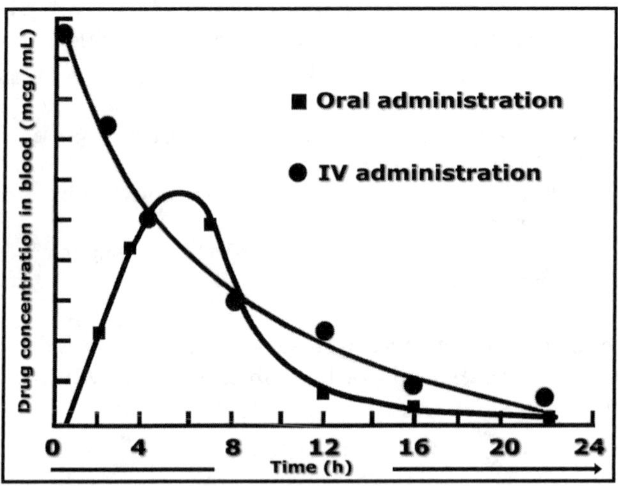

Further analysis of only these data will allow you to determine which of the following?

a. Elimination route(s)
b. Extent of plasma protein binding
c. Oral bioavailability
d. Potency
e. Therapeutic effectiveness

11. During your career you may have patients in age ranges from very young to very old, and adjustments in drug dosages or intervals between repeated doses may be required based on their age. Assume you consider only the effects of one drug; no interacting drugs or comorbidities are involved. What statement best describes the *general* relationship between chronologic age and the overall elimination plasma half-lives of drugs?

a. Depends on chemical class of drug (eg, benzodiazepine, catecholamine, dihydropyridine).
b. Depends on renal function (eg, creatinine clearance), not age per se.
c. Linear: half-life lengthens in direct proportion to age.
d. No generally applicable relationship because elimination half-life depends on the drug, not its class.
e. Peaks at around age 18 to 20 years, with half-lives being much longer at younger or older ages.

12. The elimination of a drug and its numerous metabolites is described as being heavily dependent on Phase II metabolic reactions. Which of the following is a Phase II reaction?

a. Glucuronidation
b. Decarboxylation
c. Ester hydrolysis
d. Nitro reduction
e. Sulfoxide formation

13. Instructions for administration of a hypothetical drug include the following:

- Administer only by intravenous infusion using a calibrated infusion pump; do not administer in any other way
- Dilute to a concentration of 0.5 to 5 mg/mL in sterile 0.9% NaCl before use
- Infuse at a constant rate of no less than 0.5 mcg/min (0.25 mL/min) and no greater than 2.5 mcg/min or 1 mL/min
- Use the lowest effective infusion rate for patients who may be at risk of volume overload, whether from cardiac or renal disease
- Do not exceed a total daily dose (per 24 h) of 1.5 mg (1500 mcg) in any patient; do not exceed 1 mg (1000 mcg) in patients with renal dysfunction (the manufacturer provides specific dosage recommendations based on blood creatinine levels)

Assume that throughout drug administration none of the variables given as an answer choice change. What is the main determinant of how long it will take for blood levels of this drug to reach steady-state (plateau; no change of mean blood levels over time)?

a. Bioavailability of the drug
b. Concentration of drug in the solution that will be infused
c. Half-life of the drug
d. Presence or absence of cardiovascular or renal disease
e. Plasma creatinine concentration (or creatinine clearance)
f. Total dose per 24 hours
g. Volume of drug administered per minute

14. Yee et al. Effect of grapefruit juice on blood cyclosporine concentration. Lancet. 1995;345:955-956 examined several pharmacokinetic variables related to oral cyclosporine administration with water, grapefruit juice, and orange juice:

	Grapefruit Juice	Orange Juice	Water	*p**
AUC (ng•h/mL)	7057 ± 2172	4871 ± 2045	4932 ± 1451	<0.0001
C_{max} (ng/mL)	1269 ± 381	972 ± 379	1080 ± 269	0.01
T_{max} (h)	2.86 ± 0.77	2.57 ± 0.85	2.36 ± 0.63	0.14

The numbers listed are arithmetic means ± one standard deviation of the mean. C_{max} is the peak blood concentration, and T_{max} is the time after administration at which peak plasma concentrations of the drug are reached. The *p* values (*) are based on analysis of variance corrected for repeated measures.

These data are most consistent with the hypothesis that grapefruit juice does which of the following?

a. Acidifies the urine, favoring cyclosporine's tubular reabsorption via a pH-dependent effect
b. Activates an intestinal wall transporter for cyclosporine
c. Alters the route(s) of elimination for cyclosporine
d. Inhibits metabolism of cyclosporine
e. Reduces binding of cyclosporine to plasma proteins, thereby raising free (active) drug levels in the circulation

15. A 60-year-old man with rheumatoid arthritis will be started on a nonsteroidal anti-inflammatory drug (NSAID) to suppress the joint inflammation. Published pharmacokinetic data for this drug include:

Bioavailability (*F*): 1.0 (100%)
Plasma half-life ($t_{1/2}$) = 0.5 hour
Apparent volume of distribution (V_d): 45 L

For this drug it is important to maintain an average plasma steady-state concentration of 2.0 mcg/mL in order to ensure adequate and continued anti-inflammatory activity.

The drug will be taken every 4 hours.

What dose will be needed to obtain this 2 mcg/mL average steady-state drug concentration?

a. 5 mg
b. 100 mg
c. 325 mg
d. 500 mg
e. 625 mg

16. We take a blood sample from a patient (baseline measurement) and then administer drug A intravenously. We take additional blood samples periodically thereafter and measure drug concentration in each sample. We repeat the experiment, this time giving the same drug orally. Then we plot the logarithm of drug concentration versus time with data from both administration routes to find comparable elimination "curves" indicative of first-order elimination. What do the slopes of the resulting concentration versus time curves indicate about the pharmacokinetics of drug A?

a. Area under the curve (AUC)
b. Bioavailability
c. Elimination rate constant
d. Extraction ratio
e. Volume of distribution

17. Most drugs approved by the FDA have one or several so-called "off-label" uses: uses that have not been sanctioned officially by the FDA, but for which there is reasonable evidence that the drug is both safe and effective. For which other uses can you, as a licensed physician, administer or prescribe these FDA-approved drugs?

a. Anything you wish, provided no specific laws (eg, controlled-substance laws) prohibit it
b. None—only FDA approved and written off-label uses
c. Only approved and off-label uses for older drugs in the same chemical class (eg, another thiazide diuretic, benzodiazepine)
d. Only approved and off-label uses of older drugs used for the same purpose (eg, another antihypertensive, antidepressant, or cancer chemotherapeutic agent)
e. Only uses for which there is some evidence of drug efficacy and safety in the experimental literature

18. When we evaluate new drugs in preclinical testing, one of many things we'd like to know is whether it's largely confined to the vascular compartment or distributes more widely, perhaps to specific tissues such as the lipid-rich CNS. This is, of course, ultimately important to you, the clinician, who may prescribe or administer the drug if it gets FDA approval. One way to get a handle on that is to calculate the apparent volume of distribution (V_d).

The table and graph below show some data concerning a new aminoglycoside antibiotic. We give an IV dose (5 mg/kg) of the drug to a 70-kg 21-year-old volunteer who is healthy and taking no other drugs. After allowing time for redistribution and equilibration of the drug in various body compartments, we measure plasma concentrations at various times.

Time After Dosing Stopped (h)	Plasma Aminoglycoside Concentration (mcg/mL)
1.0	5.8
2.0	4.6
3.0	3.7
4.0	3.0
5.0	2.4
6.0	1.9
8.0	1.3

Which value comes closest to the apparent V_d for this drug?

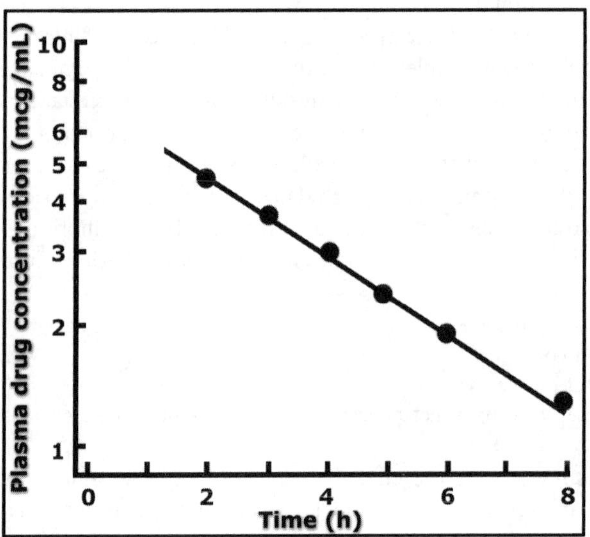

a. 0.62 L
b. 19 L
c. 50 L
d. 110 L
e. 350 L

19. You are reviewing the data from several meta-analyses that addressed the most common causes of adverse or otherwise excessive effects of prescription drugs in young adults and in the elderly (>60 years of age). Interactions between multiple drugs were not considered. Which variable would you find to be *decreased*, and be the most common general cause of these problems, in elders?

a. Body fat content
b. Lean body mass
c. Liver function
d. Renal function/clearance
e. Plasma albumin levels

20. Some texts rather emphatically state that the ability of one drug (sometimes called the "object drug") to displace molecules of another drug (the "target drug") from plasma protein binding sites, thereby raising the concentration and activity of free target drug in the blood, is not clinically relevant. The reason? Drug molecules that are displaced are rapidly eliminated and the equilibrium between bound and free drug is rapidly reestablished. This interpretation may be correct for some drugs, but not for others.

Considering only the pharmacokinetics or other relevant properties of the target drug, upon which drug-related variable does the speed of elimination and reestablishment of the bound versus free equilibrium—indeed, whether the interaction is apt to be clinically relevant—depend the most?

a. Bioavailability
b. Overall elimination $t_{1/2}$
c. p*K* (acid or base)
d. Renal clearance
e. Whether the drug is metabolized or excreted without prior metabolism

21. Upon evaluating the effects of certain sympathomimetic drugs in a variety of in vitro and in vivo models, we find that the responses exhibit the phenomenon of *tachyphylaxis*. What does the term tachyphylaxis mean?

a. An increase in the rate of the response, for example, an increase of the rate of muscle contraction
b. Immediate hypersensitivity reactions (ie, anaphylaxis)
c. Prompt conformational changes of the receptor such that agonists, but not antagonists, are able to bind and cause a response
d. Quick and progressive rises in the intensity of drug response, with repeated administration, even when the doses are unchanged
e. Rapid development of tolerance to the drug's effects

22. A postoperative patient will require prolonged analgesia. We choose a drug that has the following pharmacokinetic properties:

Half-life: 12 hours
Clearance: 0.08 L/min
Volume of distribution: 60 L

The patient has an indwelling venous catheter with a slow drip of 0.9% NaCl, and we will use this to administer intermittent injections of the drug every 4 hours. The target blood level of the drug, following each injection, is 8 mcg/mL.

With this plan in mind, and using no loading dose of the drug, which one of the following comes closest to the dose that should be administered every 4 hours?

a. 0.960 mg (or 1 mg)
b. 6.4 mg (or 6 mg)
c. 25.6 mg (or 25 mg)
d. 150 mg
e. 550 mg

23. A patient has severe postoperative pain and you plan to give a loading dose of an analgesic for prompt relief of discomfort. The drug we choose has the same pharmacokinetic properties as the one described in Question 22:

Half-life: 12 hours
Clearance: 0.08 L/min
Volume of distribution: 60 L

Our target plasma concentration for the drug is 8 mcg/mL. What number comes closest to the correct loading dose?

a. 0.48 mg (rounded to 0.5 mg)
b. 150 mg
c. 320 mg
d. 480 mg
e. 640 mg

24. We administer a highly lipid-soluble drug and monitor its elimination. All the data indicate that it is transformed to a variety of more polar and oxidized metabolites by a group of heme proteins that activate molecular oxygen to a form that is capable of interacting with organic substrates such as our test drug. What enzyme or enzyme system is most likely involved in the initial metabolism of this drug?

a. Cyclooxygenase
b. Cytochrome P450s (CYP system, mixed-function oxidases)
c. Monoamine oxidase (MAO)
d. Nicotinamide adenine dinucleotide phosphate (NADPH)
e. UDP-glucuronosyltransferase

25. We measure the heart rate of a healthy subject under the conditions noted below, allowing ample time for return to baseline conditions and full elimination of drugs between each step:

1. At rest
2. During treadmill exercise sufficient to activate the sympathetic nervous system at a time when maximum heart rate is reached
3. After administration of acebutolol, a drug with affinity for β-adrenergic receptors
4. After giving acebutolol, followed by exercise at the same level used in condition 2

Acebutolol given at rest causes a slight but consistent increase of heart rate. Give a bigger dose at rest and heart rate rises a bit more.

When the patient exercises after receiving a low-dose acebutolol, heart rate rises significantly less than it did in the absence of acebutolol. With exercise after the higher dose of acebutolol, the tachycardia is blunted even more.

The figure below summarizes the main findings. Which statement best summarizes the actions of acebutolol?

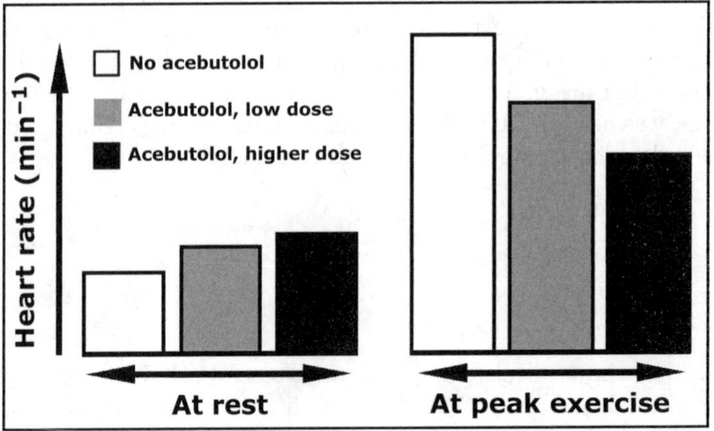

a. Has higher affinity for adrenergic receptors than the endogenous agonists, epinephrine, and norepinephrine
b. Is a partial agonist for β-adrenergic receptors
c. Is activating spare receptors on myocardial cells
d. Is an irreversible or noncompetitive β-blocker
e. Is changing conformation of the adrenergic receptors

26. We are planning to infuse a drug intravenously at a constant amount per unit time (rate). It has a first-order elimination rate constant (k_{el}) of 0.35/h. No loading dose will be given. Approximately how long will it take for blood levels to reach steady state after the infusion begins?

a. 0.7 hour
b. 1.2 hours
c. 3.5 hours
d. 9 hours
e. 24 hours

27. A patient who is supposed to be taking a drug once a day gets confused and for a couple of days takes excessive daily doses, leading to toxicity. The drug has a mean plasma half-life of 40 hours.

Right now the patient's plasma concentration of the drug is 6 mcg/mL. Although what to do next will depend on actual blood tests for drug levels, the usual plan in this case is to have the patient skip one or several daily doses of the drug until blood levels first enter the therapeutic and nontoxic range, which in this case is 0.8 mcg/mL. Assume the drug is eliminated by first-order kinetics. How many daily doses should be withheld?

a. 1
b. 2
c. 3
d. 4
e. 5

28. We want to calculate the apparent volume of distribution (V_d) for a hypothetical drug (drug A) that has a half-life of 4 hours. All (100%) of an absorbed dose of this drug undergoes Phase I oxidation, followed by conjugation (Phase II reaction) and then renal excretion.

We rapidly inject a known dose and 30 minutes later begin taking serial blood samples (30 min apart) to measure drug concentration in each sample. What one other piece of information must be measured or otherwise determined to calculate V_d in the easiest way?

a. Area under the drug concentration-time curve (AUC)
b. Bioavailability (F)
c. Clearance (Cl)
d. Elimination rate constant (k_{el})
e. Maximum blood concentration after the bolus injection (C_0)

29. A patient with a bacterial infection requires intravenous antibiotic therapy. The chosen drug has a clearance of 70 mL/min. The apparent volume of distribution is 50 L. The plan is to administer the drug intravenously every 6 hours and achieve a 4 mg/L steady-state blood level of the drug. No loading dose strategy is to be used. What maintenance dose is needed to achieve this?

a. 14 mg
b. 24 mg
c. 100 mg
d. 300 mg
e. 1200 mg

30. A pharmacologically inert but easily measured substance, X, is eliminated in a manner that follows linear kinetics (first-order; plot of log drug concentration vs time during elimination is a straight line). The plasma half-life is 30 minutes. Bolus IV doses well in excess of 100 mg must be given in order to saturate the enzymes responsible for metabolizing the drug, which will then lead to zero-order elimination kinetics.

We infuse a solution of X intravenously. The concentration of the solution is 2 mg/mL; the infusion rate is 1 mL/min and is kept constant at that. We continue the infusion for 24 hours.

After allowing ample time for the drug to be eliminated completely, we repeat the administration. This time the concentration of the solution of X is 4 mg/mL, and we infuse it at a rate of 2 mL/min.

Which other variable will also be changed as a result of the stated changes to the infusion protocol?

a. Elimination rate constant
b. Half-life
c. Plasma concentration when C_{SS} is reached
d. Time to reach steady-state concentration (C_{SS})
e. Total body clearance
f. Volume of distribution

31. A new drug, drug A, undergoes a series of Phase I reactions before its metabolites ultimately are eliminated. Which statement best describes the characteristics of drug A, or the role of Phase I reactions in its metabolism or actions?

a. Complete metabolism of drug A by Phase I reactions will yield products that are less likely to undergo renal tubular reabsorption
b. Drug A is a very polar substance
c. Drug A will be biologically inactive until it is metabolized
d. Phase I metabolism of drug A involves conjugation, as with glucuronic acid or sulfate
e. Phase I metabolism of drug A will increase its intracellular access and actions

32. Dopamine, epinephrine (or norepinephrine), and histamine are important neurotransmitter agonists. When these ligands interact with their cellular receptors, how do they mainly elicit their responses?

a. Activate adenylyl cyclase, leading to increased intracellular cAMP levels
b. Activate phospholipase C
c. Induce or inhibit synthesis of ligand-specific intracellular proteins
d. Open or close ligand-gated ion channels
e. Regulate intracellular second messengers through G protein–coupled receptors

33. The FDA assigns the letters A, B, C, D, and X to drugs it approves for human use. To which of the following does this classification refer or apply?

a. Amount of dosage reduction needed as plasma creatinine clearances fall
b. Amount of dosage reduction needed in presence of liver dysfunction
c. Fetal risk when given to pregnant women
d. Relative margins of safety (or therapeutic index)
e. The number of unlabeled uses for a drug

34. The Food and Drug Administration has broad regulatory authority over prescription drugs, OTC drugs, and nutritional supplements (herbals and other so-called nutriceuticals). Such authority includes approval, marketing (advertising), and withdrawal of drugs from the market. Which statement summarizes an element of FDA rules or guidelines?

a. Drugs approved for sale OTC first received FDA approval for sale and marketing "by prescription only"
b. If a pharmaceutical manufacturer provides data sufficient to obtain FDA approval for sale by prescription, the manufacturer is then allowed to sell the drug over-the-counter (OTC)
c. If the FDA approves a prescription drug for sale (prescribing), the physician can prescribe the drug only for the FDA-approved indication (use)
d. Nutritional supplements can be marketed without providing proof of efficacy or safety to the FDA
e. Phase III testing of prescription drugs that have been approved by the FDA gives complete information about adverse responses and pertinent drug-drug interactions

35. You have just evaluated and started treatment on a 40-year-old woman in whom you have diagnosed malignant hypertension, based on her history, her clinical presentation, and the blood pressure changes you measured over the relatively short time you've been at the bedside. You now go to the family and explain your diagnosis. You explain in simple terms what hypertension means. But when they hear the word malignant one of the family members says "Oh, her blood pressure is high because she has cancer?" How should you best explain the term malignant to the family?

a. Blood pressure is rising very quickly and dangerously
b. Cancer is present but it is not the cause of the high blood pressure
c. Her high blood pressure is, indeed, caused by a cancer ("malignancy"—in this case probably an adrenal cortical tumor—a pheochromocytoma)
d. Her high blood pressure did not fall in response to a blood pressure medication that is effective for most patients
e. The hypertension is likely to prove fatal (eg, from a ruptured aneurysm in the brain or elsewhere)

General Principles of Pharmacology

Answers

1. The answer is e. (*Brunton, pp 26-30. Katzung, pp 20-29.*) The substances and functions listed in the question provide signal transduction between ligand interactions with specific receptors, and responses that are characteristic of the agonist and the target cell(s). Suitable ligands indeed include neurotransmitters (ACh, catecholamines, various amino acids [γ-aminobutyric acid, glycine, glutamate, aspartate], opioids, serotonin, and histamine to name a few) and hormones (insulin, glucagon, thyroid hormones, etc)—or drugs with suitable structures. They are not, however, the actual receptors (b) for agonists or antagonists. These substances will also participate in ligand binding–response coupling to suitable foreign substances—drugs (c). Again, depending on the ligand and the type of cell, responses can be either excitatory or inhibitory (d), and they occur in various neural, muscle, and gland cells (a).

2. The answer is c. (*Brunton, pp 14-16. Katzung, pp 42, 48.*) For a 70-kg individual, total body water is about 40 L (0.6 L/kg); interstitial plus plasma water occupies about 12 L (0.17 L/kg).

Azithromycin, with a V_d of 30 L/kg, would be distributed in an apparent volume of about 2100 L in a typical 70-kg person.

Use simple logic to answer this question, but look at the answer to Question 18 if you wish. Even if you don't remember what total body water is (about 40 L or 0.6 L/kg), or the approximate value for interstitial plus plasma water (about 12 L or 0.17 L/kg), do the quick math. If you take the stated 30 L/kg and compute the apparent volume for a 70-kg individual, you would arrive at 2100 L. That number not only reflects distribution into a hypothetical volume far in excess of vascular and interstitial volumes, but is also far beyond what could be physically real. After all, 2100 L of water equals 2100 kg; you won't find human beings weighing that much!

Without more information, you cannot make definitive conclusions about the other properties listed as answer choices.

3. The answer is d. *(Brunton, pp 49-52. Katzung, pp 30-31.)* "Our product is the most potent pain reliever (or whatever) you can buy without a prescription," the TV ads say far too often for me. What those claims don't say is how efficacious a particular drug is, particularly compared with another (eg, a competing product). So, let's address some fundamentals.

The most basic definition of efficacy is simply the ability to cause an effect. More important is the question "how big an effect?" Aspirin, for example, will alleviate headache pain for many patients, but it simply cannot, at safe doses, alleviate severe pain from, for example, an abdominal incision. So, in the setting of severe pain, aspirin is less efficacious than, say, morphine.

If relief of simple headache pain is the goal, then such drugs as aspirin, acetaminophen, and ibuprofen, are equally efficacious. What differs is how many milligrams of each are necessary to do that. Ibuprofen is more potent than acetaminophen, which is slightly more potent than aspirin: 400 mg of ibuprofen, 600 mg of acetaminophen, and 650 mg of aspirin are reasonable dosages.

In the question provided here, drugs X, Y, and Z all have efficacy: they all increase contractile force development by the isolated cardiac muscle preparation shown and described in the question. But it should be obvious that drug Y and drug Z are more efficacious than drug X. The ED50 of drug X is lower than that of the other drugs (a), but that doesn't mean that it is more efficacious: indeed, its maximal effect on the test muscle's force of contraction is about less than half of that for drug Y and drug Z.

Answer b is incorrect: Drug Y is more potent than drug Z; its ED50 is lower than that of drug Z, but Y and Z are equally efficacious since their peak effects are identical. This also eliminates answer c as a correct answer: again, the ED50 for drug Z is higher than that of drug Y, and so Z is less potent. Answer e cannot be correct: although the ED50 of drug X is lower than the ED50s of Y and Z, the maximum intensity of drug X's response is much lower than those of Y and Z.

4. The answer is c. *(Brunton, pp 16-17. Katzung, pp 41, 46-47.)* This question, with its many variables and equations, was written intentionally to see whether you would take a needlessly complicated approach to a concept that is, when reduced to its essential point, relatively straightforward. If you give doses of a drug repeatedly at intervals that are equal to or less than the drug's overall elimination half-life, and keep every other pertinent variable constant (dose, route, elimination status, etc), you simply multiply the half-life by

4 or 5 (hence, my use of 4.5 to take a middle ground) to arrive at the approximate time until C_{SS}, the time at which "drug in = drug out" is reached.

The figure below shows what happens with repeated administration of a drug at intervals equal to the drug's half-life. Note that the average plasma concentration (C_{av}) does not appear to "flatten out," or reach a plateau, until at least 4 doses (= 4 half-lives) have been given. After that, and assuming nothing else changes (dose, dose interval, route of administration, elimination kinetics, starting or stopping other drugs), although there will still be fluctuations of peak and trough drug levels around the mean (right after each dose, right before the next), the average blood concentration does not change.

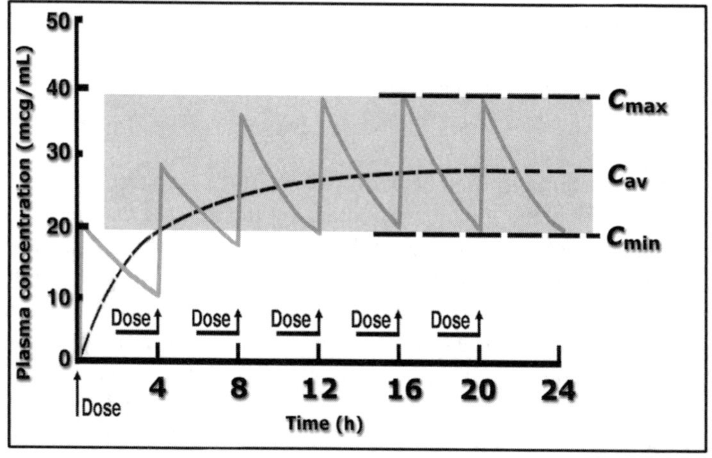

Note: the equation (0.693 × V_d)/Cl (answer a) is the equation for calculating the half-life.

5. The answer is a. *(Brunton, pp 17-21. Katzung, p 38.)* We obtain the oral AUC by measuring drug concentrations measured in sequential blood samples. However, we must compare those data to measurements of AUC obtained with giving the same drug intravenously (where bioavailability is, by definition, 1.0). The fraction of a drug dose absorbed after oral administration is affected by a variety of factors that can strongly influence the peak blood levels and the time-to-peak blood concentration. The V_d and the total body clearance also are important in determining the amount of drug that reaches a target tissue. The area under the blood concentration–time curve reflects absorption, distribution, metabolism, and excretion factors, and their interactions. It is the most reliable method of evaluating bioavailability overall.

6. The answer is d. *(Brunton, pp 17-21. Katzung, pp 38, 48-50.)* Bioavailability is defined as the fraction or percentage of a drug that becomes available to the systemic circulation following administration by any route, compared with bioavailability when the drug is given IV (since IV bioavailability is defined as 1.0 or 10%). This takes into consideration that not all of an orally administered drug is absorbed, and that a drug can be removed from the plasma and metabolized by the liver during its initial passage through the portal circulation (ie, a "first-pass" effect). An oral bioavailability of 0.25 (25%) indicates that only 20 mg of the 80-mg dose (ie, 80 mg × 0.25 = 20 mg) reached the systemic circulation. Organ clearance can be determined by knowing the blood flow through the organ (*Q*, expressed as a volume per unit time, eg, mL/min) and the extraction ratio (ER) for the drug by the organ, according to the equation:

$$\mathrm{Cl_{organ}} = Q \times \mathrm{ER}$$

The extraction ratio is a function of the amounts of drug entering the organ (arterial side; C_A) and leaving it on the venous side (C_V), and the ratio is calculated as:

$$\mathrm{ER} = (\mathrm{C_A} - \mathrm{C_V})/\mathrm{C_A}$$

In this problem, the amount of verapamil entering the liver per unit time was 76 mg (80 mg × 0.95) and the amount leaving was 20 mg. Therefore,

$$\mathrm{ER} = \frac{76\ \mathrm{mg} - 20\ \mathrm{mg}}{76\ \mathrm{mg}} = 0.74$$

$$\mathrm{Cl_{liver}} = (1500\ \mathrm{mL/min})\ (0.74) = 1110\ \mathrm{mL/min}$$

7. The answer is d. *(Brunton pp 3, 9-10, 41, 43, 49t, 66, 1297. Katzung pp 9, 10t.)* P-glycoprotein (PGP; the P stands for "permeability") is part of a superfamily of transmembrane transporter proteins, substrates for which include many xenobiotics (chemicals not found naturally in the body), including many therapeutic agents. An important member of the P-glycoprotein family is involved in an ATP-dependent (ie, active transport; this is part of the ABC—ATP-binding cassette—family) mechanism that pumps drugs and other chemically diverse xenobiotics *out* of certain cells, against the usual concentration gradient. That is, PGP serves as an ATP-driven efflux pump.

PGP does not form drug conjugates (a) or participate in other Phase II reactions; maintain membrane/receptor structure and function (b); phosphorylate any substrates (c); or play a role in signal transduction (e).

Here are some of the sites where PGP is abundant and important, and some important effects at those sites:

- in hepatocytes (where it transports substrates into the bile);
- in the intestinal epithelium (important for transporting a variety of drugs across membranes during absorption);
- in the kidneys (certain proximal tubule cells, where substrates are transported into the urine for eventual elimination); and
- in capillary endothelial cells of the "blood-brain barrier," where certain drugs that may have diffused across the barrier, into the CNS, are transported back out to the systemic circulation. This reduces exposure of the brain to the drugs.

What are some clinically relevant phenomena related to PGP activity? For starters, PGP activity is important in the development of multidrug resistance (MRP—multidrug resistance-associated protein), particularly cellular resistance to certain chemotherapeutic agents and antiviral/antiretroviral drugs. PGP promptly transports those cellular toxins out of the cells the drugs are meant to kill.

There is broader importance. Consider, for example, PGP activity in the intestinal epithelia. Many drugs that are substrates for PGP diffuse from the intestinal lumen into the epithelial cells during absorption, but PGP pumps a portion of those drug molecules right back into the lumen, from which they may not be reabsorbed to gain access to the circulation. Thus, PGP has an important role in absorption and bioavailability of many orally administered drugs.

Just as there are substrates, inducers, and inhibitors for the cytochrome P450 system, so there are substrates, inducers, and inhibitors for PGP. If PGP activity is increased by an inducer, the oral bioavailability of PGP substrates will be reduced (by virtue of greater transport back into the lumen), plasma levels in response to a dose (or doses) will be reduced (absolute decreases of plasma levels and of the "area under the time-concentration curve), and the intensity of drug responses will be reduced. Conversely, PGP inhibitors can increase oral bioavailability, plasma levels (AUC), and response intensity, of PGP substrates. Thus, there are both pharmacokinetic and pharmacodynamic consequences of PGP activity.

In some cases the clinical significance of an interaction involving PGP is weak or otherwise inconsequential; however, with many other drugs, inducers or inhibitors may cause clinically significant differences in bioavailability, drug blood levels, and the magnitude of drug responses.

The short table that follows lists some of the drugs, mentioned in this book, that are PGP substrates, inducers, or inhibitors.

SOME P-GLYCOPROTEIN SUBSTRATES, INDUCERS, AND INHIBITORS*

Substrates	Inducers	Inhibitors
Amiodarone	Rifampin	Amiodarone
Chlorpromazine	Ritonavir	Atorvastatin
Clarithromycin	St. John's wort	Chlorpromazine
Cyclosporine		Clarithromycin
Dactinomycin		Cyclosporine
Daunorubicin		Diltiazem
Digoxin		Erythromycin
Diltiazem		Hydrocortisone
Doxorubicin		Indinavir
Erythromycin		Itraconazole
Etoposide		Ketoconazole
Indinavir		Lidocaine
Itraconazole		Mifepristone
Ketoconazole		Nifedipine
Lidocaine		Propranolol
Mifepristone		Quinidine
Nifedipine		Reserpine
Ondansetron		Ritonavir
Quinidine		Saquinavir
Reserpine		Tamoxifen
Ritonavir		Testosterone
Saquinavir		Verapamil
Tamoxifen		
Testosterone		
Verapamil		
Vinblastine		
Vincristine		

*This is not a complete list, but rather one that includes drugs mentioned in this book. Note that some drugs can be a substrate, an inducer, or an inhibitor of PGP, depending on the dose of the drug and the presence of other drugs that are transported by PGP.

8. The answer is b. *(Brunton, pp 12-22. Katzung, pp 43-44.)* Among other things, knowing the AUC of a drug given intravenously (which, by definition, is associated with a bioavailability of 1.0 or 100%) is a prerequisite for knowing the bioavailability of the same drug given by any other route; bioavailability is calculated as the ratio of AUC for any non-IV route and the AUC_{IV}.

9. The answer is e. *(Brunton, pp 2-3. Katzung, pp 9-12.)* Recall the two Henderson-Hasselbach equations, which apply to how local pH affects the ionization of molecules (eg, of a drug) in an aqueous environment. And let's assume membranes are permeable only to nonionized (and more lipid-soluble) forms of a drug. Thus, we are making the assumption that ionized drugs tend to stay, or concentrate, in an environment that favors that pH-dependent ionization; conversely, in an environment that favors formation of nonionized drug molecules, a concentration gradient will favor passive diffusion of nonionized molecules to another locale.

For acidic drugs: $pH = pK_a \log [A^-]/[AH]$

For basic drugs: $pH = pK_a = \log [B]/[BH^+]$

Our drug was an acid with $pK_a = 3.4$. In the stomach (assume pH = 1.4 as noted) the ratio of nonionized to ionized molecules will be about 1:0.01. The nonionized molecules will diffuse across the membrane. Once in the plasma, pH 7.4, the ratio of HA:A^- will become 1:10,000. And the concentration ratio of total drug across the membrane will be essentially 10,000:1, with the larger amount being in the plasma.

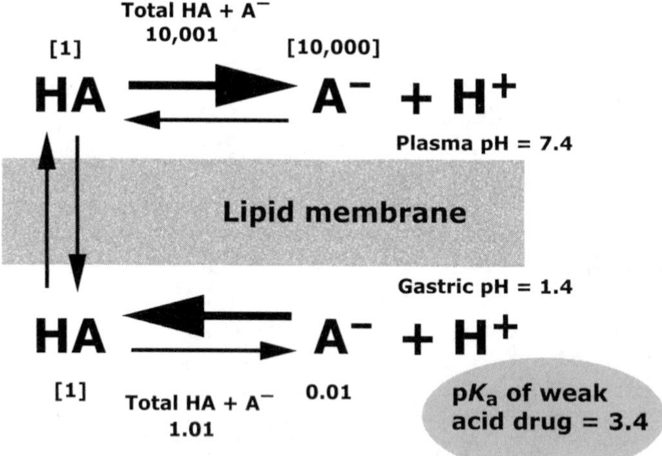

You might also want to look at the following figure to get a "big picture" of how changing pH changes the ionization of acidic and basic drugs.

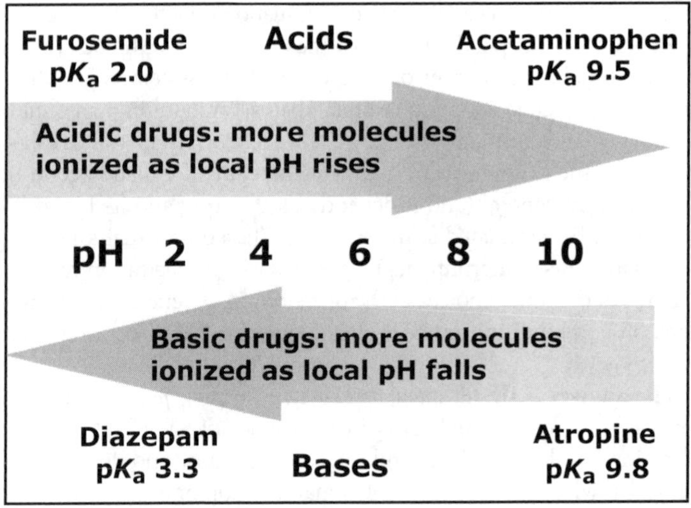

10. The answer is c. *(Brunton, pp 3-7. Katzung, p 43.)* We are making this data comparison to determine the drug's bioavailability. We define the bioavailability of a drug given intravenously as 1.0 (100%), since with IV administration we avoid all the applicable barriers to drug absorption. But, of course, it's important to know how much total drug, over a period of time, gets into the bloodstream with other administration routes that we might want to use clinically. Drugs given by routes other than IV must be absorbed (and be exposed to all the barriers that limit or slow or otherwise affect absorption). Because they might not be absorbed from their administration site, or might be susceptible to such processes as hepatic first-pass metabolism, they usually have a bioavailability of less than 1.0.

The calculation of bioavailability is based on the ratio of the area under the concentration-time curve (AUC) for the administration route being considered (oral, IM, etc) and the AUC obtained with IV administration.

Measurement of blood levels of a drug at a single time point will not give the information needed to determine bioavailability.

Note that with oral absorption there is a delay until there is some detectable drug in the blood. That reflects both the time needed for absorption of the drug and, in most cases, the sensitivity of the assay to measure the drug (which may be present, but at undetectable levels). With IV administration blood levels rise instantaneously. With oral administration you should also note that as blood levels of the drug rise toward the peak the rate of drug entry into the blood exceed the rate of elimination (whether by metabolism, excretion, or both, depending on what the drug is). Once blood concentrations start to fall, the amount of drug entering the system is less than the amount being eliminated, per unit time. That is, "amount in < amount out."

Finally—and although you can't tell precisely from the graph—the half-lives for the drug, measured under different experimental conditions, are identical: in general (and it depends on the drug and its blood level), the drug will be eliminated at the same rate (based on usual kinetic influences, such as first-order kinetics) regardless of administration route.

None of the other choices in the question (ie, potency, effectiveness, or plasma protein binding) can be evaluated using this type of comparison.

11. The answer is d. *(Brunton, pp 123-124. Katzung, pp 1029-1035, 1037-1039.)* How (or even whether) age or extremes of age affects the overall elimination half-life of a drug (and thus the right dose and dosing interval) depends on what the drug is. While renal function or a measure of it such as creatinine clearance (b) change over certain age ranges, it is not universally applicable to the elimination or elimination rates of all drugs. Remember that many drugs are completely metabolized to inactive substances, and so changes of renal function are largely unimportant in the elimination (and plasma half-lives) of such drugs.

Consider some examples, but don't try to memorize the drug-specific details.

- Theophylline's half-life is shortest between the ages of 6 months and about 9 years, being much longer at younger or older ages. That is because of differences in the rate of the drug's metabolism. Thus, the dose of this old bronchodilator, normalized to body weight, is much higher at that age range; indeed, it is likely to be excessive for and toxic to younger or older individuals. This rather odd relationship certainly does not apply to all (or even many) drugs, and so answer e is not correct for most drugs.
- When comparing the half-life of penicillin G in adults above 60 years to adults in the 20- to 30-year range, the half-life is twice as long in the older patients; it's nearly twice as long with lidocaine, too; 50% longer with digoxin; and virtually not different, age-wise, with warfarin.

Other drugs for which there are significant differences (here, in terms of hepatic clearance): most barbiturates; imipramine; meperidine; propranolol; and quinidine. And no significant age-related changes? Examples are aspirin, ethanol, prazosin, and as noted above, warfarin.

The chemical class to which a drug belongs (a) also does not invariably predict age-related changes. Consider four benzodiazepines. There are significant age-related pharmacokinetic changes with diazepam (its half-life is proportional to age) and flurazepam. In contrast, there are no significant age-related differences in the half-lives of lorazepam or nitrazepam.

12. The answer is a. *(Brunton, pp 71-80. Katzung, pp 53-60.)* Biotransformation reactions involving the oxidation, reduction, or hydrolysis of a drug are classified as Phase I (or nonsynthetic) reactions, examples of which are noted in answers b, c, d, and e. In general, these reactions may result in either the activation (as in the case of a prodrug) or, much more commonly, the inactivation of a pharmacologic agent. Phase II reactions involve conjugation of the drug (or its metabolites) with an amino acid, carbohydrate, acetate, sulfate—or glucuronic acid as noted in the question. The conjugated form(s) of the drug or its derivatives are more easily excreted than the parent compound.

13. The answer is c. *(Brunton, pp 12-18. Katzung, pp 43, 45-47.)* With intravenous infusions of a drug, only the drug's half-life determines how long it will take for blood levels to reach a steady state (on average, neither rising nor falling thereafter) so long as the infusion rate is not changed. By definition, when steady state is reached, the amount of drug entering the blood per unit time is equal to the rate at which drug is being eliminated, whether by excretion, metabolism, or a combination of both (depending on the drug).

The apparent volume of distribution has no impact on time to C_{SS}. Bioavailability does not either, because with IV drug administration the bioavailability is 1.0 (100%). Clearance, a parameter that relates elimination rate of a drug to the drug's concentration (Cl = rate of elimination [mg/h]/drug concentration [mg/mL]). Because clearance considers a rate of drug elimination, it affects the C_{SS} but it is not a determinant of it.

The infusion rate clearly affects the blood concentration reached at steady state, but it does not affect the time needed to reach it. For example, if we had a drug with a half-life of 4 hours, infused at a rate of x mg/min, and then repeated the experiment with the same drug at an infusion rate of 2*x* mg/min, blood concentrations at steady state would clearly be different. However, it would still take the same amount of time (roughly 4-5 half-lives), to reach steady state. (See the answer to Question 4 for related information.)

14. The answer is d. (*Brunton, pp 78, 88. Katzung, p 65.*) Grapefruit juice (but not most other citrus juices) and juice from Seville oranges (not others; see notes at end of answer) contain compounds (eg, naringin, furanocoumarins) that can inhibit the metabolism of several drugs, one of which is cyclosporine, via inhibitory effects on CYP3A4. The route of elimination (c) is not changed, however. (Other drugs involved in this interaction include verapamil, some of the statin-type cholesterol-lowering medications; most of the second generation antihistamines, including fexofenadine; and several antidepressants and antihypertensives.) The result of the interaction is increased bioavailability of an orally administered dose and increased area under the curve in a concentration versus time plot. The potential outcome is excessive (and, occasionally, truly toxic) effects.

The "grapefruit juice effect" does not alter the main route(s) of drug absorption or elimination, nor affect plasma protein binding capacity, because those are properties related to the drug, not how—or how well or quickly—it enters the circulation. Note that the data in the table are consistent with the hypothesis that grapefruit juice does not statistically significantly accelerate or slow entry of cyclosporine into the blood, such as by affecting intestinal transporters (b).

Changes of urine pH (a) or effects that involve drug binding to plasma proteins (e) are not applicable and can't be deduced from the data presented in the question.

Notes: (1) The fruit-derived interactants are found in the "fleshy" material under the skin and between fruit segments. (2) Seville oranges (also known as blood orange) are rarely used as juice oranges because of their very bitter taste (and so they are also called bitter oranges). However, Seville/blood orange juice is now appearing more and more in health food and retail grocery stores that sell organic or other "natural" foods. (3) There are several books, and many web sites, that state dogmatically that "ordinary" oranges or orange juices interact with many medications just as grapefruit juice does. This has, naturally, alarmed many individuals. So far, solid research evidence points to no drug interactions involving oranges other than Seville. (4) Don't be surprised to see furanocoumarin-free grapefruit juice on the market soon.

15. The answer is d. (*Brunton, pp 14-22. Katzung, pp 46-47.*) Here is how you solve the problem. Note: It's easy to be misled by inconsistent use of units of measurement (mcg vs mg, mL vs L), so be sure you first convert units as necessary for consistency.

Calculate the drug's elimination rate constant:

$$k_e = 0.693/t_{1/2} \quad \text{or}$$
$$k_e = 0.693/0.5\ \text{h} = 1.386/\text{h}$$

Then calculate the clearance:

$$\text{Cl} = k_e \times V_d, \quad \text{or}$$
$$\text{Cl} = 1.386/\text{h} \times 45\ \text{L, which equals } 62.37\ \text{L/h, or } 62{,}370\ \text{mL/h}$$

Recall that

$$C_{ave} = (\text{F/Cl}) \times (D/t)$$

where F is the bioavailability (1.0) and t is the dosing interval (given as 4 h).

Rearrange to solve for the dose.

$$D = (C_{ave} \times \text{Cl} \times t)/F, \quad \text{or}$$
$$D = [(2\ \text{mcg/mL}) \times (62370\ \text{mL/h}) \times 4\ \text{h}]/1.0$$

Thus, D = 499,000 mcg, or 499 mg (close enough to 500 mg).

16. The answer is c. (*Brunton, pp 14-22. Katzung, p 41.*) Regardless of which administration route is being used, if we plot the log of plasma concentration of a drug versus time (and assuming first-order kinetics), we get a straight line. It is described by the equation:

$$\ln C = \ln C_0 - kt$$

The slope of this line, k, is the elimination rate constant.

An arguably more useful (and familiar) measure of the rate at which a drug is eliminated is the half-life ($t_{1/2}$). It is equal to 0.693/k, and is defined as the time it takes for the concentration of a drug in the blood to fall to precisely one-half of what it is now (or at any specified time).

The area under the curve (AUC) is the integration of a time versus concentration plot for a drug. It is a linear—not a logarithmic or semilog—plot. One use for plots of AUC is to estimate one's "total exposure" to a drug, usually from "time zero" (instantaneously upon administration) until blood concentrations of drug are no longer reliably detectable or further measurements are impractical. The AUC can be used to estimate total body clearance of a drug, without the need to know the drug's volume of distribution or its half-life, since

$$\text{Clearance} = \text{Dose/AUC}$$

Determining AUC also enables us to calculate a drug's bioavailability. Bioavailability (F) is a measure of the fraction of an administered dose that is absorbed systemically and is detectable in the plasma. Note that when a drug is given intravenously, bioavailability is, by definition, 1.0 (100%), since there are no barriers that might prevent the absorption of drug from the administration site. So by administering a drug intravenously, and also giving it by another route, we can calculate bioavailability. For example, assume the other route we use is oral (PO).

$$\text{Bioavailability} = (D_{\text{IV}}/D_{\text{PO}}) \times (\text{AUC}_{\text{PO}}/\text{AUC}_{\text{IV}})$$

If we do our bioavailability determinations by giving the same dose of the drug, the dosage units in the above equation cancel out, and so

$$\text{Bioavailability} = (\text{AUC}_{\text{PO}}/\text{AUC}_{\text{IV}})$$

The extraction ratio (ER) is a measure of a drug's removal from the blood as it passes through an organ (eg, the liver) that can metabolize (or otherwise extract) it, for example, from the arterial to the venous side of that organ.

The rate of drug entry to an organ is the product of blood flow (Q) and the arterial concentration of the drug (C_A). The rate at which the drug leaves is flow × the venous concentration (C_V). If flow into and out of an organ is identical (as they often are), then the extraction ratio can be expressed as

$$\text{ER} = (C_A - C_V)/C_A$$

We can also use the extraction ratio to calculate the organ clearance of a drug—that is, the volume per unit time from which an organ removes a drug

$$\text{Organ clearance} = \text{Blood flow} \times \text{Extraction ratio}$$

The volume of distribution (V_d) relates the amount of drug in the body to its concentration in the blood (or plasma). It is typically calculated as the administered dose divided by the concentration of drug in the blood

$$V_d = D/C$$

To simplify the assessment of the kinetics we typically give the drug intravenously (so we know how much drug enters the system—the entire dose, since bioavailability = 1.0) and measure the concentration immediately thereafter (or use a plot of the log of drug concentration vs time), then extrapolate to find drug concentration at "time zero" (the y-axis intercept).

17. The answer is a. *(Brunton, pp 131-135. Katzung, pp 72-73, 1132-1134.)* Once the FDA approves a drug you, as a licensed physician, can prescribe it for anything you desire. Of course, there should be some scientific basis for your new-found or hypothesized use, hopefully backed up by supporting or other rational evidence in solid peer-reviewed clinical literature. (You probably won't, for example, see a β-blocker being used for treating anal warts, but if you wanted to use one that way you are not violating any federal laws. Just be sure you have good reason to do so, and a good attorney should something bad happen and you get sued.) And if you are conducting a clinical trial at your institution to determine new information about future clinical efficacy of a drug for which there are other approved uses, and even printed off-label uses, you'll probably need Institutional Review Board approval and will have to provide written informed consent to your study subjects.

Note: Let's consider just one drug in one drug class: fluoxetine, the prototype of the SSRI class of antidepressants. What is it approved for? Well, depression, of course. But other approved or off-label uses for this antidepressant (and the identical chemical entity, same dose as used for depression but "approved" under a different trade name for premenstrual dysphoric disorder) include the following: obsessive-compulsive disorder; bulimia nervosa; alcoholism; anorexia nervosa; ADHD; bipolar II affective disorder; borderline personality disorder; narcolepsy; kleptomania; migraine; chronic daily headaches and tension-type headache; posttraumatic stress disorder; schizophrenia; levodopa-induced dyskinesia; social phobia; chronic rheumatoid pain; panic disorder; and diabetic peripheral neuropathy. Oh, one more: trichotillomania—but don't start pulling out your own hair, or get depressed, trying to memorize this incomplete list of sometimes-odd uses.

18. The answer is c. *(Brunton, pp 14-16. Katzung, pp 37-40, 50.)* The apparent V_d is defined as the volume of fluid into which a drug appears to distribute with a concentration equal to that of plasma, or the volume of fluid necessary to dissolve the drug and yield the same concentration as that found in plasma. By convention, we use the value of the plasma concentration, based on data such as those shown here, that has been extrapolated back to "time zero." Plotting the drug concentration (y-axis) on a logarithmic scale, as shown here, allows us to do the extrapolation easily. In this example, that is about 7 mcg/mL. Therefore, the apparent V_d is calculated as:

$$V_d = \frac{\text{Total amount of drug in the body}}{\text{Drug concentration in plasma at time zero}}$$

The total amount of drug in the body initially is the dose we gave (100% bioavailability, since we gave it IV), 350 mg (ie, 5 mg/kg × 70 kg). The estimated plasma concentration at zero time is 7 mcg/mL (0.007 mg/mL). Putting these numbers in the equation yields the apparent V_d:

$$V_d = \frac{350\text{ mg}}{0.007\text{ mg/mL}} = 50{,}000\text{ mL} = 50\text{ L}$$

19. The answer is d. *(Brunton, pp 123-124. Katzung, p 1039.)* Most excessive and adverse effects from a single drug occur because of declines in renal excretory function. It affects drugs that are eliminated without prior metabolism, those for which metabolic inactivation plays a relatively small role in elimination, and those drugs that form one or more active metabolites. Declines of hepatic function (c) clearly occur in advanced age, whether in the presence or absence of other factors that might impair hepatic drug metabolism, but that does not seem to account for the majority of cases of excessive drug effects. The same applies to plasma albumin levels (e). Body fat content (a) and lean body mass (b) tend to rise, not fall, with age.

20. The answer is b. *(Brunton, pp 7-9, 121, 1788-1789, 1792. Katzung, pp 39-41, 49.)* The speed of any redistribution or re-equilibration of bound/free concentrations of the target drug depends on the drug's overall elimination half-life (which, in turn, is a composite of either or both excretion and metabolism, depending on the drug). If a drug has an overall short elimination half-life, relatively speaking, the re-equilibrium between bound and free molecules will, indeed, be reached quickly. If the drug has a relatively long half-life (and especially if relatively large amounts of the interacting drug are present and/or the interactant binds avidly to plasma proteins), then it will take longer for equilibrium to be established once again (if it occurs at all). If the drugs are in the circulation largely unbound, the consequences are less. However, consider warfarin: normally about 98% of all warfarin molecules at any given time are bound to plasma proteins. Displacement of even a small fraction of those bound molecules will have a large impact on the number of free (active) molecules, and warfarin's normal average half-life is about 2.5 days.

Bioavailability of the drug (a) is not important or relevant. No matter whether bioavailability is great (at or near 1.0) or small, once the drug is in the circulatory system the interaction will occur, and reequilibrium will be reestablished neither slower nor faster than under any other circumstances. Likewise, unless blood pH changes (I did not say it did, and there is no reason to speculate that it would), the p*K* of the drugs (c) is largely irrelevant. Renal clearance (d) may be important, but recall that many drugs are eliminated mainly or completely by metabolism, so whether clearance is important depends on the drug(s). The same reasoning applies to answer e: it is not important how the drug is eliminated, but rather the rate at which overall elimination occurs.

21. The answer is e. *(Brunton, pp 31, 162-163, 170-171. Katzung p 32.)* Tachyphylaxis is loosely defined as rapidly developing tolerance to the effects of a drug that is administered repeatedly, even if the dosages given after the first one are not changed—or even progressively increased to overcome the phenomenon. It is sometimes also called desensitization or down-regulation of the receptor(s), but those phenomena do not explain all the mechanisms by which tachyphylaxis (or tolerance in general) occurs. The mechanism behind the development of tachyphylaxis—or slower-developing drug tolerance in general—varies depending on which drug is being used, the biochemical processes by which the drug exerts its effects, and what the effector and the response(s) are. For example, consider the rapidly diminished response of a variety of cells/tissues to repeated administration of amphetamine, which acts by releasing neuronal norepinephrine. Challenge the system repeatedly and the amount of intraneuronal NE available to be released—which is essential for causing the ultimate response—goes down. Another example, with more clinical relevance, is the somewhat slower development of "tolerance" of airway smooth muscles, and their ability to relax (ie, cause bronchodilation) in response to repeated administration of β-adrenergic agonists, such as albuterol, arguably the most widely used adrenergic bronchodilator for asthma. (Note: There is no magical number that distinguishes between tachyphylaxis and "regular" tolerance. The brevity with which the tolerance develops is the key point in the working definition of tachyphylaxis.)

22. The answer is d. *(Brunton, pp 12-29. Katzung, pp 46-49.)* The dose (D) to give equals the product of the target blood concentration and the drug's clearance.

$$D = C_{\text{desired}} \times \text{Cl}$$

To simplify things, let's make the units of volume the same for both clearance and concentration. The clearance of 0.08 L/min = 80 mL/min.

Therefore

$$D = 8 \text{ mcg/mL} \times 80 \text{ mL/min} = 640 \text{ mcg/min}$$

The stated dosing interval is 4 hours, so

$$640 \text{ mcg/min} \times 60 \text{ min/h} \times 4 \text{ h} = 153{,}500 \text{ mcg}$$

which (rounded) is closest to 150 mg.

23. The answer is d. *(Brunton, pp 12-22. Katzung, p 47.)* Here the loading dose (D) equals the product of the target blood concentration (C_{desired}) and the volume of distribution (V_d).

$$D = C_{\text{desired}} \times V_d$$

As always, convert units to make things consistent. The volume of distribution, 60 L, is, of course, 60,000 mL, and so

$$\begin{aligned} D &= 8 \text{ mcg/mL} \times 60{,}000 \text{ mL} \\ &= 480{,}000 \text{ mcg} \\ &= 480 \text{ mg} \end{aligned}$$

24. The answer is b. *(Brunton, pp 72-78. Katzung, pp 54-58.)* There are four major components to this mixed-function oxidase system: (1) cytochrome P450, (2) NADPH, or reduced nicotinamide adenine dinucleotide phosphate, (3) NADPH-cytochrome P450 reductase, and (4) molecular oxygen.

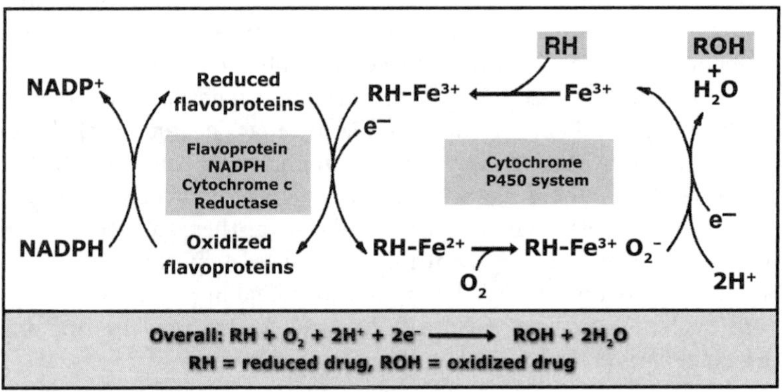

The figure shows the catalytic cycle for the general reactions dependent on cytochrome P450s. (Not all reaction steps or intermediates are shown.) In simple terms, the system acts as a monooxygenase, converting a reduced form of a drug (RH) to an oxidized form (ROH). For some drugs, those metabolic steps are followed by Phase II reactions, such as conjugation (with glucuronic acid, sulfate, etc) that further enhance the elimination of the metabolites.

Cytochrome P450s catalyze diverse reactions involved in drug biotransformation; they undergo reduction and oxidation during the catalytic cycle. A prosthetic group composed of Fe and protoporphyrin IX (forming heme) binds molecular oxygen and converts it to an activated form for interaction with the drug substrate.

NADPH gives up protons to the flavoprotein NADPH-cytochrome c reductase. The reduced flavoprotein transfers these reducing equivalents to cytochrome P450. The reducing equivalents are used to activate molecular oxygen for incorporation into the substrate, as described in the preceding paragraphs. Thus, NADPH provides reducing equivalents, and

NADPH-cytochrome P450 reductase passes them on to the catalytic enzymes that comprise cytochrome P450.

Cyclooxygenase (COX; answer a) is a general term for two main enzymes, COX-1 and -2, that metabolize endogenous arachidonic acid to prostaglandins, prostacyclins, and other eicosanoids. Its substrate specificity is largely limited to the endogenous molecules derived from arachidonic acid, not xenobiotics. A good example of a COX-1 and COX-2 is aspirin. Most other nonsteroidal anti-inflammatory drugs are also COX-1 and COX-2 inhibitors. The exemplar of a selective COX-2 inhibitor is celecoxib.

Monoamine oxidase (MAO; c) is a flavoprotein enzyme that is found on the outer membrane of mitochondria in certain neurons, and also in hepatocytes. It oxidatively deaminates short-chain monoamines only. ATP is involved in the transfer of reducing equivalents through the mitochondrial respiratory chain, not the microsomal system. There are various forms of MAO, distinguished mainly by their cellular locations, their substrates, and their inhibitors. MAO-A, for example, is found in rather diverse locations, such as in the liver and other cells. MAO-B is the predominant form in certain parts of the brain (thus, the appended letter B).

UDP-glucuronosyltransferase, along with such enzymes as glutathione-S-transferase, methyltransferases, and *N*-acetyltransferases, are important in Phase II metabolism of various drugs. Substrates for these enzymes generally are drugs or other xenobiotics that were previously transformed by Phase I reactions, such as the actions of the CYP450 mixed-function oxidases. These enzymes add a functional group to a substrate, rather than chemically modifying the original substrate via oxidation, reduction, deamination, and the like—all of which are responsibilities of the mixed-function oxidase systems.

25. The answer is b. *(Brunton, pp 24-26, 33-38, 272, 274t, 285. Katzung, pp 18-19.)* Partial agonists have both the ability to bind to receptors (affinity), and the ability to evoke a response by activating those receptors (efficacy), albeit weakly, under basal conditions. Thus, when acebutolol is administered at rest (a condition under which endogenous catecholamine levels are low), heart rate rises slightly due to β_1-receptor activation via weak agonist activity. However, the occupation of adrenergic receptors by this weak agonist reduces the number of receptors available to bind and respond to stronger agonists (epinephrine, norepinephrine). As a result, the magnitude of the response to stronger agonists in the presence of the partial agonist is lower than in the absence of it (all other things being equal).

26. The answer is d. *(Brunton, pp 14-17. Katzung, pp 38-42, 46.)* With first-order elimination of a drug, we get a straight line if we plot the log of drug concentration in the blood versus time once dosing has stopped. The slope of the line is the elimination rate constant (k_{el}). The drug's half-life—a value we will need to use momentarily—is related to k_{el} as follows: $t_{1/2} \times (k_{el})/0.693$. So, for the drug noted in the question, $t_{1/2} = 0.693/0.35$, or approximately 2 hours. It takes approximately 4 to 5 half-lives to reach a steady-state blood concentration. Do the math and you'll see that the time for this drug to reach steady state is approximately 8 to 10 hours.

27. The answer is e. *(Brunton, 14-17. Katzung, pp 41-42.)* After a 40-hour (about 1.67 days) drug-free interval passes the concentration of the drug will fall, as predicted by the half-life, to 3 mcg/mL; to 1.5 mcg/mL 40 hours after that; and to 0.75 mcg (now in the nontoxic range) after yet another 40 hours pass. Thus we have to wait 120 hours, or 5 daily doses skipped, to achieve our goal.

28. The answer is e. *(Brunton, pp 14-17. Katzung, pp 37, 39.)* You should recall that $V_d = D/C_0$. We know what the dose is. What we must calculate is the initial drug concentration (C_0)—the peak drug concentration that is reached "instantaneously" after giving the IV bolus dose. Unfortunately, we've waited 30 minutes before taking our first blood sample, but that is not a significant problem: plot the log of drug concentration versus time and extrapolate to where the line intercepts the log-concentration axis (t_0). This gives us a good estimate of C_0. Plug the extrapolated C_0 into the equation and you have your answer.

Note that bioavailability is not a factor in this instance, because with IV administration bioavailability is, by definition, 1.0 (100%). Knowing or calculating the elimination rate constant won't help either, because it is inextricably linked to the half-life, which we already know as $k_{el} = 0.693/t_{1/2}$ (and you can rearrange the equation easily).

Calculating the AUC (concentration vs time integral) with a bolus injection will give us no information more useful than what we already have. Clearance (generally referring to renal clearance) is irrelevant in this situation. I've stated that the drug is completely metabolized to other products; thus, there is no drug A to measure in the urine.

29. The answer is c. *(Brunton, pp 18-22. Katzung, p 46.)* The scenario in Question 28 makes calculations relatively straightforward, particularly because no loading dose therapy will be used.

Steady-state blood levels occur when the rate of "drug in" equals the rate of "drug out." The volume of distribution, given in the question, is irrelevant for the calculations.

The rate of drug out is given as a Cl = 70 mL/min.

Recall that the dose $(D) = \text{Cl} \times C_{SS}$

Therefore, with a little rearranging, the dose can be computed as:

$$\text{Desired plasma level} = V_d \times \text{Cl, or } 4 \text{ mg/L} \times 70 \text{ mL/min.}$$

Convert the units so they're consistent for both variables, and don't forget to calculate how many minutes there are in the dosing interval, cited as 6 hours. Now, the rest of the math:

The target blood level of 4 mg/L is the same as 4 mcg/mL, and this is a reasonable change of volume units to make for subsequent calculations, since clearance is given in units of mL/min

$$4 \text{ mcg/mL} \times 70 \text{ mL/min} = 280 \text{ mcg/min} = 0.28 \text{ mg/min}$$

And since the drug will be given every 6 hours:

$$0.28 \text{ mg/min} \times 60 \text{ min/h} \times 6 \text{ h} = 100.8 \text{ mg}$$

(closest answer is 100 mg) every 6 hours.

30. The answer is c. *(Brunton, pp 18-22. Katzung, pp 46-49.)* Only the drug concentration at steady state will change: it will be greater with this altered protocol. Do not be misled by the numbers. The time to reach C_{SS} with a constant drug infusion is a function of half-life (or the elimination rate constant, which is related to it: $k_{el} = 0.693/t_{1/2}$), and that will not change under the conditions stated. Likewise, with the vast majority of drugs eliminated by first-order kinetics, there will be no change of total body clearance or of volume of distribution. (Note: I described substance X as being pharmacologically inert. That's so you didn't conjure up confounding but largely irrelevant issues, such as a drug that caused long-lasting induction of hepatic drug-metabolizing enzymes.)

31. The answer is a. *(Brunton, pp 72-77. Katzung, pp 54-57.)* Phase I metabolic reactions generally convert (via addition or unmasking of such polar functional groups as $-NH_2$ or $-OH$ through, say, oxidations, reductions, or deamination) very nonpolar (ie, very lipid-soluble) drugs into more polar (more water-soluble) metabolites. Among other things, polar metabolites of drugs, in general, are less likely to undergo tubular reabsorption. We can generalize by saying that Phase I reactions play a role in forming metabolites that are "more easily excreted." If drug A, the parent drug, was already very polar (answer b), there would be little need for Phase I metabolism. There is no reason to assume that drug A will lack intrinsic biological activity (answer c); and because it is quite lipid-soluble to begin with, once in the circulation it should have good ability to diffuse across membranes and reach intracellular sites (hence, e is incorrect). Finally, note that those reactions described as Phase II that further increase polarity (water-solubility) of some drugs via forming conjugates with glucuronic acid or sulfate.

32. The answer is e. *(Brunton, pp 28, 49-56, 323-326, 334. Katzung, pp 24-29, 82-83.)* The general issue of ligand-receptor-response coupling involves signal transduction and is addressed in Question 1. The specific agonists noted in the question transduce their signals and eventually cause a response by processes involving G proteins—a family of guanine nucleotide-binding proteins. These ligands bind to the extracellular face of the transmembrane protein. The various G proteins (eg, G_i, G_q, G_s) bind to intracellular portions of the receptor. They then couple the initial ligand interaction to the eventual response through a series of effector enzymes or enzyme systems that are G protein-regulated.

For example, adenylyl cyclase can be activated, catalyzing the formation of cAMP that then activates a particular kinase that phosphorylates specific intracellular proteins. But the actual steps that occur after ligand binding depend on what the ligand is, what specific G protein is involved, which kinases are activated, and what proteins they phosphorylate. And what happens (ie, what the response is) depends on all of the above and, of course, which cell type is being affected.

Activation of adenylyl cyclase and increased cAMP levels may occur in one system, but the opposite may occur in another. Some signal transduction pathways involve phospholipase C, others do not. A calcium channel may be affected in one system and a potassium channel (or no ion channel at all) in others.

By way of review, recall that there are three other main mechanisms or pathways for signal transduction about which we have reasonable knowledge.

One uses a receptor protein that spans the cell membrane, but G proteins are not involved. On the inner membrane face the protein possesses enzymatic activity that is regulated by the presence or absence of ligand bound to the extracellular face. The tyrosine kinase pathway is an example, and the overall pathway is responsible for the activity of various growth factors and insulin (which is also a growth-regulating hormone).

Another mechanism is used by very lipid-soluble ligands that cross cell membranes easily and act on some intracellular receptor. For example, glucocorticosteroids ultimately act in the nucleus and, through interaction with heat-shock protein (hsp90), eventually alter transcription of specific genes.

The third involves transmembrane ion channels, the "open" or "closed" states of which are controlled by ligand binding to the channel. This process applies to some of the important neurotransmitters, especially those in the brain (GABA, the main inhibitory neurotransmitter) and such amino acids as glycine, which exert "excitatory" actions. The nicotinic receptor for ACh fits in this category too.

33. The answer is c. *(Katzung, pp 1026-1029.)* These are FDA "pregnancy categories." The short table presented below summarizes what each of the five FDA pregnancy classes means. The actual adverse fetal effect(s), and the trimester(s) of pregnancy at which their risks are greatest, depend on the drug class or, in many instances, on the actual drug. The adverse effects may include teratogenesis, fetal death, or such other responses as endocrine imbalances (eg, neonatal hypothyroidism—cretinism—if mother received certain antithyroid drugs). You can look up information for specific drugs, and the trimester(s) at which the fetal risk is greatest or applicable (eg, the main risks of embryopathy from warfarin, a widely used oral anticoagulant, apply to the first 12 or so weeks of gestation), as the need arises (eg, during your ob-gyn and perhaps other clerkships).

Notes: Some drugs and/or their active metabolite(s) are excreted in breast milk and may adversely affect the nursing child. If the mother

FDA Category	Basis for Classification—Interpretation
A	Remote risk of fetal harm. Well-controlled studies in pregnant women have not found an increased risk of fetal abnormalities in any trimester of pregnancy.
B	Slightly more risk than category A. Animal studies have found no evidence of fetal harm, but there are no adequate or well-controlled studies in pregnant women.... *or* Animal studies have shown an adverse fetal effect, but adequate and well-controlled studies in pregnant women have not demonstrated a fetal risk in any of the trimesters.
C	Greater risk than category B. Animal studies have shown adverse fetal effect(s) and there are no adequate and well-controlled studies in pregnant women.... *or* No animal studies have been conducted and there are no adequate and well-controlled studies in pregnant women.
D	Proven risk of fetal harm. Adequate well-controlled or observational studies in pregnant women have demonstrated a risk to the fetus. However, the benefits of therapy may outweigh the potential risk. For example, the drug may be acceptable if needed in a life-threatening situation or serious disease for which safer drugs cannot be used or are ineffective.
X	Proven risk of fetal harm. Adequate well-controlled or observational studies in animals or pregnant women have demonstrated positive evidence of fetal abnormalities or risks. Use of the drug or product containing it is contraindicated in women who are, or may become, pregnant because risks outweigh benefits.

requires one or more of those drugs, she should be instructed not to breast-feed, or a suitable alternative drug that is not excreted in maternal milk (if one is available) might be prescribed instead. Providing a list of such drugs is beyond the scope of this review book; many professional texts and on-line resources are available for you to get more information. Drugs that pose or have fetal risks (from maternal use) are not necessarily ones that should be avoided by breast-feeding women; the converse also applies. Finally, expect that the FDA will largely abandon its pregnancy classifications, and substitute more descriptive information for drugs, in the next few years.

34. The answer is d. *(Brunton, pp 131-135. Katzung, pp 70-72, 1113-1114.)* One of the most controversial (if not mind-boggling) aspects of marketing herbals, nutritional supplements, and other "nutriceuticals" is that manufacturers and sellers have to provide no proof of safety or efficacy to the FDA—something that must be provided, and with abundant and scientifically sound data, before the FDA will approve a drug for sale by prescription. Herbals, for example, came under the umbrella of the Dietary Supplement Health and Education Act (DSHEA) of 1994.

Such products, you may have noted, come with labels that state "serving size," rather than dose, as if we are going to be ingesting some carrots instead of a potentially active or dangerous drug.

Sellers of such products as herbals cannot make explicit claims that their products will prevent, diagnose, treat, or cure any disease. DHSEA allows a seller of a nutritional supplement to say such obtuse things as "boosts your memory," or "improves urinary tract health," but they cannot state "helps prevent or treat Alzheimer disease" or "reduces urinary frequency and nocturia if you have benign prostatic hypertrophy." In fact, DSHEA simply requires that the label on or advertisements for the product state, in essence, that the FDA hasn't evaluated any of the claims the manufacturer has made, explicitly or implicitly.

Moreover, while a drug company must provide and pay for the obligatory preclinical and clinical studies before a prescription drug gets the OK, if there is a reason or attempt to pull a nutriceutical from the market the FDA must do the work and pay the costs to prove that the product is unsafe or ineffective.

Drugs needn't be approved by the FDA as prescription drugs (answer a) before they can be sold OTC. While such prior approval is the norm (eg, consider many antihistamines for allergy or insomnia; or drugs that inhibit gastric acid secretion being marketed for "heartburn" or "acid indigestion"), consider aspirin. It's been available OTC for decades and for its common uses (pain, fever, inflammation) it never got an FDA blessing as a prescription drug. Indeed, some say that if aspirin were being considered for approval as a prescription drug today, it might not be approved because of the risks of serious adverse responses (eg, bleeding tendencies from antiplatelet effects, bronchospasm in many asthmatics), numerous drug-drug interactions, and so on. But aspirin is a glaring example of how things were done, not how they're done today. The many OTC drugs now a days first got approval for sale by prescription only, for example, antihistamines, inhibitors of gastric acid secretion (noted above), and others. Approval for OTC sale is petitioned by the manufacturer, and then approved only after reviews by, and recommendations from, FDA's expert advisory panels.

Answer c is incorrect. Once a drug gets approval for sale is used as a prescription drug, and for a given indication (or more, depending on data submitted and approved), the physician can prescribe that drug for any reasonable purpose that he or she thinks is appropriate, safe, and effective. Physicians and scientists learn or hypothesize about new uses for a drug, conduct clinical studies, and overall can legally prescribe drugs for the off-label or unlabeled uses.

Phase III testing of drugs is conducted in usually no more than 5000 patients with a disease for which the drug is to be marketed. The main goal is to assess effectiveness for the stated use and for overall safety. These are rather tightly controlled studies. The number of subjects, and the conditions in which the drug is given, are quite different from what happens in the "real world" where tens or hundreds of thousands of patients may get the drug in largely uncontrolled circumstances. Many drugs have come (been FDA-approved) and gone (pulled from the market because of adverse reactions or interactions, including those leading to death) because of what we've learned after the drugs were approved by the FDA.

35. The answer is a. You probably won't find the definition of malignant in a pharmacology book, but you ought to know what it is. (Many of my M1 and M2 students thought "malignant" only meant "the big C" until I told them otherwise.) Malignant hypertension, malignant hyperthermia, neuroleptic malignant syndrome, malignant cancer, etc. The term simply means a condition is rapidly getting worse. Nothing necessarily linked to cancer; no implication that the condition will not respond to usually effective (or even second- or third-line) therapies and medications (refractory is the term for resistance to intervention); no guarantee, or even a likelihood, that the condition will be fatal if it is treated properly.

The Peripheral Nervous Systems: Autonomic and Somatic Nervous System Pharmacology

Acetylcholine synthesis, fates, and actions
Acetylcholinesterase and its inhibitors
Adrenergic receptor subtypes
Adrenergic agonists and antagonists
Catecholamine synthesis, fates, and actions
Cholinergic receptor subtypes
Cholinergic agonists and antagonists
Ganglionic stimulants and blockers
Peripheral nervous system structure and function
Skeletal muscle relaxants (centrally acting)
Skeletal neuromuscular blockers

Questions

Questions 36 to 42

Questions 36 to 42 are based on a schematic diagram of the peripheral nervous system. I think this is a suitable and efficient way to help you assess, or clarify, some fundamental and essential aspects of peripheral nervous system anatomy, physiology, and pharmacology based on a few main "rules" and key exceptions to them. I hope this approach will be beneficial.

The diagram on the next page shows the main efferent pathways in the peripheral nervous systems—the autonomic (parasympathetic and sympathetic; PNS, SNS, respectively) and somatic nervous systems—from the CNS/spinal cord (at the far left, not labeled) out to peripheral targets (effectors). The sweat glands shown in the figure represent eccrine sweat glands. The arrector pili muscles (plural is arrectores pilorum) are innervated in the same manner as the sweat glands, but they are not labeled in the diagram.

Those nerves (and answer choices) are:

a. Preganglionic parasympathetic
b. Postganglionic parasympathetic
c. Preganglionic sympathetic
d. Postganglionic sympathetic to structures other than sweat glands and arrector pili muscles
e. "Preganglionic" (functional equivalent) sympathetic to the adrenal (suprarenal) medulla
f. Preganglionic sympathetic, eccrine sweat gland (and arrector pili) innervation
g. Postganglionic sympathetic to eccrine sweat glands and arrector pili muscles
h. Motor nerve, somatic nervous system

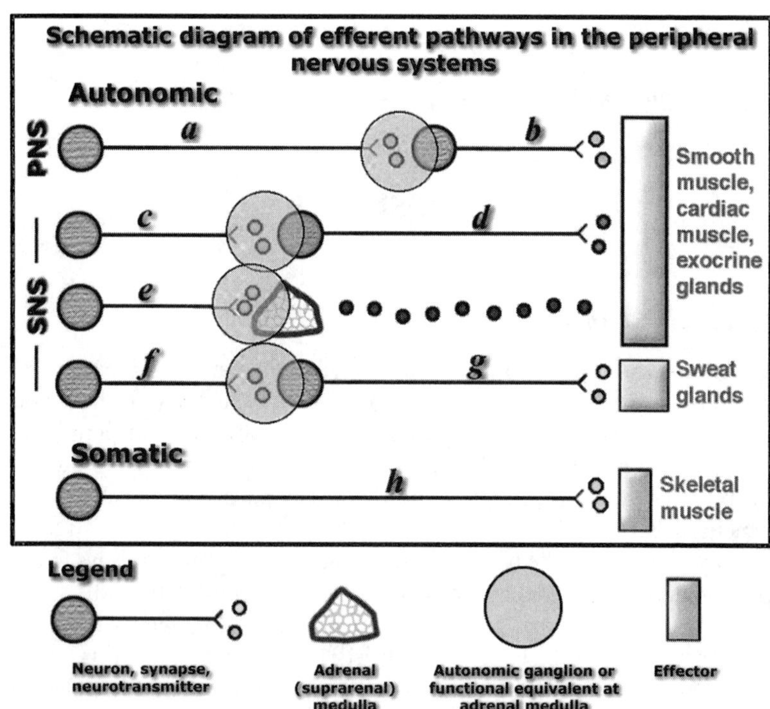

36. Anatomic, neurochemical, and pharmacologic studies of *nerves a, c, e, f,* and *h* indicate that they share one common property. Which statement correctly summarizes what that is?

a. Are cholinergic, activate postsynaptic muscarinic receptors
b. Are cholinergic, activate postsynaptic nicotinic receptors
c. Cannot release their neurotransmitter(s) in the presence of atropine
d. Have the ability to activate all the adrenergic and all the cholinergic nerves
e. Recycle their neurotransmitter after each action potential, rather than synthesizing new transmitter de novo

37. Multidisciplinary assessments of *nerve d,* a "typical" postganglionic sympathetic nerve, indicate that it is quite different from all the other nerves shown in the peripheral nervous system schematic. Which statement describes that difference?

a. Atropine selectively blocks activation of receptors by the neurotransmitter released from *nerve d.*
b. It causes bronchodilation (airway smooth muscle relaxation) when it is activated.
c. It is adrenergic (or noradrenergic if you wish to use that term instead).
d. The primary neurotransmitter synthesized by *nerve d* is epinephrine.
e. When *nerve d* is physiologically activated by an action potential, actions of its released neurotransmitter are terminated mainly by hydrolysis in the synaptic cleft.

38. Reuptake (into the nerve) is the main physiologic process for terminating the postsynaptic activity of a peripheral nervous system neurotransmitter. To which nerve does this process apply?

a. *Nerve a*
b. *Nerve b*
c. *Nerve c*
d. *Nerve d*
e. *Nerve e*
f. *Nerve f*
g. *Nerve g*
h. *Nerve h*

39. *Nerve d*, the more typical postganglionic sympathetic nerve, is activated by a normally generated action potential followed by neurotransmitter release into the synapse. On which receptor type does the neurotransmitter it releases act? Remember: you can select only one answer.

a. α_1 Adrenergic
b. α_2 Adrenergic
c. β_1 Adrenergic
d. β_2 Adrenergic
e. Muscarinic
f. Nicotinic
g. It depends on what the target tissue (effector) is

40. Which statement correctly describes what is rather unique about *nerve g*, the postganglionic sympathetic fibers that innervate eccrine sweat glands and arrector pili muscles, compared with virtually all other postganglionic sympathetic nerves?

a. Cocaine blocks release of its neurotransmitter.
b. Is cholinergic.
c. Is stimulated by preganglionic adrenergic nerves (*nerve f*).
d. Its released neurotransmitter acts on nicotinic receptors.
e. Uses epinephrine as its neurotransmitter.

41. *Nerve g*, the postganglionic nerve innervating eccrine sweat glands and arrector pili muscles, is activated by a normally generated action potential and subsequent release of neurotransmitter from *nerve f*. On which receptor type does the neurotransmitter released by *nerve g* act?

a. α_1 Adrenergic
b. α_2 Adrenergic
c. Muscarinic
d. Nicotinic
e. β_1 Adrenergic
f. β_2 Adrenergic

42. Assume that all the efferent autonomic pathways in the schematic are tonically active (a reasonable assumption), even if at low or quantitatively different levels. We add tubocurarine or pancuronium to the system and, as expected, it blocks neurotransmitter activation of certain structures. Which nerve innervates those structures and normally would activate them in the absence of tubocurarine, pancuronium, or similar drugs?

a. *Nerve a*
b. *Nerve b*
c. *Nerve c*
d. *Nerve d*
e. *Nerve e*
f. *Nerve f*
g. *Nerve g*
h. *Nerve h*

Questions 43 to 47

The figure below shows some of the main elements of norepinephrine (NE) synthesis, release, actions, and other steps in adrenergic neurotransmission. You do not need the diagram to answer this series of questions, but seeing it may aid your answering or reviewing. Note that the effector (target) cell on the far right has either an α-adrenergic receptor *or* a β-adrenergic receptor. (There are a few structures, important ones too, where both types of adrenergic receptors are present. I'll get to that later.)

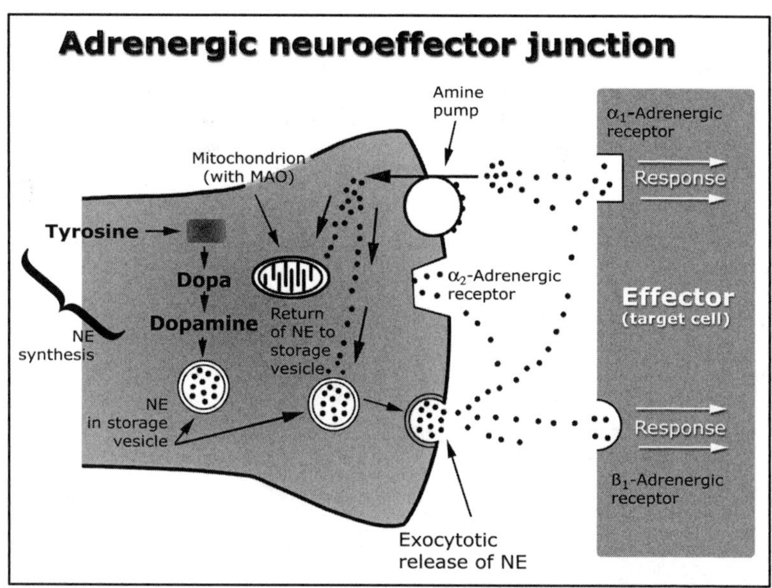

43. Mitochondria in the terminus of adrenergic nerve "endings" contain an abundance of monoamine oxidase (MAO). What best summarizes the biological role of the MAO in these adrenergic nerves?

a. Drives storage vesicles that contain NE to the nerve "ending" so that exocytotic release can occur in response to an action potential
b. Metabolically degrades NE that is free (not stored in vesicles) in the nerve terminal
c. Metabolizes dopamine to NE
d. Provides metabolic energy for nonexocytotic release of NE in response to amphetamines and other catecholamine-releasing drugs
e. Synthesizes ATP that is required to transport free intraneuronal NE into the storage granules/vesicles

44. Ultrastructural studies, combined with suitable histochemical techniques, show that the bulk of norepinephrine (NE) in the normal resting adrenergic neuron is stored in membrane-bound vesicles or granules. We administer a drug that, over time, depletes this supply of neurotransmitter and decreases the intensity of responses to sympathetic nerve activation. In vitro studies reveal that the drug acts by inhibiting uptake of intraneuronal NE into the vesicles; it has no direct effect on catecholamine synthesis, release, or interactions with its receptors. Which drug fits this description best?

a. Pargyline
b. Prazosin
c. Propranolol
d. Reserpine
e. Tyramine

45. A substance abuser self-administers cocaine and experiences a variety of significant changes in cardiovascular function, in addition to the CNS-stimulating effects for which the drug was used. What statement describes the mechanism by which the cocaine caused its main peripheral and CNS effects?

a. Activates α_2-adrenergic receptors, leading to increased NE release
b. Blocks NE (and dopamine, in the CNS) reuptake via the amine pump
c. Directly activates postsynaptic α- and β-adrenergic receptors, leading to sympathomimetic (adrenomimetic) responses
d. Inhibits monoamine oxidase, leading to increased intraneuronal NE levels
e. Prevents NE exocytosis

46. We administer a drug that is a selective antagonist at the presynaptic α-receptors (α_2) in the peripheral nervous systems. It has no effect on α_1 receptors, β-receptors, or any other ligand receptors that are important in peripheral nervous system function. What is the main response that is likely to occur following administration of the α_2-blocker?

a. Activation of the amine pump, stimulation of NE reuptake
b. Inhibition of dopamine β-hydroxylase, the enzyme that converts intraneuronal dopamine to NE
c. Increased NE release in response to each action potential
d. Inhibition of NE exocytosis
e. Stimulation of intraneuronal monoamine oxidase activity

47. Not shown in the diagram is an enzyme that has the ability to metabolically inactivate NE that has diffused away from the synapse. It is also present in the liver (as is monoamine oxidase) and in the intestinal walls. Among other things, the rapidity with which this enzyme catabolizes its substrates accounts for why NE, dopamine, and dobutamine have extraordinarily short half-lives, must be given intravenously in order to cause meaningful effects, have negligible effects when given by other parenteral routes, and are ineffective when given by mouth. An inhibitor of this drug is used therapeutically, but not for its autonomic effects. What is the name of this enzyme?

a. Aromatic L-amino acid decarboxylase
b. Catechol *O*-methyltransferase (COMT)
c. Dopamine β-hydroxylase
d. Phenylethanolamine *N*-methyltransferase
e. Tyrosine hydroxylase

48. We administer a therapeutic dose of a drug that selectively and competitively blocks the postsynaptic α-adrenergic receptors (α_1). It has no effects on presynaptic α-adrenergic receptors (α_2) or β-adrenergic receptors found anywhere in the periphery, whether as an agonist or antagonist. What is the most likely drug?

a. Ephedrine
b. Labetalol
c. Phentolamine
d. Phenylephrine
e. Prazosin

49. Festoterodine is a newly approved drug that is being heavily marketed to prescribers and directly to consumers. It is indicated for the treatment of an overactive urinary bladder to reduce urge incontinence, urinary urgency, and frequent urination. It prevents physiologic activation of the bladder's detrusor and simultaneously prevents relaxation of the sphincter. Side effects include constipation, dry mouth, blurred vision, photophobia, urinary retention, and slight increases of heart rate. An advisory for the drug states: "Heat stroke and fever due to decreased sweating in hot temperatures have been reported." Festoterodine has no direct effects on blood vessels that might change blood pressure. Based on this information, what prototype drug is most like festoterodine?

a. Atropine
b. β-Adrenergic blockers (eg, propranolol)
c. Isoproterenol
d. Neostigmine
e. Phentolamine

50. A morbidly obese person visits the local bariatric (weight loss) clinic seeking a pill that will help shed weight. The physician prescribes dextroamphetamine. In addition to causing expected centrally mediated anorexigenic (appetite-suppressant) and cortical-stimulating effects, it causes a host of peripheral adrenergic effects that, for some patients, can prove fatal. What best summarizes the main mechanism by which dextroamphetamine, or amphetamines in general, cause their peripheral autonomic effects?

a. Activates monoamine oxidase
b. Blocks NE reuptake via the amine pump/transporter
c. Displaces, releases, intraneuronal NE
d. Enhances NE synthesis, leading to massive neurotransmitter overproduction
e. Stabilizes the adrenergic nerve ending by directly activating α_2 receptors

51. We administer a pharmacologic dose of epinephrine and observe (among other responses) a direct increase of cardiac rate, contractility, and electrical impulse conduction rates. Which adrenergic receptor is responsible for these direct cardiac effects?

a. α_1
b. α_2
c. β_1
d. β_2
e. β_{3a}

52. A patient with a history of narrow-angle (angle-closure) glaucoma experiences a sudden rise of intraocular pressure that is sufficiently severe. In addition to pain, it poses an imminent risk of permanent vision loss. The patient requires immediate treatment, one element of which is administration of echothiophate. What enzyme is affected by this autonomic drug?

a. Tyrosine hydroxylase—stimulated
b. Acetylcholinesterase (AChE)—inhibited
c. Catechol *O*-methyltransferase (COMT)—inhibited
d. Monoamine oxidase—stimulated
e. DOPA decarboxylase—stimulated

53. We plan to prescribe scopolamine, as a transdermal drug delivery system (skin patch), for a patient who will be leaving for an expensive cruise and is very susceptible to motion sickness. What comorbidity would weigh against prescribing the drug because it is most likely to pose adverse effects—or be truly contraindicated?

a. Angle-closure (narrow-angle) glaucoma
b. Bradycardia
c. History of allergic reactions to uncooked shellfish
d. Resting blood pressure of 112/70
e. Hypothyroidism, mild
f. Parkinson disease (early onset, not yet treated)

54. A patient has essential hypertension, and lab tests would show that their circulating catecholamine and plasma renin levels are unusually high. The chosen therapeutic approach for this patient is to give a single drug that blocks both α- and β-adrenergic receptors, thereby reducing blood pressure by reducing both cardiac output and total peripheral resistance (systemic vascular resistance). What drug is most capable of doing that?

a. Labetalol
b. Metoprolol
c. Nadolol
d. Pindolol
e. Timolol

55. A man who has been "surfing the Web" in search of an aphrodisiac or some other agent to enhance "sexual prowess and performance" discovers yohimbine. He consumes the drug in excess and develops symptoms of toxicity that require your intervention. You consult your preferred drug reference and learn that yohimbine is a selective α_2-adrenergic antagonist. What would you expect as a response to this drug?

a. Bradycardia
b. Bronchoconstriction
c. Excessive secretions by exocrine glands (salivary, lacrimal, etc)
d. Reduced cardiac output from reduced left ventricular contractility
e. Rise of blood pressure

56. A patient with Alzheimer disease is taking an acetylcholinesterase inhibitor specifically approved for that indication, primarily because it is quite lipophilic and so enters the CNS well. What drug is this patient most likely receiving?

a. Ambenonium
b. Edrophonium
c. Neostigmine
d. Pyridostigmine
e. Tacrine

57. A child overdoses on a drug that affects both the autonomic and somatic nervous systems. As blood levels of the drug rise he experiences hypertension and tachycardia, accompanied by skeletal muscle tremor. Further elevations of blood levels of the drug cause all the expected signs and symptoms of autonomic ganglionic blockade, plus weakness and eventual paralysis of skeletal muscle. Which drug did the child most likely ingest?

a. Bethanechol
b. Nicotine
c. Pilocarpine
d. Scopolamine
e. Tubocurarine

58. Many clinical studies have shown that propranolol will lower blood pressure to varying degrees in nearly every patient with essential hypertension (ie, high BP of unknown etiology or identifiable causes, such as pheochromocytoma or vasopressor drug overdose). What is the most likely—and physiologically, most important—mechanism for propranolol's pressure-lowering effect?

a. Induced a baroreceptor reflex that reduces vasoconstriction usually caused by activation of the sympathetic nervous system
b. Inhibited catecholamine release from adrenergic nerves and the adrenal medulla (suprarenal medulla)
c. Reduced heart rate and left ventricular contractility
d. Reduced total peripheral resistance via direct vasodilator actions involving nitric oxide synthesis in endothelial cells
e. Stimulated renin release, ultimately leading to enhanced synthesis of vasodilator chemicals such as bradykinin

59. A 35-year-old man who weighs 70 kg and is 5 ft 10 in tall is transported to the emergency department in severe distress. He complains of episodes of severe, throbbing headaches, profuse diaphoresis, and palpitations. Eighteen months ago his physician told him he is healthy except for essential hypertension, but he refused medication and has not seen a health care provider until today's ED visit. He denies use of any drugs, whether prescription or over-the-counter, legal or otherwise.

Assessment reveals that he is tachycardic and has an irregular pulse (occasional premature ventricular beats are noted on his ECG). Heart rate at rest is approximately 130 beats/min, sometimes more. His resting blood pressure is 200/140 mm Hg. These cardiovascular findings are shown in the figure on the next page.

The first-year house officer who is caring for this patient knows that all the orally effective β-adrenergic blockers are approved for use to treat essential hypertension, and concludes that prompt lowering of blood pressure is essential for this patient. Therefore, he orders intravenous administration of propranolol, and a large dose of it because the symptoms seem severe. Unknown to the physician is the fact that the patient's signs and symptoms are due to a pheochromocytoma (epinephrine-secreting tumor of the adrenal/suprarenal medulla).

What is the most likely ultimate outcome of administering this β-blocker (or any other β-blocker that lacks α blocking or other vasodilator activity), supplemented with no other medication?

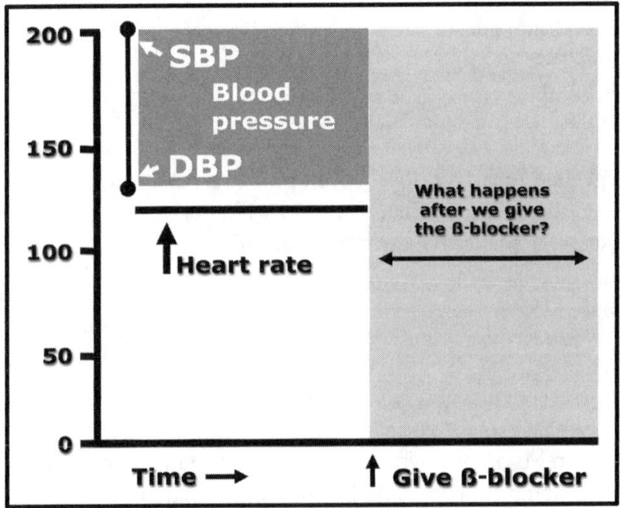

a. Heart failure, cardiogenic shock, death
b. Long-lasting normalization of heart rate, contractility, and blood pressure
c. Normalization of blood pressure, but persistence of tachycardia
d. Restoration of normal sinus rate and rhythm, but no change of blood pressure from predrug levels
e. Sudden and significant rise of systolic blood pressure and heart rate

60. The house officer considers prescribing nadolol for a 53-year-old patient. What preexisting condition (comorbidity) would most likely contraindicate safe use of this drug?

a. Angina pectoris, chronic-stable ("effort-induced")
b. Asthma
c. Essential hypertension
d. Heart failure, mild
e. Sinus tachycardia

61. A variety of ophthalmic drugs, working by several main mechanisms of action, are useful for managing chronic open-angle glaucoma. Which one reduces intraocular pressure by decreasing the formation of aqueous humor, rather than by changing the size of the pupil(s)?

a. Timolol
b. Echothiophate
c. Isoflurophate
d. Neostigmine
e. Pilocarpine

62. We give an "effective dose" of atropine to a person who was poisoned with an AChE inhibitor. What structure will continue to be overactivated by the excess ACh after the atropine is given?

a. Airway smooth muscle
b. SA node
c. Salivary and lacrimal glands
d. Skeletal muscle
e. Vascular smooth muscle

63. Guanadrel is an antihypertensive drug: it reduces arteriolar constriction and, in doing so, lowers BP by reducing the amount of NE in peripheral adrenergic nerves. Lowered blood pressure is not accompanied by reflex tachycardia, and in fact a reduction of heart rate from predrug levels is the more common outcome. The main ocular effect of guanadrel is miosis. The widespread abolition of sympathetic influences throughout the body often causes diarrhea and urinary frequency. Based on this description, to which prototypic drug is guanadrel most similar in terms of its ultimate qualitative autonomic effects, and in terms of overall mechanism of action?

a. Acetylcholine
b. Atropine
c. Epinephrine
d. Isoproterenol
e. Norepinephrine
f. Propranolol
g. Reserpine

64. A patient with chronic obstructive pulmonary disease (COPD, eg, emphysema, chronic bronchitis) is receiving an orally inhaled muscarinic receptor-blocking drug to maintain bronchodilation. What drug belongs to that class?

a. Albuterol
b. Diphenhydramine
c. Ipratropium (or tiotropium)
d. Pancuronium
e. Pilocarpine

65. A 48-year-old female patient has a history of myasthenia gravis. She has been treated with an oral acetylcholinesterase (AChE) inhibitor for several years, and has done well until now. Today she presents in your clinic with muscle weakness and other signs and symptoms that could reflect either a cholinergic crisis (excess dosages of her maintenance drug) or a myasthenic crisis (insufficient treatment). We will use a rapidly acting parenteral acetylcholinesterase inhibitor to help make the differential diagnosis. Which drug would, therefore, be most appropriate to use?

a. Edrophonium
b. Malathion
c. Physostigmine
d. Pralidoxime
e. Pyridostigmine

66. It is common to include small amounts of epinephrine (EPI) in solutions of local anesthetics that will be administered by infiltration (injection around sensory nerve endings), as when a skin laceration needs suturing. What is the most likely reason for, or outcome of, including the EPI?

a. To antagonize the otherwise intense and common vasoconstrictor and hypertensive effects of the anesthetic
b. To counteract cardiac depression caused by the anesthetic
c. To prevent anaphylaxis in patients who are allergic to the anesthetic
d. To reduce the risk of toxicity caused by systemic absorption of the anesthetic
e. To shorten the duration of anesthetic action

67. A patient presents with an anaphylactic reaction following a wasp sting. What is the drug of choice for treating the multiple cardiovascular and pulmonary problems that, if not promptly corrected, could lead to the patient's death?

a. Atropine
b. Diphenhydramine
c. Epinephrine
d. Isoproterenol
e. Norepinephrine

68. Cardiac output improves when dobutamine is given, by IV infusion, to a 60-year-old man with acute heart failure. By what adrenergic receptor-mediated actions, and through which ultimate effects of it, do therapeutic doses of dobutamine mainly raise cardiac output?

a. α-Adrenergic agonist
b. α-Adrenergic antagonist
c. β_1-Adrenergic agonist
d. β_1-Adrenergic antagonist
e. Mixed α and β agonist
f. Mixed α and β antagonist

69. It's fair to say that epinephrine, norepinephrine, and acetylcholine play the most important roles as endogenous agonists for the various receptors under control of the peripheral nervous systems. However, dopamine also plays a small but important therapeutic role, particularly when administered IV at low doses. What other peripheral effects can dopamine cause at usual therapeutic doses?

a. Bronchodilation via relaxation of airway smooth muscles
b. Direct activation of pressure receptors (eg, baroreceptors) in response to blood pressure changes triggered by other agonists
c. Direct activation of the juxtaglomerular apparatus leading to aldosterone release
d. Inhibition of epinephrine release from chromaffin cells (catecholamine-producing cells of the adrenal/suprarenal medulla)
e. Regulation of renal blood flow *via* control of renal arterial tone

70. We are conducting a study on similarities and differences between two prototypic drugs, phentolamine and prazosin, as they affect cardiovascular responses. We have selected two identical twins to ensure their pharmacogenetics make up, and so their responses to drugs, is identical. One twin will get the phentolamine, the other gets prazosin.

Their cardiovascular parameters at baseline (rest) are identical and normal, and everything else that might have an impact on their drug responses is normal and, well, identical. They aren't taking any other drugs.

One twin gets an IV injection of phentolamine. His mean blood pressure falls 20 mm Hg in 20 seconds.

The other gets an IV injection of prazosin at an equally effective dose in terms of the blood pressure response. His mean BP falls by an identical amount, 20 mm Hg, over the same time period, 20 seconds.

What is the most likely difference you will find in the responses of these two boys, one who got phentolamine and the other who got an equivalent pressure-lowering dose of prazosin?

a. Phentolamine will trigger a greater baroreceptor-mediated reflex increase of heart rate and contractility than the prazosin will
b. Prazosin will lead to a bigger reflex positive inotropic and chronotropic response than phentolamine
c. Prazosin will block all reflex cardiac responses because it also has strong β-blocking activity
d. Prazosin will lead to a greater rise of cardiac output than phentolamine by selectively blocking norepinephrine-mediated vasodilation
e. Phentolamine will reduce left ventricular afterload, prazosin will raise it

71. We are using novel in vitro methods to investigate the fate and postsynaptic actions of NE, released upon an action potential generated in an adrenergic nerve. An action potential is generated and the postsynaptic effector briefly responds. Almost instantaneously the response is over. What process mainly accounted for the brevity of the response, and termination of the released NE's actions?

a. Metabolism by enzyme(s) located near the postsynaptic receptor(s) and/or in the synaptic cleft
b. Reuptake into the nerve ending
c. Metabolism by catechol *O*-methyltransferase (COMT)
d. Degradation by mitochondrial monoamine oxidase
e. Conversion to a "false neurotransmitter" in the nerve ending

72. We are contemplating administration of a nonselective β-adrenergic blocker to a patient. In which of the following conditions is this considered generally acceptable, appropriate, and safe?

a. Angina, vasospastic ("variant"; Prinzmetal angina)
b. Asthma
c. Bradycardia
d. Diabetes mellitus, insulin-dependent and poorly controlled
e. Heart block (second degree or greater)
f. Hyperthyroidism, symptomatic and acute
g. Severe congestive heart failure

73. A patient presents in the emergency department in great distress and with the following signs and symptoms:

bizarre behavior, delirium	distended abdomen, full bladder
facial flushing	hot, dry skin
clear lungs, no wheezing, rales, etc	no lacrimal or salivary secretions
high heart rate	very high fever
absence of bowel sounds	dilated pupils

Which drug most likely caused these signs and symptoms?

a. AChE inhibitor
b. α-Adrenergic blocker
c. Antimuscarinic
d. β-Adrenergic blocker
e. Parasympathomimetic (muscarinic agonist)
f. Peripherally acting (neuronal) catecholamine depletor

74. Acebutolol and pindolol are classified as β-adrenergic blockers with intrinsic sympathomimetic activity (ISA). In a practical sense, what does ISA mean apropos the actions of these two drugs?

a. Are partial agonists (mixed agonist/antagonists)
b. Cause norepinephrine and epinephrine release
c. Induce catecholamine synthesis
d. Potentiate the actions of norepinephrine on α-adrenergic receptors
e. Useful when cardiac positive inotropic and chronotropic effects are wanted

75. A 10-year-old boy is diagnosed with attention deficit/attention deficit-hyperactivity disorder (ADD/ADHD). Which drug is most likely to prove effective for relieving the boy's main symptoms?

a. Dobutamine
b. Methylphenidate
c. Pancuronium
d. Prazosin
e. Scopolamine
f. Terbutaline

Questions 76 to 82

The table below shows the perioperative medication administration record (MAR) for an otherwise healthy 50-year-old woman. (To make things interesting I'll deviate from her actual MAR and ask a few questions about relevant but hypothetical scenarios.) She is a nonsmoker, consumes no more than four glasses of wine per week, and has no personal or familial risk factors for heart disease or diabetes. She is taking no other medications. This patient had two scheduled (nonemergent) laparoscopic abdominal surgeries done back to back in the OR. The first was to remove an adnexal (ovary and/or fallopian tube) mass that had been present for a couple of years and grew slowly and irregularly over a couple of years, and to get a pathology report to see whether it is cancerous. Her pathology affected one ovary. Once the ovary was removed a different surgeon performed a second procedure, through the same belly incisions, to alleviate some inconvenient urinary bladder problems.

Her MAR is very typical of what you would find for many otherwise healthy patients undergoing the same or similar surgeries. The first drug listed, midazolam, was given in the preop area right before she was transported to the OR (and I will address its use in the CNS questions; the abbreviation IVP next to midazolam means "IV push," ie, a bolus injection). All the rest were given in the OR by a CRNA (certified registered nurse anesthetist).

Use the table's data, or what you should be able to infer from it, to answer the next seven questions.

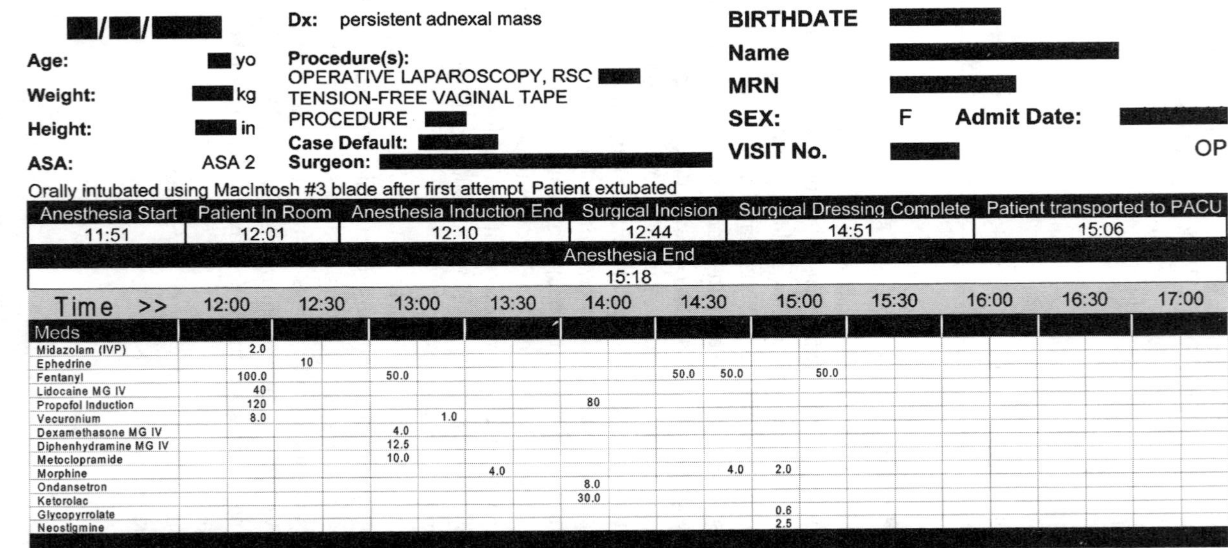

■/■/■

Age:	■ yo	**Dx:** persistent adnexal mass	**BIRTHDATE**	■
Weight:	■ kg	**Procedure(s):** OPERATIVE LAPAROSCOPY, RSC ■ TENSION-FREE VAGINAL TAPE PROCEDURE ■	**Name**	■
Height:	■ in	**Case Default:** ■	**MRN**	■
ASA:	ASA 2	**Surgeon:** ■	**SEX:**	F **Admit Date:** ■
			VISIT No.	■ OP

Orally intubated using MacIntosh #3 blade after first attempt Patient extubated

Anesthesia Start	Patient In Room	Anesthesia Induction End	Surgical Incision	Surgical Dressing Complete	Patient transported to PACU
11:51	12:01	12:10	12:44	14:51	15:06

Anesthesia End
15:18

Time >>	12:00		12:30		13:00		13:30		14:00		14:30		15:00		15:30		16:00		16:30		17:00	
Meds																						
Midazolam (IVP)		2.0																				
Ephedrine			10																			
Fentanyl		100.0			50.0						50.0	50.0		50.0								
Lidocaine MG IV		40																				
Propofol Induction		120							80													
Vecuronium		8.0				1.0																
Dexamethasone MG IV					4.0																	
Diphenhydramine MG IV					12.5																	
Metoclopramide					10.0																	
Morphine							4.0					4.0	2.0									
Ondansetron									8.0													
Ketorolac									30.0													
Glycopyrrolate													0.6									
Neostigmine													2.5									

76. Ephedrine was the first drug administered after anesthesia premedication and induction with several parenteral drugs. What best describes ephedrine's mechanism of action?

a. Directly, selectively, strongly stimulates α-adrenergic receptors in the peripheral vasculature
b. Enhances NE release by blocking presynaptic α-receptors
c. Increases NE synthesis
d. Inhibits NE's intraneuronal metabolic inactivation
e. Releases intraneuronal NE into the synapse, weakly but directly activates all adrenergic receptors

77. Ephedrine and drugs that act in similar ways or cause similar effects have a variety of therapeutic uses. Given the background information provided for this patient and the timing of ephedrine administration on the medication administration record, what is the most likely reason why the ephedrine was given?

a. Cause bronchodilation so mechanical support of ventilation would be easier
b. Counteract CNS depression caused by the induction agents
c. Inhibit sinoatrial and atrioventricular nodal automaticity to terminate or prevent anesthesia-related cardiac arrhythmias
d. Lower heart rate that was raised excessively by the anesthetic drugs
e. Raise blood pressure that was lowered excessively by the induction agents

78. Assume, hypothetically, that the surgery had to be done emergently. The patient had been taking another drug—still in her circulation at usually effective concentrations—that weakened but did not completely eliminate all of ephedrine's peripheral autonomic effects. Which drug(s) would be most likely to do that?

a. Atenolol (or metoprolol)
b. Cocaine or a tricyclic antidepressant (eg, imipramine)
c. Trimethaphan (or hexamethonium)
d. Pargyline (or a similar nonselective MAO inhibitor)
e. Propranolol

79. Shortly after the surgical wounds were closed and dressed, and right before the patient was transferred to the postanesthesia care unit she received neostigmine. What was the reason for which it was given?

a. Raise and support blood pressure during recovery.
b. Raise or otherwise control bradycardia upon recovery from anesthesia.
c. Restore normal neurotransmission in the brain, since it had been suppressed by the induction and anesthetic agents.
d. Reverse skeletal neuromuscular blockade/paralysis.
e. Suppress urinary bladder function to reduce the risk of postoperative bladder incontinence.

80. The patient got her dose of glycopyrrolate mere seconds before the neostigmine was injected. This is done routinely in thousands of surgeries in which the drugs used, and the timing of their administration, are identical to what was done here. To which pharmacologic class does glycopyrrolate most likely belong?

a. α-Adrenergic agonist
b. Antimuscarinic (atropine-like)
c. Cholinesterase inhibitor
d. Muscarinic receptor agonist
e. Nicotinic receptor (skeletal muscle; N_M) agonist

81. The patient in the case presented here was not facing any emergent or imminently life-threatening problems, so skeletal muscle paralysis and intubation were relatively straightforward procedures, not at all rushed. Now assume, hypothetically, that emergency intubation was required, and succinylcholine (SuCh) was used because of its very rapid onset of action. Assume also that a slow infusion of SuCh was used to maintain paralysis throughout the procedure; blood levels of the drug were kept well in the therapeutic range such that no so-called "Phase 2" block occurred; no curare-like (nondepolarizing) blocker was used; and the patient had no genetic or other factors that would affect the pharmacokinetics or action of SuCh. When the surgery is done, what drug would be given to reverse the neuromuscular blockade caused by SuCh?

a. Atropine
b. Bethanechol
c. Neostigmine
d. Physostigmine
e. Nothing

82. Now assume this patient received bethanechol several hours after her abdominal surgery, after effects of all the drugs used intraoperatively, except for morphine and ketorolac (analgesics), had worn off. The bethanechol caused her heart rate to fall slightly and she experienced some wheezing. Which word or phrase most likely accounts for or describes these cardiac and pulmonary responses to bethanechol?

a. Expected side effects
b. Idiosyncrasy
c. Parasympathetic ganglionic activation
d. Reflex (baroreceptor) suppression of cardiac rate
e. Undiagnosed asthma

83. Terbutaline is indicated for suppressing uterine contractions in some women who are in premature labor. Side effects of the drug include increases of heart rate and of the force of left ventricular stroke volume. High-output heart failure (caused by excessively increased cardiac output) and pulmonary edema have occurred, and in some cases the outcome has been fatal. Terbutaline also causes bronchodilation and can be used for that purpose in patients with asthma. It has no vasoconstrictor effects, nor any effects on the size of the pupil(s) of the eye(s). The description most closely fits the characteristics of what class of drugs?

a. α-Adrenergic agonist
b. Atropine-like/antimuscarinic drug
c. β-Adrenergic agonist
d. β-Adrenergic blocker
e. Muscarinic receptor agonist (parasympathomimetic)

84. A patient with a history of asthma experiences significant bronchoconstriction and urticaria, and drug-induced histamine release is a main contributor to these responses. Which drug is most likely to have caused these problems, not because it has any intrinsic bronchoconstrictor or histamine agonist effects but because it quite effectively releases histamine from mast cells?

a. Atropine
b. Neostigmine
c. Pancuronium
d. Propranolol
e. *d*-Tubocurarine

85. During surgery we administer trimethaphan to an anesthetized patient. What would you expect in response to this drug?

a. Bradycardia mediated by activation of the baroreceptor reflex
b. Increased GI tract motility, possible spontaneous defecation
c. Increased salivary secretions
d. Miosis
e. Vasodilation

86. We administer an "effective" dose of a drug and observe the following responses:

- Stimulates the heart
- Dilates some blood vessels but constricts none
- Dilates the bronchi (relaxes airway smooth muscles)
- Raises blood glucose levels
- Neither dilates nor constricts the pupil of the eye

Which of the following drugs is capable of causing all these responses?

a. Atropine
b. Epinephrine
c. Isoproterenol
d. Norepinephrine
e. Phenylephrine

87. "First-generation" (older) histamine H_1 blockers such as diphenhydramine, phenothiazine antipsychotic drugs (eg, chlorpromazine), and tricyclic antidepressants (eg, imipramine) have pharmacologic actions, side effects, toxicities, and contraindications that are very similar to those of which other drug?

a. Atropine
b. Bethanechol
c. Isoproterenol
d. Neostigmine
e. Propranolol

88. A 6-year-old is transported to the emergency department by a parent, who says the boy took a large amount of an allergy medication. The sole active ingredient in the product the parent mentions is diphenhydramine, and it is clear the child is experiencing toxicity from an overdose. The intern, fresh out of medical school, orders parenteral administration of neostigmine, and the medication order is not questioned. What adverse effect of the diphenhydramine will persist following neostigmine administration?

a. Bronchoconstriction and wheezing
b. Delirium, hallucinations, and other CNS manifestations of toxicity
c. Profuse secretions from lacrimal, mucus, and sweat glands
d. Skeletal muscle tremor or fasciculations
e. Tachycardia

89. In between your first and second years of medical school you are volunteering in a hospital in a very poor part of the world. Their drug selection is limited. A patient presents with acute cardiac failure, for which your preferred drug is dobutamine, given intravenously. However, there is none available. Which other drug, or combination of drugs, would be a suitable alternative, giving the pharmacologic equivalent of what you want the dobutamine to do? (All these drugs are available in parenteral formulations.)

a. Dopamine (at a very high dose)
b. Ephedrine
c. Ephedrine plus propranolol
d. Norepinephrine plus phentolamine
e. Phenylephrine plus atropine

90. In general, structures that are affected by sympathetic influences respond to both sympathetic neural activation and to the hormonal component, epinephrine released from the adrenal medulla. Which structure/function is unique in that it responds to epinephrine, but not norepinephrine, and has no direct sympathetic neural control?

a. Airway (tracheal, bronchiolar) smooth muscle: relaxation
b. Atrioventricular node: increased automaticity and conduction velocity
c. Coronary arteries: constriction
d. Iris of the eye: dilation (mydriasis)
e. Renal juxtaglomerular apparatus: renin release

91. The figure below shows several responses measured in a subject (healthy; receiving no other drugs) at rest (before) and after receiving a dose of an unknown drug.

Note: The blood pressures shown can be considered mean blood pressure; the fall caused by the unknown drug was mainly due to a fall of diastolic pressure.

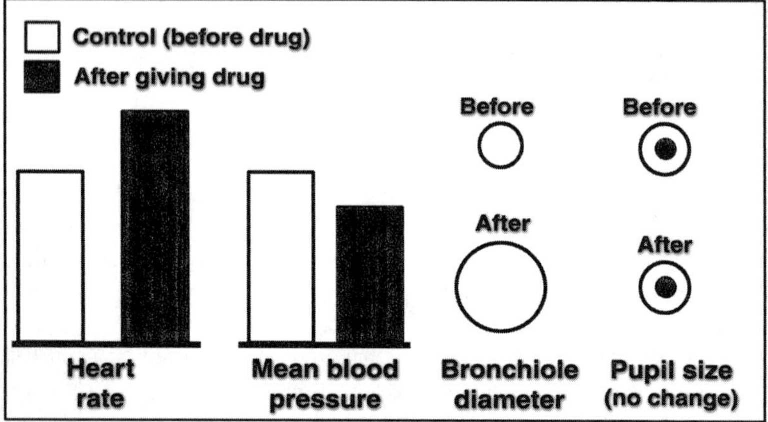

Which of the following drugs most likely caused the observed responses?

a. Atropine
b. Isoproterenol
c. Neostigmine
d. Phenylephrine
e. Propranolol

92. Adrenergic nerves to the heart are activated, leading to a reflex increase of heart rate and cardiac contractility, in response to a sudden and significant fall of blood pressure. Those sympathetic nerves release norepinephrine (NE). What is the main physiologic mechanism by which the actions of the released NE are terminated?

a. Diffusion away from postsynaptic receptors
b. Hydrolysis by nonspecific deaminases
c. Metabolic inactivation by MAO
d. Metabolic inactivation by catechol *O*-methyltransferase
e. Reuptake into the adrenergic nerve from which the NE was released

93. A 59-year-old man has a history of emphysema from 40 years of cigarette smoking; hypercholesterolemia that is being managed with atorvastatin; and Stage II essential hypertension for which he is taking metolazone. He presents in clinic today with his main new complaints: nocturia, urinary frequency, and an inability to urinate forcefully and empty his bladder. Following a complete workup, the physician arrives at a diagnosis of benign prostatic hypertrophy (BPH). The physician starts daily therapy with tamsulosin. What is the most likely side effect the patient may experience from the tamsulosin, and about which he should be forewarned?

a. Bradycardia
b. Increased risk of statin-induced skeletal muscle pathology
c. Orthostatic hypotension
d. Photophobia and other painful responses to bright lights
e. Wheezing or other exacerbations of the emphysema

94. A patient walks out of the ophthalmologist's office and into bright sunlight after a comprehensive eye examination, for which he received a topical ophthalmic drug. The drug has not only dilated his pupils but also impaired his ability to focus his eyes up close.

The drug this patient received was most likely classified as, or worked most similar to, which prototype?

a. Acetylcholine
b. Epinephrine
c. Homatropine
d. Isoproterenol
e. Pilocarpine
f. Propranolol

95. The Institutional Review Board approved a study of the in vitro (tissue bath) responsiveness of isolated human arteriolar segments (obtained during surgery) to a variety of pharmacologic and other interventions. The tissue samples are 1-cm-long "cylinders" of otherwise-normal (but now denervated) arterioles obtained from the lower legs of patients undergoing amputation surgery.

The experimental model allows us to perfuse the vessels with a solution that will keep the tissue functionally and structurally intact for many hours; to monitor and change perfusion pressure (mm Hg; analogous to "blood pressure" in the intact organism) and perfusate flow (mL/min); and to assess the effects of various vasoactive drugs on the system.

We add ACh to the perfusate to give a concentration identical to the plasma concentration of ACh that causes "expected responses" in an intact human.

Under this experimental setup, adding ACh causes a rise of perfusion pressure and a decrease of flow, both of which basically reflect vasoconstriction.

What is the most likely explanation for these findings?

a. ACh released norepinephrine from the endothelium, which caused vasoconstriction
b. Atropine was added to the tissue bath before adding the ACh
c. Botulinum toxin was added to the bath before adding the ACh
d. The vascular endothelium has been damaged or removed (denuded)
e. This response is precisely what we'd expect with injection of ACh into the intact human

96. A 33-year-old woman becomes poisoned after receiving an injection of illicitly prepared and overly concentrated botulinum toxin. What is the main neurochemical mechanism by which this *Clostridium* toxin causes its effects?

a. Directly activates all muscarinic and nicotinic receptors
b. Inhibits ACh release from all cholinergic nerves
c. Prevents neuronal NE reuptake
d. Releases NE via a nonexocytotic process
e. Selectively and competitively blocks nicotinic receptors

97. A patient takes a massive overdose of diphenhydramine, suffering not only significant CNS depression but also numerous and serious peripheral autonomic side effects. By what mechanism did diphenhydramine exert its untoward peripheral autonomic actions?

a. Activation of both β_1 and β_2 adrenoceptors
b. Blockade of α-adrenergic receptors
c. Competitive antagonism of ACh actions on muscarinic receptors
d. Massive, direct overactivation of ganglionic nicotinic receptors
e. Sudden release of epinephrine from the adrenal medulla (suprarenal medulla)

98. A patient with a recent drug poisoning is transported to the emergency department. The physician orders (correctly, in this case) administration of pralidoxime as part of the comprehensive emergency treatment plan. Which best describes who the patient was?

a. A 13-year-old boy who took an overdose of methylphenidate for his ADD/ADHD
b. A 43-year-old who took an overdose of neostigmine, prescribed for her myasthenia gravis, in a suicide attempt
c. A 6-year-old who got into the family medicine cabinet and took 10 "adult doses" of her dad's prazosin
d. A farm/field worker accidentally doused with insecticide from an overflying crop-duster plane
e. An asthma patient who accidentally gave himself an intravenous injection of epinephrine in an attempt to self-treat a developing anaphylactic reaction

99. To facilitate a certain eye examination we want to cause mydriasis, but not alter normal control of accommodation. All of the following drugs are available as topical ophthalmic formulations. Which one will dilate the pupil without altering accommodation?

a. Atropine
b. Epinephrine
c. Homatropine
d. Isoproterenol
e. Pilocarpine
f. Timolol

100. A 26-year-old woman has rhinorrhea, excessive lacrimation, and ocular congestion from a bout with the common cold. Diphenhydramine provides symptomatic relief. What is the most likely mechanism by which this drug relieved her symptoms?

a. α-Adrenergic activation (agonist, vasoconstrictor)
b. β-Adrenergic blockade
c. Calcium channel blockade
d. Histamine (H_2) receptor blockade
e. Muscarinic receptor blockade

101. You have treated dozens of patients with acute hypotension from various causes, including overdoses of antihypertensive drugs, all of which can cause hypotension. Your usual approach to restoring blood pressure, and one that has worked well every time before, is to inject *x* mg of phenylephrine intravenously. Today a patient with severe drug-induced hypotension presents in the emergency department. He has been taking this drug for many months. He is not volume-depleted, nor hemorrhaging. You give the phenylephrine at the same dose and by the same route as you always have. It causes no change of blood pressure. Which drug did the patient most likely take and overdose on?

a. Atenolol
b. Bethanechol
c. Prazosin
d. Propranolol
e. Reserpine

102. This is a strange day for you in the emergency department. Now you have to treat another normovolemic patient with acute drug-induced hypotension, and so you give the usually correct and effective dose of phenylephrine. This time the drug causes a vasopressor response that is far greater than you've ever encountered when giving the very same dose: systolic pressure rises dramatically, if not dangerously. What drug did the patient most likely take?

a. Atenolol
b. Bethanechol
c. Prazosin
d. Propranolol
e. Reserpine

103. A 43-year-old woman with diagnosed myasthenia gravis, and taking pyridostigmine daily, presents in the neurology clinic with profound skeletal muscle weakness. You are unsure whether she is experiencing a cholinergic crisis or a myasthenic crisis, so you administer a usually appropriate diagnostic dose of parenteral edrophonium. Assume the patient was actually experiencing a cholinergic crisis. What is the most likely response to the edrophonium?

a. Hypertensive crisis from peripheral vascular constriction
b. Myocardial ischemia, and angina, from drug-induced tachycardia and coronary vasoconstriction
c. Premature ventricular contractions from increased ventricular automaticity
d. Prompt improvement of skeletal muscle tone and function
e. Ventilatory distress or failure

104. A patient who will be new to your practice makes an appointment for their first visit. Your nurse asks them to bring in all their current prescribed medications and any OTC drugs they take regularly. They comply. One OTC drug is a popular brand-name product that contains doxylamine as its sole active ingredient. Which property or characteristic best describes this drug?

a. Likely to lower heart rate excessively
b. May be a cause of diarrhea that the patient says he often gets
c. Should not be used by patients with prostatic hypertrophy or angle-closure glaucoma
d. Tends to raise blood pressure through a typical catecholamine-like vasoconstrictor (α adrenergic) mechanism
e. Used during the day, helps them keep awake and alert via a weak amphetamine-like action in the CNS

The Peripheral Nervous Systems: Autonomic and Somatic Nervous System Pharmacology

Answers

I've reproduced the figure presented in the questions section here, but modified it to show the nerve types and locations, and the receptors, to save you a bit of page-flipping when you review your answers.

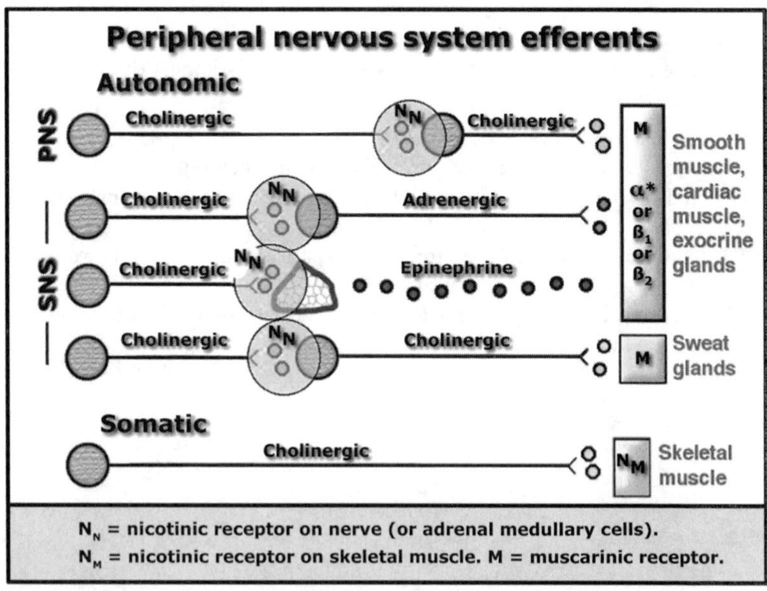

*Note: Whether a structure under the influence of the sympathetic nervous system has an α_1, β_1, or β_2 receptor depends on what the structure is. Recall, also, that adrenergic nerves release norepinephrine, which only activates α_1 and β_1 receptors. Not shown are presynaptic α receptors (α_2).

36. The answer is b. *(Brunton, pp 137-142. Katzung, pp 78-80.)* Here's a simple rule: in the peripheral nervous systems—that is, the somatic nervous system and both branches of the autonomic nervous system—"the first nerve 'out' of the CNS (in this diagram, *a*, *c*, *e*, *f*, and *h*) is always cholinergic and the ACh released from those nerves always activates the nicotinic subtype of cholinergic receptor on the postsynaptic target cell(s)."

37. The answer is c. *(Brunton, pp 137-142. Katzung, pp 78-80.)* Another rule, with one important exception: "all the efferents in the peripheral nervous systems are cholinergic *except* postganglionic sympathetics going to structures other than sweat glands and arrector pili muscles." There are 8 nerves in the schematic. Seven of them—all except the majority of postganglionic sympathetics (*nerve d*)—are cholinergic (synthesize and release ACh as their neurotransmitter). The main postganglionic sympathetic fibers (except those innervating eccrine sweat glands and arrector pili muscles) synthesize and release norepinephrine (NE; not epinephrine; answer d) as their neurotransmitter, and so are adrenergic (or noradrenergic if you prefer) nerves. What else can you call *nerve d*? A postganglionic sympathetic nerve to certain smooth muscles, to cardiac muscle, and certain exocrine glands except sweat glands.

Atropine (a) is incorrect. It selectively and competitively blocks the effects of ACh (and other muscarinic agonists) on muscarinic receptors. In the preceding diagram, those receptors are found on structures innervated by *nerves b* and *g*.

Answer b is incorrect. NE, *nerve d*'s neurotransmitter, is an effective agonist for α-adrenergic receptors (α_1 and α_2) and for β_1 receptors. Bronchodilation caused by sympathetic activation requires activation of β_2 receptors; NE cannot do that but EPI, released from the adrenal (suprarenal) medulla, certainly can. And once NE has been released from its neurons and activates its postsynaptic receptors, its actions are promptly terminated by reuptake via an "amine pump" that can be blocked by cocaine or tricyclic antidepressants. Hydrolysis in the synaptic cleft (e) is the mechanism by which the actions of ACh, released from cholinergic nerves, is terminated.

38. The answer is d. *(Brunton, pp 146-150. Katzung, pp 78-80.)* The actions of NE, released from adrenergic nerves, are terminated by neuronal reuptake. (Don't forget that this reuptake process is inhibited by cocaine and tricyclic antidepressants, and the outcome is increased and more prolonged effects of NE because it lingers longer and accumulates in the synapse, exposed to its postsynaptic targets.) All the other nerves shown in the diagram are cholinergic; the actions of the ACh they release are terminated promptly by hydrolysis (via acetylcholinesterase).

39. The answer is g. *(Brunton, pp 139-141. Katzung, pp 78-80.)* The neurotransmitter released from *nerve d*, the postganglionic sympathetic fibers (to structures other than sweat glands and arrector pili muscles), is norepinephrine. NE can activate α-adrenergic receptors (both α_1 and α_2), and β_1 receptors (not β_2). Of course, different structures have different subtypes of these receptors: such structures as arterioles and the iris dilator muscle have α_1 receptors; β_1 receptors are found in the heart and in the juxtaglomerular apparatus (kidneys), while β_2 receptors (remember, they are *not* activated by NE) are found on various smooth muscles, mainly in the airways. So, the only correct response to the question "which receptors are activated?" really depends on which structure is being innervated. As a final note, NE cannot activate cholinergic receptors, and so answers e and f are incorrect.

40. The answer is b. *(Brunton, 138-140, 140f, 144t. Katzung, pp 75-76, 78-80.)* The postganglionic sympathetic fibers innervating sweat glands and arrector pili muscles are cholinergic. That is the exception to the rule that "all postganglionic sympathetic fibers are adrenergic." How do you know it's cholinergic? A variety of biochemical and histochemical methods can prove that ACh is the neurotransmitter. They also show that there is abundant acetylcholinesterase (AChE), which hydrolyzes ACh, in the synaptic cleft. Pharmacologically we can prevent release of neurotransmitter from *nerve* g with botulinum toxin, which affects only (and all) cholinergic nerves. We can prevent the response of the sweat glands and the arrectores pilorum innervated by *nerve* g with atropine, the prototype muscarinic receptor antagonist—a drug that has no effects on nicotinic (or other) receptors (eg, answer d) at usual doses. Likewise, nicotinic receptor blockers (or nicotine itself) have no effect at this site—another reason why answer d is incorrect. And how do you know it's part of the SNS? Sweat glands are activated (secretions are increased) when the rest of the SNS is activated during the fight or flight response, and if you trace the origins of the preganglionic nerves that activate the postganglionic ones, they emanate from the same regions of the spinal cord from which all other sympathetic preganglionic fibers arise—the thoracic and lumbar regions of the cord. Innervation of the arrectores pilorum, leading to "hair standing on end," is similar.

Cocaine (a) is incorrect. It, and tricyclic antidepressants (eg, amitriptyline, imipramine), block neuronal reuptake of NE. That is, its site of action is at the neuroeffector junction of postganglionic sympathetic neurons (*nerve d*)—all of them except those that innervate most sweat glands, of course.

41. The answer is c. *(Brunton, pp 138-141, 150-153. Katzung, pp 78, 81t.)* The nerve is cholinergic, so the neurotransmitter it acts on, postsynaptically, must be either nicotinic or muscarinic. Nicotinic receptors are found on cell bodies of all postganglionic nerves (in both SNS and PNS; N_N receptors), on the adrenal medulla (also N_N), and on skeletal muscle (somatic nervous system, N_M)—at the "first synapses out of the CNS." Cholinergic receptors at all other sites are muscarinic, "defined" by the fact that those receptors are competitively blocked by atropine. Be sure to see the explanation for Question 36.

42. The answer is h. *(Brunton, pp 220-225. Katzung, pp 78, 452-460.)* Pancuronium and tubocurarine (as well as, metocurine, vecuronium, and several related drugs) are nondepolarizing skeletal neuromuscular blockers (quite different, mechanistically, from succinylcholine, a depolarizing blocker). They specifically and competitively block activation of nicotinic receptors (N_M) on skeletal muscle by ACh, thereby preventing skeletal muscle depolarization and subsequent contraction; and have no effect on muscarinic receptors or any of the adrenergic receptor subtypes. (Remember something about the natives of the Amazon obtaining a poisonous substance from the skin of certain species of frogs, putting it on the tips of their darts, and using that to kill their dinner with a blow-gun? That was curare, *d*-tubocurarine, the prototype nondepolarizing skeletal neuromuscular blocker, as we've come to know it.)

Here again is the diagram to which Questions 43 to 47 referred.

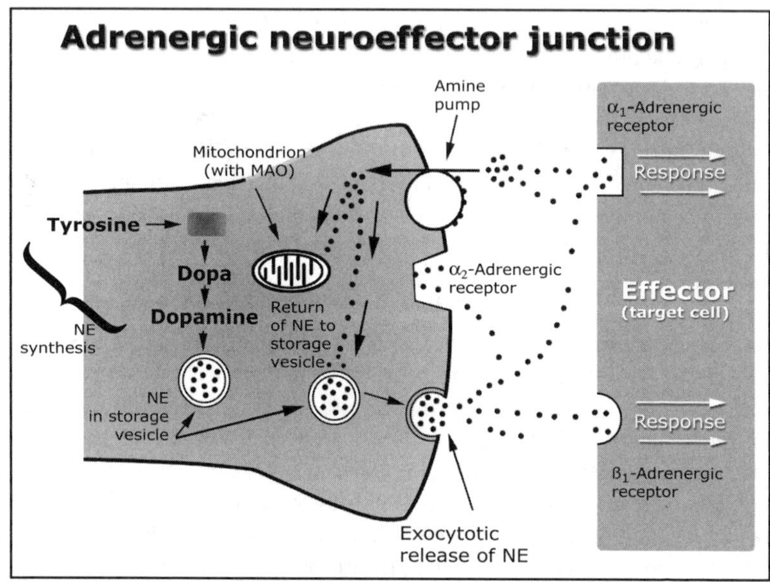

43. The answer is b. *(Brunton, pp 158-164. Katzung, pp 84, 86f, 92t, 517-520.)* While mitochondria in virtually all cells in which they are found are important for oxidative phosphorylation and ATP synthesis, I asked about the mitochondrial MAO that is rich in adrenergic neurons. There MAO degrades NE that is free (ie, not safely stored away in the storage vesicles). If that intravesicular uptake is inhibited, as with occurs with reserpine and a few other drugs like it, NE stores will be depleted as the result of MAO-mediated NE breakdown.

None of the structures or processes shown in the diagram is responsible for intraneuronal movement of NE-containing storage vesicles to, and ultimate fusion with, the nerve "ending" (a). Metabolism of dopamine to NE (c) occurs in the storage vesicles via the enzyme dopamine β-hydroxylase. MAO does not provide "energy" for nonexocytotic NE release (d), and plays no role in ATP synthesis (e).

44. The answer is d. *(Brunton, pp 158-164, 171t, 172t. Katzung, pp 81-82, 90.)* Reserpine blocks intraneuronal storage of NE, thereby exposing the free NE to degradation by intraneuronal MAO. This is important because the final synthesis of NE from its precursor occurs in the vesicles; if dopamine entry is blocked, NE synthesis is thereby inhibited. Reserpine also blocks vesicular uptake of dopamine in parts of the CNS.

Pargyline (a) is a nonselective MAO inhibitor. Note that unlike reserpine, MAO inhibitors do not inhibit intraneuronal storage of NE. Rather, they prevent metabolic inactivation of NE (or, at other sites, other monoamines). Prazosin (b) and propranolol (c) are adrenergic receptor blockers (α_1 and $\beta_{1,2}$, respectively) and have no direct effect on NE storage. Tyramine (e) is an indirect-acting sympathomimetic that displaces and releases neuronal NE.

45. The answer is b. *(Brunton, pp 158-162, 171t, 239, 377, 620. Katzung, pp 82-84, 92t, 142.)* Cocaine (and tricyclic antidepressants such as imipramine) are classic examples of drugs that inhibit catecholamine reuptake by the "amine pump," which is the main process by which released NE (or dopamine) reenters the neuron and its receptor-mediated effects are terminated physiologically. In the presence of cocaine or a tricyclic, released neurotransmitter lingers and accumulates in the synapse (neuroeffector junction), and so pertinent adrenergic responses appear heightened or more intense, and prolonged. The pump is also important for the neuronal uptake, and ultimate effects, of such catecholamine-releasing drugs as ephedrine, pseudoephedrine, amphetamines, methylphenidate, and tyramine.

As long as an adrenergic synapse is present (as it is in the diagram) and exposed to cocaine or a tricyclic antidepressant, the drugs' effects are not dependent on whether the effector (target) is smooth muscle, cardiac muscle, or an exocrine gland of any sort.

Cocaine has no direct effect on α_2-adrenergic receptors (a), nor on any of the postsynaptic adrenergic receptors (c). Likewise, the drug has no effect on MAO (d) nor on the exocytotic release of NE in response to an action potential (e).

There is no direct functional link between the amine pump and such processes as NE release (exocytotically or otherwise) or activation of presynaptic (α_2) adrenergic receptors.

46. The answer is c. *(Brunton, pp 167-170, 172t. Katzung, pp 24-26.)* The adrenergic neuronal α_2 (presynaptic) receptor, like other adrenergic receptors, is G-protein-coupled. When the receptor is activated by a suitable agonist, it signals the neuron to stop further NE release following an action potential. Norepinephrine itself is one such agonist; its activation of the presynaptic α_2-receptor, which occurs concomitant with activation of postsynaptic [α_1 or β_1] adrenergic receptors (depending on what the distal target cell is), provides a physiologic "feedback" signal that halts further NE release. That is, released NE regulates the release of more NE from the very neuron from which the neurotransmitter came.

Although activation of both the presynaptic α_2 receptors and NE reuptake by the amine pump/transporter occurs almost simultaneously, there is no direct functional or biochemical linkage between the two. That is, blocking (or stimulating) the α_2 receptor will not directly affect NE reuptake (a), nor will drugs that affect the amine pump necessarily have any direct effect on the α_2 receptors and the function they serve. There is no effect on norepinephrine synthesis (b, whether by dopamine β-hydroxylase or other enzymes involved in neurotransmitter synthesis), nor on MAO (d).

Note: Clonidine, which you typically (and correctly) think of as a centrally acting antihypertensive drug, acts as an α_2 agonist in the periphery. It's "turning off" of NE release, then, can contribute to reduced vasoconstriction (and other adrenergic processes mediated by NE), which in turn helps lower blood pressure. However, clonidine is a very lipophilic drug. When it is given in usual doses, by the usual route (oral or transdermal), the drug enters the CNS well, and rather promptly, and it acts there (in the cardiovascular control center of the brain's medulla) to inhibit sympathetic outflow. It is that central effect that accounts for the drug's main antihypertensive mechanism.

47. The answer is b. *(Brunton, pp 163-165f, 172t, 174. Katzung, pp 84, 86t, 476.)* Only COMT has the properties noted in the question. Entacapone is an example of a COMT inhibitor that is used therapeutically. It is given mainly to manage Parkinson disease, in conjunction with levodopa. It inhibits the peripheral (eg, intestinal) conversion of levodopa to dopamine (recall that dopamine itself does not cross the blood-brain barrier), and is an alternative to carbidopa, which inhibits DOPA decarboxylase. (See Questions 113, 136, 149, and 165 in the CNS chapter for more on entacapone, carbidopa, and drugs for parkinsonism in general.)

The other enzymes listed in the question are involved in catecholamine synthesis. Aromatic L-amino acid decarboxylase (a) converts DOPA to dopamine, which is then converted to norepinephrine by dopamine β-hydroxylase (c). In the adrenal medulla phenylethanolamine *N*-methyltransferase (d) converts some norepinephrine to epinephrine. Tyrosine hydroxylase (e) converts tyrosine to DOPA.

48. The answer is e. *(Brunton, pp 144-145, 172t, 269-270, 246-247. Katzung, pp 150-152, 177.)* Prazosin selectively blocks α_1-adrenergic receptors and, unlike many other α-blockers (phentolamine, phenoxybenzamine), has virtually no presynaptic (α_2) effects at usual doses.

None of the other drugs fit the bill: ephedrine (a) exerts sympathomimetic (adrenomimetic) effects in part by releasing intraneuronal NE, and in part by directly but weakly acting as an agonist on all the adrenergic receptors. It has no antagonist activity with respect to any adrenergic (or cholinergic) receptors. (Related drugs are pseudoephedrine and phenylpropanolamine, the latter [now off the market]; and the lesser-known drug metaraminol.) Labetalol (b) blocks both α- and β-adrenergic receptors, and is an agonist for neither. (A mechanistically related and important drug is carvedilol.) Phentolamine (c) nonselectively blocks both α_1 and α_2 receptors, has no β-blocking activity, and is an agonist for none of the adrenergic receptors. Phenylephrine (d) is a strong agonist for all the α-adrenergic receptors, has no α-agonist activity, and exerts no effects of any type on β-receptors.

49. The answer is a. *(Brunton, pp 166t, 189-195, 197. Katzung, pp 116-122.)* You probably never learned or read about festoterodine (it's too new), but that makes no difference in terms of being able to answer this question. The description of this drug is, in reality, also an excellent description of many of the properties of atropine, the prototype muscarinic receptor blocking drug, and of nearly a dozen other antimuscarinics marketed for "overactive bladder." In terms of bladder function, parasympathetic influences tend to promote urine flow; antimuscarinics, then, tend to suppress that effect. (Conversely, sympathetic influences, via α-adrenergic receptor activation, tend to suppress urine flow and α-adrenergic blockers cause the opposite.)

You should be able to spot incorrect answers by a simple process of elimination. For example, do β-blockers (b) cause the visual, urinary tract, sweat gland, or cardiovascular responses noted in the question? Not at all, nor do isoproterenol (c; $\beta_{1,2}$ agonist), neostigmine (d; cholinesterase inhibitor, which produces precisely the opposite responses that atropine, festoterodine, and all the other antimuscarinics used for bladder overactivity do), or phentolamine (e; nonselective α-blocker).

Note: The mechanism of action of festoterodine, its indications, side effects and adverse responses—and just about any other relevant property you can imagine, including the dose—are exactly the same as those of an older and widely advertised brand name drug, tolterodine. Coincidental? Not at all. Both drugs have the same active metabolite.

50. The answer is c. *(Brunton, pp 161-163, 171t-172t, 257-259. Katzung, pp 134, 141, 144-145.)* Amphetamines (dextroamphetamine, methamphetamine, amphetamine, and several related drugs) can be classified as indirect-acting sympathomimetics (adrenomimetics). They are transported into the adrenergic nerve ending by the amine pump, displace NE from its storage vesicles (*via* processes that are not dependent on an action potential) and cause the stored neurotransmitter to be released into the synaptic space. At that point, all the expected effects of NE on its receptors and effectors occur. These drugs have no direct effects, whether as an agonist or antagonist, on the adrenergic receptors. Their actions are wholly dependent on intraneuronal catecholamine stores.

Amphetamines and related drugs have no ability to directly activate (or inhibit) MAO (a); to affect intraneuronal NE stores (c); or stimulate (or inhibit) intraneuronal NE synthesis (d). The amine pump upon which cocaine and related drugs mainly act is located on the presynaptic adrenergic nerve "ending," as are the main populations of α_2 receptors; however, these drugs do not directly affect, either by stimulating or blocking, those α_2 receptors (e).

51. The answer is c. *(Brunton, pp 243-246. Katzung, pp 136-139, 143-144, 343.)* The inotropic (contractility), chronotropic (rate), and dromotropic (conduction velocity-related) effects of epinephrine on the heart are mediated through activation of β_1-adrenergic receptors. These receptor sites mediate an epinephrine-induced increased firing rate of the SA node (spontaneous, or Phase 4, depolarization), increased conduction velocity through the AV node and the His-Purkinje system, and increased contractility and conduction velocity of atrial and ventricular muscle. Epinephrine activation of α-adrenoceptors does not affect cardiac function in any physiologically or therapeutically important way—except for the crucial role of α-adrenoceptors as mediators of coronary artery vasoconstriction (clearly a vascular smooth muscle, not cardiac muscle, phenomenon). The β_2-adrenergic receptors play no direct role in cardiac stimulation. They are more important in the relaxation of airway smooth muscle, dilation of arterioles that serve skeletal muscles, increased secretion of insulin by the pancreas, and to a lesser degree relaxation of the detrusor of the urinary bladder. (Lipolysis in fat cells and melatonin secretion by the pineal gland appear to involve stimulation of β_3-adrenergic receptors. However, we do not have any clinically useful drugs that selectively activate or block the β_3 receptors, and so you might not want to spend your time learning about the β_3 receptors.)

52. The answer is b. *(Brunton, pp 205, 207t, 1720t, 1723. Katzung, pp 103-109.)* Echothiophate is an "irreversible" which basically means "very long acting" in terms of the duration of effects) acetylcholinesterase inhibitor. It is used topically on the eye, as a miotic, to treat various types of glaucoma. By increasing synaptic levels of ACh it increases contraction of the circular muscles of the eye, causing the pupils to constrict (miosis). That reduces mechanical obstruction of aqueous humor outflow via the Canal of Schlemm and the trabecular "meshwork" in the angle of the anterior chamber. (In contrast, sympathetic activation causes mydriasis by activating the radial muscles through α-agonist effects, and can lead to increased intraocular pressure due to reduced aqueous humor drainage.) Maximum reduction of intraocular pressure occurs within 24 hours, and the effect may persist for several days. The drug is water-soluble, which affords a practical advantage over the lipid-soluble isofluorphate (another cholinesterase inhibitor used to treat glaucoma).

Note: Had I listed a drug with a generic name ending in the suffix "-stigmine," you no doubt would have answered correctly and immediately. However, echothiophate is one of those cholinesterase inhibitors that is not a stigmine. If you're unfamiliar with the drug, by all means look it up!

Tyrosine hydroxylase (a) is involved in the biosynthesis of catecholamines. COMT (c) is involved in extraneuronal metabolism of catecholamines, while MAO (d) is the major intraneuronal enzyme that degrades NE in adrenergic nerves. Forms of MAO are also found in, and important in, the liver and parts of the CNS. DOPA decarboxylase (e) catalyzes the metabolism of DOPA (dihydroxyphenylalanine) to dopamine as part of the catecholamine biosynthetic pathway.

53. The answer is a. *(Brunton, pp 192, 196, 1711, 1722. Katzung, pp 116-120.)* With any antimuscarinic drug—and scopolamine certainly is one—narrow-angle glaucoma (which accounts for about 10% of all glaucomas) is the biggest concern (assuming no relevant comorbidities). The drug might provoke significant rises of intraocular pressure as it further reduces aqueous humor drainage, causing not only pain but vision problems that might be severe or permanent. Bradycardia (b) is not a concern; if anything, usual doses of scopolamine may increase heart rate a bit. Should the patient eat some shellfish or other allergy-provoking food (c), the incidence or severity of diarrhea might be reduced or prevented altogether by the scopolamine, due to its effects on longitudinal muscles in the gut (inhibited) and on sphincters (activated). A resting blood pressure of 112/70 or thereabouts (d) is not at all uncommon or worrisome, and not likely to be changed at all by the drug. Hypothyroidism (e) typically is associated with slight bradycardia; again, no likely problem with scopolamine. And if our patient had mild Parkinson disease (f), we might actually, eventually, see a little improvement with this drug. Recall, one strategy to manage parkinsonism—basically a central imbalance between dopamine and ACh, the latter appearing to be acting in relative excess—is to block central muscarinic receptors with such drugs as benztropine or trihexyphenidyl (see CNS chapter).

54. The answer is a. *(Brunton, pp 283t, 285. Katzung, pp 153-157, 159, 177.)* Labetalol is a competitive antagonist at both α- and β-adrenergic (both β_1 and β_2) receptors. (Here is a "trick" that might help you remember that labetalol blocks both main types of adrenergic receptors: take the first two letters in "labetalol" and reverse them—*la* transposes to *al*, as in *alpha*—and then add the next four letters—*beta*. You'll simply have to memorize the name of another important α-/β-blocker, carvedilol.) Note, too, that the generic names of all the drugs listed end in *-olol*—a great tip-off that a drug has β-blocking activity. In fact, every drug with a generic name that ends in *-olol* is a β-blocker.

Labetalol's α-blocking actions are relatively weak compared with its actions at the β-receptors, but they are clinically important in terms of lowering total peripheral resistance and blood pressure nonetheless. This relative difference is somewhat concentration-dependent: at relatively low blood levels, as might be achieved with typical oral doses, labetalol is about three times more potent as a β-blocker than as an α-blocker (do not commit this number to memory!). With higher concentrations, such as those often achieved with parenteral (eg, IV) dosing, the intensity of β-blockade increases considerably with little increase in α-blocking efficacy. One of labetalol's main uses is for managing essential hypertension (all the orally administered β-blockers are indicated for essential hypertension and for chronic-stable angina). It lowers pressure in three ways: reduces heart rate, reduces contractility, and also reduces renin release, thereby reducing the formation of angiotensin II and, indirectly, release of aldosterone. All these effects are mediated by β_1 blockade. Given parenterally (IV), labetalol is often a first-choice agent for managing urgent hypertensive crises when more efficacious (and potentially more dangerous) IV drugs aren't indicated or cannot be given safely.

Metoprolol (b; and atenolol and acebutolol, not listed) have a preferential (but certainly not absolute!) and dose-dependent effect on β_1 receptors ("cardioselectivity") versus β_2, and have no α-blocking actions. Relatively high doses of those drugs can (and often do) block β_2 receptors, and any dose may pose serious risks of bronchoconstriction or bronchospasm for patients with asthma. Nadolol (c) and timolol (d) are nonselective β-blockers. (One property to remember for nadolol is its relatively long half-life; for timolol you might want to recall that a topical ophthalmic dosage form is often used for chronic open-angle glaucoma.) Pindolol (d) is a nonselective β-blocker and also exerts strong intrinsic sympathomimetic activity (ISA; ie, partial agonist-antagonist activity).

55. The answer is e. *(Brunton, pp 166t, 174, 264, 264f, 271. Katzung, pp 152-153.)* Whether you memorize that yohimbine is a selective α_2 antagonist is up to you (I think you have far more important drugs to learn about), but you should know what the main effects of a drug described as a selective α_2 antagonist are. That, of course, depends on knowing what α_2 receptors—at least in the peripheral autonomic nervous system—does in the physiological sense. Recall that the preponderance of physiologically important α_2 receptors are located on adrenergic nerve terminals (or nerve "endings"). When stimulated by a suitable agonist, the response is a turning-off of further NE release. Because NE is the neurotransmitter released from adrenergic nerves and it is an excellent α agonist, the presynaptic α_2 receptors upon which NE acts serve as the main physiologic mechanism for regulating neurotransmitter release.

So, when we block those receptors with yohimbine, we enhance the apparent overall activity of the sympathetic nervous system on its effectors by interfering with norepinephrine's ability to turn-off its own release. Of the responses listed, only hypertension (owing to the vasoconstrictor effects of NE on postsynaptic α-adrenergic receptors) occurs as a result of yohimbine (or of NE excess). The other main effects you should anticipate would be cardiac stimulation (rate, contractility, electrical impulse conduction rates; all β_1-mediated effects) and, usually of less clinical consequence, mydriasis (α).

In terms of the aphrodisiac effects, the drug probably increases arousal via an action in the CNS, but the mechanism isn't known for sure; and it increases the vigor of ejaculation, which is predominantly an α-mediated effect. (Recall that erection primarily involves muscarinic-cholinergic vascular effects, mediated by enhanced production of endothelium-derived relaxing factor ie, nitric oxide.)

56. The answer is e. *(Brunton, pp 204, 211, 214, 538-540. Katzung, pp 98, 108, 1041.)* Patients with Alzheimer disease present with progressive impairment of memory and cognitive functions such as a lack of attention, disturbed language function, and an inability to complete common tasks. Although the exact defect in the central nervous system (CNS) has not been elucidated, evidence suggests that a reduction in cholinergic nerve function or receptor activation plays an important role in the etiology. At the very least, increasing central cholinergic receptor activation seems to reduce symptom severity.

Tacrine mainly acts in the CNS. It has been found to be somewhat effective in patients with mild-to-moderate symptoms of this disease for improvement of cognitive functions. The drug is primarily a reversible cholinesterase inhibitor that increases the concentration of functional ACh in the brain. However, the pharmacology of tacrine is complex; the drug also acts as a muscarinic receptor modulator in that it has partial agonistic activity, as well as weak antagonistic activity on muscarinic receptors in the CNS. In addition, tacrine appears to enhance the release of ACh from cholinergic nerves, and it may alter the concentrations of other neurotransmitters such as dopamine and NE.

Of all of the reversible cholinesterase inhibitors, only tacrine and physostigmine cross the blood-brain barrier in sufficient amounts to make these compounds useful for disorders involving the CNS. Physostigmine has been tried as a therapy for Alzheimer disease; however, it is more commonly used to antagonize the effects of toxic concentrations of drugs with strong antimuscarinic properties, including atropine, antihistamines, phenothiazines, and tricyclic antidepressants.

Ambenonium (a), neostigmine (c), and pyridostigmine (d) are used mainly in the treatment of myasthenia gravis; edrophonium (b), a very fast but short-acting cholinesterase inhibitor is mainly used to help differentiate between myasthenic and cholinergic crises in patients who are being treated for myasthenia gravis and present with unexplained muscle weakness or paralysis. Since these other cholinesterase inhibitors work mainly in the periphery, both unwanted or excessive muscarinic effects and skeletal muscle stimulation (nicotinic receptors) are important accompaniments of their use.

57. The answer is b. *(Brunton, pp 152-154, 231-233. Katzung, pp 108-109.)* Nicotine initially stimulates and then blocks nicotinic-skeletal muscular (N_M) and nicotinic-neural (N_N; in autonomic ganglia and on adrenal medullary cells) cholinergic receptors. (Both effects involve depolarization of the target cells, and in many ways it is comparable to the depolarizing blockade of skeletal muscle activation by succinylcholine—initial stimulation followed by inhibition.) Initial ganglionic stimulation leads to vasoconstriction and hypertension, both of which are manifestations of sympathetic activation. Heart rate changes can vary. Parasympathetic ganglionic activation is likely to increase the normally predominant parasympathetic (bradycardic) tone on heart rate, but sympathetic ganglion activation may cause the opposite effect. Initial stimulation of skeletal muscle N_M receptors would account for the tremor. As nicotine's blood levels rise we get autonomic ganglionic blockade, leading to hypotension and bradycardia. Subsequent blockade at the skeletal neuromuscular junction leads to muscle weakness and respiratory depression caused by interference with the function of the diaphragm and intercostals. Bethanechol (a) and pilocarpine (c) are cholinomimetics that, at usual blood levels, exert their primary effects as direct agonists on muscarinic receptors for ACh, not on nicotinic receptors. Scopolamine (d) is a muscarinic blocker with virtually no effects on skeletal muscle (nicotinic responses). Tubocurarine (e) is a competitive nicotinic receptor antagonist, acting almost exclusively on skeletal muscle. It is not at all likely to cause direct autonomic effects, whether by blocking muscarinic receptors or by other likely mechanisms.

58. The answer is c. *(Brunton, pp 275-276, 850-851. Katzung, pp 155-158.)* Recall that the basic "equation" for blood pressure is

$$BP = \text{cardiac output} \times \text{total peripheral resistance } (CO \times TPR)$$

and since CO = heart rate × stroke volume, then

$$BP = HR \times SV \times TPR$$

If you wish to use the term systemic vascular resistance instead of total peripheral resistance, that's fine.

Propranolol is, of course, a nonselective (β_1 and β_2) β-adrenergic blocker that lacks any α-blocking or other vasodilator effects (eg, due to nitric oxide generation), regardless of the dose. So to answer the question, given the above equation, you simply ask "which of the variables—HR, SV, TPR—is reduced by a nonselective β-blocker?" The answer, of course, is both HR and SV.

Rapid parenteral administration of propranolol or another β-blocker in the same class will lower blood pressure, and if that occurs quickly enough (eg, with rapid and brief-acting β-blocker esmolol) and blood pressure falls by a sufficient magnitude, a baroreceptor reflex (answer a) will be activated. This reflex sympathetic activation will lead to increased peripheral vasoconstriction, since α-adrenergic receptors are not blocked by propranolol or any other β-blockers except for labetalol or carvedilol (therefore answer a is incorrect), but this will not lead to reflex-mediated increases of either HR or SV. No β-blocker has the ability to inhibit catecholamine release, whether from adrenergic nerves or from the adrenal (suprarenal) medulla (b). As noted above, there is no mechanism by which a β-blocker such as propranolol will lower TPR (d). (Labetalol and carvedilol can, by α-blockade; and nebivolol does by a nitric-oxide mediated mechanism.) Finally, β-blockers reduce renin release (a β_1-mediated effect) from the kidneys' juxtaglomerular apparatus, and so answer e is incorrect.

59. The answer is a. *(Brunton, pp 164, 269-270, 855, 857. Katzung, pp 153-154, 160.)* The figure, below, approximates what is likely to happen following administration of a β-blocker to a patient with a pheochromocytoma.

To answer this question correctly you must integrate your basic knowledge of both autonomic pharmacology and cardiovascular physiology. With a pheochromocytoma we have what might be described as "massive" amounts of catecholamines—mainly epinephrine—being released from the tumor into the bloodstream. Germane to our problem, then, are excessive stimulation of cardiac rate, contractility, impulse conduction and automaticity (β_1); intense vasoconstriction (α); and vasodilation in some vascular beds (β_2).

Nonetheless, while the patient I've described is not at all healthy, he is still alive before we give the β-blocker. But what happens after we give the β-blocker is critical. The β-blocker does nothing to block the α-mediated

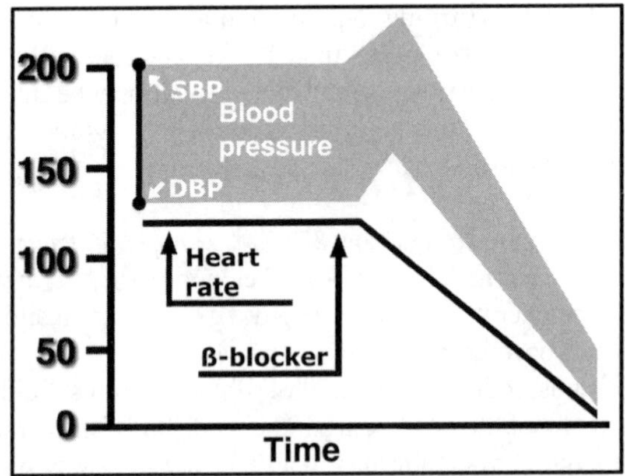

vasoconstriction, so in terms of only vascular effects BP will remain very high. If you wish to opine that blocking β_2-mediated vasodilation will raise BP a bit, that's fine; I've shown that in the figure above. (Remember: Usually effective doses of a β-blocker will either lower BP [most common response], or not affect it at all, in patients with essential hypertension. If pressure rises in response to a β-blocker, suspect pheochromocytoma.)

Nonetheless, there will not be a sudden and significant rise or normalization of BP and/or cardiac function (b, c, d). Likewise, heart rate will not rise significantly (e); it can't: the β_1 receptors necessary for that to occur are blocked.

Next you must recall that the inotropic state of the heart (ie, of the left ventricle, LV) is critical. This is critical because LV peak systolic pressure must exceed aortic pressure in order to establish the LV-aortic pressure gradient to expel blood into the aorta, and propel blood throughout the circulation. If aortic diastolic pressure exceeds LV peak systolic pressure, blood will not flow out of the heart. But until we give the β-blocker, the heart can maintain (for a while) its function thanks to catecholamine-mediated stimulation.

But when we give just a β-blocker to the pheochromocytoma patient we have done little if anything to lower the already high aortic pressure and TPR, and simultaneously have inhibited cardiac contractility and rate. The function of the heart as a pump is suppressed. It now faces a very high aortic pressure and TPR, and ultimately it fails. Cardiac output falls; the patient develops cardiogenic shock, and is then likely to die.

This is why, when treating hypertension associated with a pheochromocytoma, we give an α-blocker first. Blood pressure will fall. We then deal with the excessive cardiac stimulation (which may be intensified, via the baroreceptor reflex, in response to a sudden and significant BP fall) by giving a suitable β-blocker immediately thereafter.

60. The answer is b. *(Brunton, pp 272-278, 287-288. Katzung, p 158.)* You probably learned that nadolol is a β-blocker, and perhaps that it's a nonselective (β_1/β_2) blocker with a rather long duration of action and half-life. If not, you should have been able to recognize that since the generic name ends in "-olol" it is, indeed, some kind of β-blocker. You should also know that asthma is one of the main contraindications for β-blocker administration. β-Adrenergic blockade results in an increase in airway resistance (by antagonism of bronchodilation mediated by epinephrine) that can be fatal in some asthmatic patients. Nadolol, and all the other orally effective β-blockers, are approved for treating chronic-stable angina (a) and essential hypertension (c). They are critical elements in contemporary therapy of heart failure (d; except when it is severe and cardiac output is profoundly depressed); and have beneficial effects to control heart rate in such conditions as sinus tachycardia (e).

61. The answer is a. *(Brunton, pp 186-188, 207-208, 212, 1720-1722; Katzung, pp 103-106.)* When applied topically to the eye, both the direct-acting cholinomimetic agents (eg, pilocarpine) and those that act by inhibition of AChE (eg, echothiophate, isoflurophate, and physostigmine) cause miosis by contracting the sphincter muscle of the iris and reducing intraocular pressure by contracting the ciliary muscle, allowing better drainage of aqueous humor. In patients with glaucoma, this latter effect permits greater drainage of the aqueous humor through the trabecular meshwork in the canal of Schlemm and a reduction in resistance to outflow of the aqueous humor. Certain β-adrenergic blocking agents (eg, timolol and levobunolol), applied to the eye(s), are also very useful in treating chronic wide-angle glaucoma. These drugs appear to act by decreasing the secretion (or formation) of aqueous humor by antagonizing the effect of circulating catecholamines on β-adrenergic receptors in the ciliary epithelium. Echothiophate (b), isoflurophate (c), and neostigmine (e) are acetylcholinesterase inhibitors and all constrict the pupil. Pilocarpine (d) is muscarinic receptor agonist; it, too, causes miosis.

62. The answer is d. *(Brunton, pp 209-211. Katzung, pp 103-106, 108-109, 993-994.)* In cholinesterase poisoning we are dealing with overstimulation (from accumulated ACh) of both peripheral muscarinic and nicotinic receptors. Recall that atropine is a specific muscarinic receptor blocker, and the muscarinic receptors are the ones found on such structures as smooth muscle, cardiac nodal tissue, and exocrine glands. In contrast, the cholinergic receptor on skeletal muscle is nicotinic, so skeletal muscle isn't affected by atropine. If one receives a lethal dose of a cholinesterase inhibitor, he or she may be a little more comfortable (less defecation, urination, respiratory tract mucus hypersecretion and bronchoconstriction, and all that, after the atropine is given), but they are still likely to die from skeletal muscle (N_M nicotinic) overstimulation and then paralysis. Paralysis of the diaphragm and intercostals muscles are the most lethal consequences.

63. The answer is g. *(Brunton, pp 161-162, 171t, 173-174, 855-856. Katzung, pp 174-175.)* The qualitative and mechanistic effects of guanadrel are very similar to those of reserpine. Both drugs cause what has been called a "chemical sympathectomy," gradually but eventually markedly reducing sympathetic (adrenergic) influences on all the usual target structures and thereby exposing or unmasking opposing parasympathetic influences. (The resulting syndrome is sometimes called "parasympathetic predominance" because attenuating adrenergic influences leaves PNS tone on a host of structures unopposed and now exposed.) For example, in the presence of guanadrel miosis, diarrhea, and urination develop; and arterioles dilate and blood pressure falls (because there's little/no norepinephrine to be released, since it has been depleted from adrenergic nerve endings). Heart rate does not increase reflexly (via the baroreceptor reflex mechanism) for two main reasons. First, heart rate cannot rise because after a sufficient duration of treatment there is little or no NE to be released. The second reason for no baroreceptor reflex is that guanadrel (and reserpine) cause BP to fall so slowly that the baroreceptors simply do not respond to any BP changes. Indeed, heart rate falls markedly during treatment as sympathetic influences decline and parasympathetic control is unmasked. Reserpine causes its effects mainly by interfering with intraneuronal storage of NE, exposing the neurotransmitter to metabolic inactivation by MAO and ultimately depleting the NE. Guanadrel releases NE directly, and gradually, eventually leading to a state of intraneuronal NE depletion with signs and symptoms very similar to those caused by reserpine.

None of the other drugs listed will have any effects on the levels of NE in adrenergic nerves. Acetylcholine (a), the agonist for both muscarinic and nicotinic receptors, will cause many of the responses described for guanadrel, but, again, does not do so by reducing catecholamine levels in adrenergic neurons. It's also worth noting that ACh is not classified—and certainly not used—as an antihypertensive drug. The peripheral autonomic effects of atropine (b) administration would be the opposite of those described for guanadrel. Usual parenteral doses of epinephrine (c; α and β agonist) or norepinephrine (e; α and β_1 agonist) tend to raise blood pressure and peripheral resistance (the effects clearly are dose-dependent), and if there were any changes in pupil size it would be manifest as mydriasis due to activation of α-receptors on iris dilator muscle cells. Isoproterenol (d; β agonist with no direct effects on α-receptors) also tends to raise BP by increasing cardiac output (via increased heart rate and stroke volume). Propranolol (f) certainly is an antihypertensive drug, but it and most other β-blockers do not affect intraneuronal NE levels; do not cause any change in pupil size (ie, no mydriasis nor miosis); and do not typically unmask parasympathetic influences on such structures as the gut and urinary tract musculature.

64. The answer is c. *(Brunton, pp 189-190, 194-196. Katzung, pp 119, 347, 351.)* Ipratropium, a quaternary antimuscarinic drug, is FDA-approved, for use as an inhaled bronchodilator for COPD. (It is used, but not FDA-approved, for some cases of asthma.) Its action involves blockade/antagonism of ACh-mediated bronchoconstriction, and it is often used adjunctively with albuterol or other β_2 agonists. A related drug is tiotropium.

Albuterol (a) is an inhaled bronchodilator for asthma or COPD, but it works, of course, as a β_2-adrenergic agonist. Diphenhydramine (b) has bronchodilator activity (by blocking both histamine H_1 and muscarinic receptors), but it is not given by inhalation; moreover, for ambulatory patients with asthma the mucus-thickening effects of muscarinic receptor blockade can do more harm than good. Pancuronium (d) is a curare-like skeletal neuromuscular blocker (competitive antagonist of ACh at N_M receptors). Pilocarpine (e) is a muscarinic agonist, used mainly for causing miosis in patients with angle-closure glaucoma. It will cause bronchoconstriction—an effect that may be harmful for patients with COPD and certainly would be harmful for asthmatics.

65. The answer is a. *(Brunton, pp 203-204, 211-213, 1724. Katzung, pp 105-107.)* Although several of the listed drugs inhibit the activity of AChE, only edrophonium is used in the diagnosis of myasthenia gravis. The drug has a more rapid onset of action (1 to 3 min following intravenous administration) and a shorter duration of action (~5 to 10 min) than pyridostigmine. This fast acting/short duration profile is precisely what we want in this situation. We can quickly get our diagnostic answer, yet not have to deal too long with adverse responses (such as ventilatory paralysis) if the patient was experiencing a cholinergic crisis (excessive doses of oral cholinesterase inhibitor) and we've now worsened the situation by inhibiting the metabolic inactivation of ACh even more with our diagnostic medication. (The short duration and the need for parenteral administration preclude use of edrophonium as a practical drug for long-term treatment of myasthenia gravis.)

Malathion (b) is used topically to treat head lice and is never used internally (intentionally). Pyridostigmine (e) is used orally for maintenance therapy of myasthenia gravis. Physostigmine (c) is indicated for treatment of glaucoma (given topically), and is also a valuable parenteral drug for treating toxicity of anticholinergic drugs such as atropine. They are all cholinesterase inhibitors. Pralidoxime (d) is a "cholinesterase reactivator" and is used adjunctively (with atropine) in the treatment of poisonings caused by "irreversible" cholinesterase inhibitors, such as the "nerve gases" used as bioweapons and some commercial insecticides.

66. The answer is d. *(Brunton, pp 247, 375. Katzung, pp 136t, 146, 446-450.)* There are several reasons for and outcomes of adding a vasoconstrictor (usually epinephrine) to some local anesthetics given by infiltration. The vasoconstrictor confines the local anesthetic to the desired site of action (basically the site of administration) by reducing local blood flow and the rate of anesthetic entry into the bloodstream. It is the bloodstream (or, more precisely, it is the presence of anesthetic in the systemic circulation) that delivers the drug to sites where signs and symptoms of toxicity occur. Slow down anesthetic absorption rates and the drug will enter the circulation slowly enough that it can be metabolized (inactivated) fast enough to prevent accumulation to toxic levels. That is, we reduce the risk of systemic toxicity with added vasoconstrictor.

Another outcome of including a vasoconstrictor is to prolong (and certainly not shorten) the duration of local anesthetic effect. That occurs also because reduced local blood flow keeps the anesthetic in the vicinity of sensory nerves longer (since the anesthetic is not being removed as quickly by blood flow).

More on this issue will be presented in the CNS questions. But for now: Local anesthetics (except cocaine) can cause vasodilation (not vasoconstriction; a), but unless the local anesthetic dosages are quite high (toxic), the vasodilation is not intense; hypotension is uncommon with usual dosages. Likewise, cardiac depression can occur, but again that is a manifestation of overdose. We don't routinely include epinephrine in a local anesthetic to combat or prevent these cardiac-depressant problems (b), and the amount of epinephrine found in these preparations is far too low to do anything meaningful to remedy these adverse responses should they occur. Likewise, the amounts of vasoconstrictor are far too low to prevent (or treat) anesthetic-induced anaphylaxis (c)—a reaction that requires only a few molecules of antigen to occur.

So what the vasoconstrictor does is essentially cause a pharmacologic tourniquet, reducing regional blood flow that otherwise would quickly "wash away" the anesthetic. This essentially confines the anesthetic to the desired site longer (not shorter; e) than otherwise, and decreases the potential systemic reactions (d). Some local anesthetics cause vasodilation, which allows more compound to escape the tissue and enter the blood.

Two final notes: In plastic surgery and many other types of surgery the direct vasoconstrictor effects of EPI not only antagonize the local vasodilator effects of a local anesthetic, but also cause direct vasoconstriction in the region, and thereby limit blood loss further. It is also important to note that epinephrine (or other vasoconstrictors) should not be used in or as a supplement to parenteral local anesthetics being used to relieve or prevent pain in "end organs"—fingers, toes, penis, tip of the nose, earlobes, etc. Such structures have relatively discrete blood supplies, and blocking blood flow to distal tissues can lead to ischemia and tissue damage.

67. The answer is c. *(Brunton, pp 244-247, 262, 640. Katzung, p 138.)* Epinephrine, an excellent agonist for all the adrenergic receptors, is the drug of choice for managing the symptoms of an acute, systemic, immediate hypersensitivity reaction to an allergen (anaphylactic shock), all of which result from the release or production of various substances (eg, histamine, kinins) that contribute to cardiac, vascular, and pulmonary dysfunction. Death can occur because of several main adverse responses: profound hypotension and angioedema (which can be reversed by epinephrine's α-agonist/vasoconstrictor effects); cardiac depression (reversed by epinephrine's β_1 actions); and laryngospasm and bronchospasm (reversed by the β_2 effects of epinephrine).

Atropine (a), the prototype muscarinic receptor blocker, will have modest effects to counteract airway smooth muscle contraction caused by acetylcholine, but no effect on the strong adverse cardiovascular or airway effects of histamine, kinins, and other mediators that play a critical role in anaphylaxis. Diphenhydramine (b) has strong histamine H_1 and muscarinic receptor blocking actions, but it, too, cannot block all the adverse and potentially lethal cardiovascular and pulmonary effects of anaphylaxis-associated mediators. (Diphenhydramine clearly can alleviate bothersome urticaria and other cutaneous manifestations of allergic or anaphylactic reactions, but those actions are rather trivial compared with other life-threatening responses that it cannot beneficially affect.) No antihistamine can be considered a life-saving substitute for epinephrine. Isoproterenol (d), the prototype β_1 and β_2 agonist will counteract airway smooth muscle contraction and help restore cardiac function, but because it lacks any vasoconstrictor (ie, α agonist) activity it will not counteract widespread vasodilation and the hemodynamic consequences of it. Norepinephrine (e) has beneficial cardiac and peripheral vasoconstrictor activity, but since it lacks β_2-bronchodilator activity it is not an acceptable alternative to epinephrine. Its bronchodilator effects are relatively weak, and it lacks any vasopressor effects that are needed to help restore blood pressure.

68. The answer is c. *(Brunton, pp 250-251, 890. Katzung, pp 140, 216-217.)* Dobutamine is mainly a β_1-selective agonist that causes a positive inotropic effect and in turn raises stroke volume, leading to increased cardiac output. Dobutamine has some positive chronotropic activity (also β_1 mediated) that also contributes to a rise of cardiac output, but the drug's effects on the heart's inotropic state predominate.

Note: The best way to characterize the receptor-mediated effects of dobutamine are as a "selective β_1 agonist," but dobutamine's actions (in the form available for therapeutic use) are a bit more complex. It is actually a racemic mixture of two isomers: the (+) isomer is the potent β_1 agonist that causes the predominant cardiac and hemodynamic effects, but it also has some weak α_1 antagonist (vasodilator) effects; the (–) isomer is an efficacious and potent α_1 agonist (vasoconstrictor). The opposing vasoconstrictor effects of one isomer essentially cancel-out the vasodilator effects of the other. Regardless, it would not be correct to characterize the drug's *predominant* cardiovascular actions as involving α agonist or antagonist effects (a, b, e, f), and the drug certainly has no β-blocking actions (d).

69. The answer is e. *(Brunton, pp 248-250. Katzung, pp 78f, 80, 82t, 133, 139, 645.)* Infusing low doses of dopamine activates D_1 receptors, raises vascular smooth muscle cAMP levels, and causes vasodilation in the kidneys and mesentery. (Clinicians often refer to these as "renal doses" because, in such conditions as low cardiac output the drug is given not only as a cardiac stimulant but also to increase renal blood flow and urine output.) The outcome of the increased renal blood flow is increased glomerular filtration and sodium excretion. A similar D_1/cAMP-mediated effect also occurs in the renal tubules (particularly the proximal tubules and the medullary region of the thick ascending limb in the Loop of Henle). This inhibits a Na^+-K^+-ATPase, which further increases renal sodium loss by inhibiting sodium reabsorption.

70. The answer is a. *(Brunton, 172t, 268-270. Katzung, 150, 152, 177.)* First you need to know that prazosin and phentolamine are α-adrenergic blockers. Then you need to know upon which α-adrenergic receptors they act, and what responses they elicit. Phentolamine is a nonselective α-adrenergic blocker, acting at both α_1 (postsynaptic) and α_2 receptors (presynaptic). Prazosin selectively blocks α_1 receptors. Activating the postsynaptic receptors, on vascular smooth muscle cells, causes contraction (vasoconstriction); block those receptors and vasodilation (that is, the fall of blood pressure we noted) occurs. Both phentolamine and prazosin do this.

The blood pressure fall upon drug administration is of a sufficient magnitude (20 mm Hg), and occurs sufficiently quickly (20 sec or less), that the baroreceptor reflex is activated. This leads to increased sympathetic "outflow" to the periphery as part of the body's attempt to maintain the cardiovascular status quo. Sympathetic stimulation of vascular smooth muscle normally will cause vasoconstriction, but since the α-adrenergic receptors that must be activated to cause it are blocked (by phentolamine or prazosin), vasoconstriction will not occur (or be very much reduced).

Increased baroreceptor-mediated sympathetic stimulation of the heart also occurs, and neither phentolamine nor prazosin blocks the β_1 receptors on which released NE exerts its cardiac-stimulating effects.

But what else occurs at the adrenergic neuroeffector junctions, such as at the heart? Normally, some of the released NE acts on the presynaptic α-receptors. The result of that interaction is a physiologic "turning off" or feedback-inhibition of further NE release in response to each action potential. Phentolamine blocks the presynaptic α-receptors, thereby blocking what amounts to the ability of released NE to suppress further NE release.

The consequence of this? Significant increases in the amount of NE released into the synapse, and prolonged presence of NE in the synapse, and significantly increased cardiac stimulation. Prazosin, however, does not block the presynaptic α-receptors, and in doing so does not interfere with the normal feedback-inhibitory effects of released NE. And the obvious difference? Much less intense reflex cardiac stimulation with prazosin than with phentolamine—not the opposite (b).

Prazosin and phentolamine have no β-blocking activity (c). Neither drug blocks NE-mediated vasodilation (d). And neither will reduce LV afterload (e): as noted in the question, both drugs lowered arterial pressure and so afterload is obviously decreased too.

71. The answer is b. *(Brunton, pp 163-164. Katzung, pp 82-84, 92t.)* Norepinephrine (and other monoamine neurotransmitters such as dopamine) is removed from its receptors by an "amine pump" located in the neuronal membrane. Recall that this reuptake process can be blocked by (among other drugs) cocaine and tricyclic antidepressants. (You might ask "what about 'stimulation' of presynaptic α_2 receptors?" Well, that answer might work, but it wasn't one of the choices here. Moreover, presynaptic α_2 receptor activation only inhibits release of additional NE; it does not stop the effects of NE that has already been released.)

Monoamine oxidase (MAO; answer d), and to a lesser degree catechol *O*-methyltransferase (COMT; answer c), are enzymes responsible for metabolic degradation of NE (the former intraneuronally as far as monoaminergic nerves go, the other extraneuronal). However, they are not important in terminating the immediate actions of released NE, which is a process dependent mainly on neuronal reuptake following each action potential and which is not affected by MAO or COMT inhibitors.

Answer a, which cites metabolic inactivation of neurotransmitter in the synaptic cleft, is a good description of what happens to neuronally released ACh. Answer e, which mentions formation of a "false neurotransmitter" does not explain the physiologic termination of released norepinephrine's actions. That concept, however, has been mentioned as a potential mechanism by which monoamine oxidase inhibitors alter the adrenergic responses when MAO inhibitors are administered.

72. The answer is f. *(Brunton, pp 290, 1522-1523, 1530. Katzung, pp 162, 677.)* The tachycardia associated with symptomatic hyperthyroidism reflects, to a great degree, thyroid hormone-related hyperreactivity of β-adrenergic receptors to drugs that have β-agonist activity. Of most concern in this situation is hyperreactivity of β_1 receptors, which accounts for the untoward and potentially dangerous cardiac responses that usually occur. These can be managed, symptomatically, with a β-blocker. Indeed, during an acute and life-threatening episode of hyperthyroidism (thyrotoxicosis or "thyroid storm") a β-blocker is not only indicated but also may be life-saving. Of all the conditions listed, this is the only indication for propranolol or virtually any other β-blocker; and the only one that is not likely to worsen some aspect of the current clinical presentation.

β-Blockers may be safe and effective for chronic-stable angina—and they are often used prophylactically in that condition—but they may worsen and so are generally contraindicated in patients with vasospastic (variant, or Prinzmetal) angina (a). In situations of coronary vasospasm, α-mediated vasoconstrictor/spasm-provoking influences tend to be opposed by β_2-mediated vasodilator influences. Block the β_2 effects and the constrictor or spasm-favoring α influences are unmasked, leading to increased frequency and severity of angina and myocardial ischemia.

Asthma (b) is an important and common condition that relatively or absolutely contraindicates the use of a β-blocker, regardless of its spectrum of activity or administration route. Even very small doses of a β-blocker—even a topical β-blocker that might be used for glaucoma, and even the so-called selective β_1 blockers such as atenolol or metoprolol—can prove lethal for some asthmatics. That is because the airways of asthmatic individuals depend greatly on β_2 activation (and other influences) to prevent bronchoconstriction or bronchospasm. Block those effects, and serious or even fatal consequences may arise.

β-Adrenergic blockers lower heart rate and slow AV nodal conduction velocity. Thus, preexisting bradycardia (c) or heart (AV nodal) block (e) tend to weigh against, if not contraindicate, safe use of any β-blocker. A working definition of heart block is, of course, an abnormally prolonged PR interval, which can be detected easily on an electrocardiogram. If the patient has first-degree heart block (PR intervals are prolonged, but all supraventricular electrical activity passes through the AV node to activate the ventricles), a β-blocker may cause second-degree heart block (some supraventricular impulses are not conducted through the AV node). If the patient has second-degree heart block, a β-blocker may cause complete (third degree) block, which can have dire consequences because the ventricular myocardium loses all control by impulses passing through the AV node, and so ventricular activity is likely to fall to dangerous levels.

β-Blockers may pose significant problems for some patients with severe, poorly controlled diabetes mellitus (d). These drugs can, for example, prevent tachycardia that is one signal to the patient that blood glucose levels are too low, and they can delay the recovery of blood glucose levels following an episode of hypoglycemia. However, for many patients with mild and well-controlled diabetes (especially Type 2), in such conditions as mild-to-moderate heart failure (and others) the judicious use of a β-blocker probably provides more benefit than harm.

73. The answer is c. *(Brunton, p 198. Katzung, pp 114-118, 122.)* These are among the classic signs and symptoms of atropine (antimuscarinic) poisoning. The antimuscarinic drug-poisoned patient often can be described as:

- red as a beet (characteristic facial flushing; a so-called "atropine flush");
- dry as a bone (no exocrine gland secretions, no fecal or urinary output because bowel and bladder motility are inhibited);
- hot as a furnace (profound fever; a CNS "problem" compounded by a lack of body heat loss normally afforded by sweating);
- blind as a bat (paralysis of accommodation and dilated pupils do not respond to even very bright light);
- mad as a hatter (as in the Mad Hatter from Lewis Carroll's *Alice in Wonderland:* CNS problems, including delirium and hallucinations).

You may never see true atropine poisoning. As you know, that prototype antimuscarinic drug is not used clinically all that often, except in some particular specialties or situations. However, you should realize that many common groups of drugs (see Question 87), some of which are available over-the-counter (specifically, diphenhydramine), exert strong antimuscarinic effects. The signs and symptoms of "atropine poisoning" are an important component of their overdose syndromes, and you should be able to recognize them.

74. The answer is a. *(Brunton, pp 23-25, 272, 274t, 276, 282t. Katzung, pp 7, 19, 159, 177.)* The β-blockers with intrinsic sympathomimetic activity (ISA) are partial agonists—they act simultaneously as both β agonists and competitive β-blockers. How can that be? At usual doses, and in the presence of low (eg, resting) sympathetic tone, they act as weak agonists for β-adrenergic receptors. Under these conditions, then, they may actually but slightly increase such β-mediated responses as heart rate. However, while these drugs are occupying the β-adrenergic receptors, they simultaneously block (antagonize) the effects of more efficacious ("stronger") β agonists, for example, epinephrine and norepinephrine, or such exogenous agents (drugs) as isoproterenol. Thus, although they weakly increase resting heart rate, when catecholamine levels are high (as with stress, or exercise), such β-mediated responses as acceleration of heart rate and contractility are less intense than they would be had these drugs with ISA not been present. See Question 25 (in the General Principles chapter) for more information, because it was based on the effects of a β-blocker with ISA/partial agonist activity.

Acebutolol and pindolol—indeed, all drugs classified as β-blockers—have no ability to cause release of norepinephrine (from adrenergic nerves) or epinephrine (from the adrenal medulla), and so answer b is incorrect. Likewise, these drugs do not induce (stimulate; nor inhibit) catecholamine synthesis (c); do not potentiate the actions of norepinephrine on α- (or on β-) adrenergic receptors (d); and cause negative inotropic and chronotropic effects (not positive; answer e).

75. The answer is b. *(Brunton, pp 257-259, 263. Katzung, pp 134f, 141, 145, 1020.)* Methylphenidate is pharmacologically similar to amphetamine. In the context of ADD/ADHD therapy it works as a CNS stimulant, with more pronounced effects on mental than on motor activities. It does so by releasing neuronal norepinephrine and dopamine via a nonexocytotic (not dependent on action potentials) mechanism. It is also used to treat narcolepsy. Dobutamine (a) is a β_1-adrenergic agonist. Pancuronium (c) is a nondepolarizing skeletal neuromuscular blocker (nicotinic receptor competitive antagonist). Prazosin (d) is a competitive and selective α_1-adrenergic blocker. Scopolamine (e) is an antimuscarinic (atropine-like) drug with greater efficacy for causing sedation and antimotion sickness effects. Terbutaline (f) is an agonist predominantly selective for β_2-adrenergic receptors at "low" doses, but it can exert nonselective (isoproterenol-like) β_1- and β_2-agonist effects at high doses, including doses that may commonly be given therapeutically.

76. The answer is e. *(Brunton, pp 237-238, 259-260, 262. Katzung, p 141.)* Ephedrine (and pseudoephedrine) are classified as mixed-acting sympathomimetics, meaning that their overall actions are a mixture or combination of two mechanisms. They mainly release intraneuronal norepinephrine, and so the predominant effects you see in the periphery are quite similar to those of NE itself (α and β_1 activation) because they are caused by NE. They also directly, but relatively very weakly, activate all the adrenergic receptors—alphas and the betas. Ephedrine and pseudoephedrine also exert similar effects in the CNS, leading to such effects as greater alertness (and difficulty falling asleep) and appetite-suppression (anorexigenic effect). The intensity of these effects is greater than those of typical direct-acting adrenergic agonists (EPI, NE, etc) but much weaker than those of indirect-acting sympathomimetics such as the amphetamines.

Ephedrine's actions are not at all selective for α-receptors on vascular smooth muscle, or anywhere else. So, answer a is incorrect. The mixed-acting (and indirect-acting) sympathomimetics have no α- (or β- or cholinergic) blocking activity (b); do not enhance NE synthesis (c); and do not inhibit NE's metabolism in any other way (d).

77. The answer is e. *(Brunton, pp 237-238, 259-261. Katzung, p 141-142.)* Ephedrine's mechanisms of action were addressed in the previous answer. There I noted that ephedrine's direct vasoconstrictor effects are "weak," and they are not at all limited to α-adrenergic receptors (vascular or elsewhere). Nonetheless, the weak direct vasoconstrictor effect combined with the predominant NE-releasing action leads to clinically useful vasopressor effects. The preanesthetic and induction drugs given to this patient (and many others) are likely to produce some cardiodepressant effects (central, cardiac, and vascular), one manifestation of which is an excessive fall of blood pressure. Restoring blood pressure is the main purpose for which the ephedrine is given here.

Ephedrine does cause CNS-stimulating effects (b), but it is generally weak and certainly insufficient to overcome (let alone affect) the CNS depression caused by several other drugs the patient received (midazolam, propofol, morphine). Moreover, the patient is supposed to be anesthetized; why would we want to give a drug to counteract this so early into surgery? Ephedrine does not inhibit SA and AV nodal electrophysiology (c), nor heart rate (d), or contractility. If anything, through its indirect and NE-releasing effects it would be much more likely to stimulate the heart.

Many years ago ephedrine was used as an oral bronchodilator, mainly for patients with asthma. Having no oral or inhaled "selective" β_2 agonists as we have today, it was basically the "only game in town" for chronic management of airway smooth muscle constriction. Its bronchodilator effects were, at best, weak. The direct actions on β_2 receptors are intrinsically weak; and since NE does not activate β_2 receptors, NE release that occurs elsewhere does nothing in the way of causing bronchodilation. Again, there was nothing in the patient's history of bronchoconstriction, nor did she receive any drugs that were likely to cause bronchoconstriction. (Yes, morphine can release histamine, which can cause bronchoconstriction, but this patient was described as otherwise healthy; and she was not a smoker, which might have put her at slightly greater risk of bronchoconstriction.)

Note: Some texts and lecturers downplay the clinical importance of ephedrine. To a large degree that is because it is a largely outmoded and rather poor bronchodilator. Nonetheless, the intraoperative use of injected ephedrine to raise/normalize blood pressure is exceedingly common. Thus, I think you need to know about this drug.

78. The answer is b. *(Brunton, pp 259-260. Katzung, pp 141-142.)* In order for ephedrine to exert its predominant NE-releasing effects, it must be taken up from the synapse, into the adrenergic nerve "ending." Cocaine and the tricyclic antidepressants inhibit ephedrine transport, just as they inhibit reuptake of NE that has been released from adrenergic nerves in response to an action potential (or in response to other NE-releasing drugs).

Atenolol and metoprolol (a) relatively selectively block β_1 receptors (at usual therapeutic doses; at high doses they also block β_2 receptors—important if the patient has asthma, for example). They have no α-blocking activity at all. Thus, they don't weaken all the effects of ephedrine. (If I had listed labetalol or carvedilol, which block all the α- and β-receptors, I'd give you your "two points" if you picked that answer.) Hexamethonium and trimethaphan (c) are autonomic (PNS and SNS) ganglionic (N_N receptor) blocking drugs. They have no effect on ephedrine's direct receptor-mediated actions, nor on ephedrine's NE-releasing effects, both of which occur distal to the ganglia. (They would, of course, reduce or eliminate baroreceptor reflex responses that might arise if ephedrine suddenly and markedly raised blood pressure.) Pargyline (d), arguably the prototypic nonselective monoamine oxidase inhibitor, would intensify the responses to ephedrine or other sympathomimetics that work in part or in whole by releasing intraneuronal NE. Remember that MAO inhibitors cause a gradual but eventually dramatic rise in intraneuronal NE levels by inhibiting NE degradation by the enzyme; and although that NE is not released by a normal action potential, catecholamine-releasing sympathomimetics (ephedrine, pseudoephedrine, amphetamines, and even dietary tyramine) certainly, suddenly, and massively do so. Propranolol (e), of course, blocks all β-adrenergic receptors, but has no α-blocking activity and so does not affect any α-mediated responses to ephedrine.

79. The answer is d. *(Brunton, pp 203-205, 211-214, 222. Katzung, pp 103-107.)* In the vast majority of situations in which we give a patient a nondepolarizing (curare-like) neuromuscular blocking drug (vecuronium in this case), we will also be giving the patient two other drugs. One, the focus of this question, is an acetylcholinesterase (AChE) inhibitor (neostigmine, listed here, is the most common one). It is given to reverse the competitive skeletal neuromuscular blockade: cause a build-up of ACh at the synapse by inhibiting its enzymatic hydrolysis by AChE), and the ACh can now overcome the blockade of the N_M receptors on skeletal muscle.

As explained more fully in other questions, the AChE inhibitor will cause build-up of ACh at all peripheral cholinergic synapses by inhibiting ACh's metabolic inactivation. This leads to a variety of usually unwanted muscarinic effects. (Neostigmine does not enter the CNS, as does physostigmine [which is not at all appropriate for this indication], and so answer c is incorrect.) If the neostigmine (alone) does anything to blood pressure it will cause a fall (not a rise, a) due to the drug's indirect (via increased ACh) negative chronotropic effect on the heart (thus, b is also incorrect). The secondary rise of ACh will also stimulate the bladder's detrusor and trigone, and relax the sphincter, and so there will be no reduced risk or severity of urinary incontinence (e).

80. The answer is b. *(Brunton, pp 189-190, 197. Katzung, pp 107, 453, 455, 461-462.)* The patient will receive neostigmine, and as explained in the previous question it will act at all cholinergic synapses in the peripheral nervous system—the N_M receptors on skeletal muscle that we want to reactivate, and the muscarinic receptors that we don't. If we didn't block the muscarinic responses first, the patient is likely to experience ACh-mediated suppression of heart rate and nodal automaticity and conduction; stimulation of various gut and urinary tract muscles and relaxation of sphincters;

bronchoconstriction; and increases in the secretory activity of a host of exocrine glands (salivary, lacrimal, mucous, gastric acid/parietal cell). As a result, and routinely, we give an antimuscarinic drug right before giving the stigmine, and that is what you need to know (and should have been able to deduce, even though you might not be familiar at all with glycopyrrolate.)

Note: Glycopyrrolate is yet another drug that seems to get relegated to miscellaneous or unimportant status in texts and lectures (in which it might not be mentioned at all). However, it is used routinely in many hospitals as the go-to antimuscarinic in situations such as described here. Why not atropine, which you obviously know about? The effects of atropine tend to last much longer than what is needed here. Glycopyrrolate's onset and duration of action is shorter than atropine's—indeed, a rather close match to the pharmacokinetics of neostigmine, and so it is an excellent choice for this use.

81. The answer is e. *(Brunton, pp 220-226. Katzung, pp 454-460.)* At usual therapeutic (ie, nontoxic) doses, succinylcholine (SuCh) causes rapid, brief (with a single dose), and noncompetitive depolarizing blockade of N_M receptors on skeletal muscle. Even if skeletal muscle paralysis is maintained longer by continuous infusion of the drug (it is sometimes done), skeletal muscle function will return spontaneously—due to rapid metabolic inactivation of the drug by cholinesterases—without the need to administer any "reversal" drug. Indeed, for all practical purposes there is no clinically useful SuCh reversal drug (but see the following note). Succinylcholine has no effect on muscarinic receptors, and so atropine (a) or any other antimuscarinic drug will do nothing in terms of skeletal muscle function. Bethanechol (b) activates only muscarinic receptors (at all but extraordinarily high doses). Stigmines (neostigmine, physostigmine, or any other AChE inhibitors) will theoretically add to skeletal muscle paralysis, not reverse it. (I say theoretically because if skeletal muscle is now paralyzed by SuCh, it's not likely that making more ACh available at the skeletal neuromuscular junction will intensify an already "maximum" response.)

Note: You may have learned about so-called Phase II neuromuscular blockade caused by SuCh, and that it can be reversed with such drugs as atropine. It is not a part of the "normal pharmacology" of SuCh unless a frank overdose occurs and toxicity develops. If it does occur all one needs to do is keep the patient on mechanical ventilation for as long as necessary, simply wait for the drug to be eliminated, and be as sure as possible before extubating the patient and/or stopping mechanical ventilation that spontaneous respiration is adequate and not likely to be compromised again.

82. The answer is a. *(Brunton, pp 186-189. Katzung, pp 95-102.)* These are expected side effects (not at all idiosyncratic, b) from bethanechol, a muscarinic agonist (parasympathomimetic drug). They occur even though the effects of the drug—the ones for which it is given—are "predominately" on the bladder musculature: contraction of the detrusor and relaxation of the sphinchter to enable (if not cause) urination. The side effects noted in the question nonetheless are common and dose- (and patient-) dependent, and not at all idiosyncratic reactions. Moreover, although we could inhibit those side effects with an atropine-like (antimuscarinic) drug, doing so would simultaneously inhibit the drug's intended effects on the bladder. Bethanechol has no sympathetic (or parasympathetic) ganglionic activating (c) or blocking actions at usual doses.

The potential cardiac/cardiovascular effects of bethanechol used at usual doses are not so simple to explain, but certainly would not involve baroreceptor reflex-mediated suppression of cardiac rate (d). In order for the baroreceptors to reflexly suppress heart rate, blood pressure would have to go up quite a bit, and quite quickly. Bethanechol is a vasodilator, and so would lower BP (quickly, if injected too fast). The expected baroreceptor response to that would be increased sympathetic "outflow" from the CNS to the periphery, and that in turn would favor reflex tachycardia. However, bethanechol simultaneously will directly suppress spontaneous depolarization (Phase IV of the action potential) of the SA node, attempting to slow heart rate via direct muscarinic receptor agonist activity. So, what happens to heart rate? So the chronotropic effects depend on whether the direct bradycardic effect "wins out" or the reflex tachycardic influences do.

If the patient had undiagnosed asthma (e; the presence of asthma would contraindicate use of the drug), the pulmonary response would be much more significant than "some wheezing." Potentially fatal bronchospasm could occur because the airway smooth muscles of asthmatic individuals are exquisitely (hyper)sensitive to muscarinic agonists, with even small doses of those drugs capable of causing a lethal outcome.

83. The answer is c. *(Brunton, pp 251-254. Katzung, pp 135t, 136, 138, 144.)* Terbutaline is a relatively selective β_2-adrenergic agonist that relaxes uterine smooth muscle (called a tocolytic effect). Note the word "relatively;"

the preferential β_2 effects (vs β_1) are not absolute, and they are dose-dependent. Yes, terbutaline, the uterine-relaxing drug is classified mechanistically the same as, for example, albuterol, salmeterol, or terbutaline, and several other drugs typically used as adrenergic bronchodilators for asthma. Will, or can, terbutaline cause bronchodilation? Absolutely, even at the relatively low doses used for uterine-relaxing effects! And when blood levels become sufficiently high (and perhaps even still in the therapeutic range for uterine effects) the preferential activation of β_2 receptors is lost, and the drug behaves just like isoproterenol, the prototype β_1/β_2 agonist, to cause not only bronchodilation but also cardiac stimulation, enhanced renin secretion, hyperglycemia, and more. This dose-dependent loss of β_2-adrenergic agonist "selectivity" is a property of all the drugs classified, inappropriately and imprecisely, as selective β_2 agonists or selective adrenergic bronchodilators.

Note: A similar drug, ritodrine, was widely used as an adrenergic uterine-relaxing drug, but it is no longer available in the United States.

84. The answer is e. *(Brunton, pp 154-158, 172t, 220-226. Katzung, p 460.)* Tubocurarine, arguably the prototypic nondepolarizing skeletal neuromuscular blocker (competitive antagonist of the effects of ACh on skeletal muscle nicotinic receptors—N_M), differs from most of the other nondepolarizing neuromuscular blockers (including pancuronium, c) because it triggers histamine release. It exerts a "direct" degranulating effect on mast cells, an antigen-mediated process involving activation of antibodies on mast cells. This histamine-releasing effect is not clinically significant for patients who do not have asthma, but for many who do the bronchoconstriction can be intense and problematic (even though the patient is intubated). In the absence of (released) histamine, curare and the other neuromuscular blockers would have no effect on airway smooth muscle activity, since these drugs block only nicotinic receptors on skeletal muscle and have no effects on muscarinic receptors found on smooth and cardiac muscle cells. Tubocurarine is not an agonist for histamine—or other—receptors.

Atropine (a) causes bronchodilation by blocking muscarinic receptors on airway smooth muscle cells. Propranolol (d) can provoke severe and sometimes fatal airway smooth muscle contraction in asthmatics, but that is due to blockade of epinephrine's agonist (bronchodilator) actions on β_2 receptors. The same outcome can be caused by neostigmine (b), but that occurs because the drug inhibits metabolic inactivation (by AChE) of acetylcholine—another bronchoconstrictor agonist to which the airways of asthmatics are exquisitely sensitive.

85. The answer is e. *(Brunton, pp 142-145, 233-235. Katzung, pp 122-123, 174.)* Answering this question requires knowledge of two things: how trimethaphan is classified (what it does); and which branch of the autonomic nervous system, parasympathetic or sympathetic, exerts "predominant resting tone" over various structures and their functions. Trimethaphan is an autonomic ganglionic blocking drug, preventing activation of N_N receptors found on all postganglionic nerves (and on the adrenal/suprarenal medulla). Upon giving this drug we essentially denervate distal structures by a pharmacologic means. (If you have not specifically learned or read about trimethaphan, perhaps you know about other and very old ganglionic blocking drugs such as hexamethonium. It's OK to consider these ganglionic blockers equivalent for the purpose of answering this question.) Now, we observe how things change.

For all the structures and functions listed (and several others that weren't), with the exception of controlling vascular smooth muscle and peripheral resistance (vasomotor tone), it is the parasympathetic nervous system that exerts the predominant resting tone. In contrast, control of vascular smooth muscle tone (and, therefore, of peripheral resistance and blood pressure) is primarily regulated by the sympathetic nervous system. Block all ganglionic transmission and vasodilation will occur as predominant SNS influences on the vessels are removed.

As far as the other structures go—all of which, I said, have predominant PNS tone at rest—we would observe a rise of heart rate (not bradycardia, a); decreases of bladder and gut tone (eg, reduced tone of the bladder detrusor and longitudinal muscles of the gut), not increases (b); contraction of sphincters in the GI and urinary tracts; mydriasis; and reduced salivary secretions (xerostomia), not increases (c). Eccrine sweat gland secretions, which are mainly under sympathetic-cholinergic influences, would decrease too. In terms of pupil size, ganglionic blockade would lead to mydriasis, not miosis (d).

Finally, realize that in the presence of an autonomic ganglionic blocking drug no autonomic reflexes (eg, baroreceptor reflexes; pupillary constriction in response to bright light) can occur. Although the afferent pathways that are important in eliciting those reflexes are unimpaired, responses such as changes in heart rate or pupil size depend on intact efferent pathways, and ganglionic blockade interrupts those pathways and the reflex responses that otherwise might occur.

86. The answer is c. *(Brunton, pp 143t-144t, 250. Katzung, pp 88t-89t.)* Piece things together. Some tip-offs to help arrive at the correct answer: no effect on the size of the pupil, so rule out any drug that has effects on the "parasympathetic" side, whether as an agonist or antagonist (here, atropine), and rule out any drug with α effects. (As noted above, no β-receptors control the size of the pupil of the eye.)

Does isoproterenol fit all the other criteria/properties? Yes. And none of the other choices have all the stated properties, only some of them.

87. The answer is a. *(Brunton, pp 191-194, 198. Katzung, pp 114-118, 493t, 527t.)* These drugs all possess antimuscarinic (atropine-like) actions that often are sufficiently strong to cause all the side effects and adverse responses associated with atropine itself. Likewise, it is prudent to assume they share all the contraindications and precautions associated with atropine and that managing severe overdoses of those drugs or drug groups will resemble (and need to be treated) in quite the same way as those of the prototype antimuscarinic. That would include the potential need to administer physostigmine, the acetylcholinesterase inhibitor that plays an important role in managing atropine poisoning.

Note that of all the drugs with atropine-like actions, diphenhydramine (and, to a somewhat lesser extent the other first-generation antihistamines) are available over-the-counter. Although you may do your best to avoid prescribing drugs with atropine-like actions for patients who should not receive them, atropine-like problems can arise in patients who self-prescribe these nonprescription medications.

Clearly, the effects of bethanechol (muscarinic agonist) and neostigmine (acetylcholinesterase inhibitor) are the opposite of those you'd expect to see with atropine (muscarinic receptor blocker). You might argue that isoproterenol (β_1 and β_2 agonist) causes some effects (eg, tachycardia) that you would expect with atropine. True. However, despite any similarities in appearance, the mechanism is quite different, the spectrum of all effects caused by the drug is different, and certainly most contraindications and toxic manifestations are very different. Propranolol (prototype nonselective β-blocker) is radically different from atropine in nearly every important way.

88. The answer is b. *(Brunton, pp 198, 211-214. Katzung, pp 103-107.)* The major signs and symptoms of diphenhydramine toxicity are attributable to its strong antimuscarinic (atropine-like) effects in both the peripheral and central nervous systems. Neostigmine—unlike the preferred antidote, physostigmine—is a quaternary compound and does not enter the CNS. Thus, delirium, hallucinations, and other CNS manifestations of diphenhydramine poisoning will persist. Physostigmine is the preferred antidote specifically because it is not a quaternary (ionized) at physiologic pH, and will readily cause desired antidotal effects in the CNS as well as in the periphery.

Bronchoconstriction and wheezing (a) are not expected outcomes of diphenhydramine toxicity; the antimuscarinic effects of the drug will cause bronchodilation by blocking the bronchoconstrictor influences of endogenous ACh. Likewise, toxic (or even therapeutic) blood levels of diphenhydramine will inhibit—not stimulate—exocrine gland secretions (c). Excesses of diphenhydramine (or atropine itself) will have no significant effects on skeletal muscle activation (d) because these drugs only affect muscarinic receptors; skeletal muscle activation by ACh involves nicotinic receptors. Overdoses of diphenhydramine or any other drugs with strong peripheral muscarinic receptor-blocking effects certainly will cause tachycardia by blocking muscarinic receptor activation of the sinoatrial node. That effect can be reversed by acetylcholinesterase inhibitors, even those that work only in the peripheral nervous systems, such as neostigmine.

You won't encounter too many patients overdosed on atropine itself, but you'll see many people suffering toxicity from older antihistamines (eg, diphenhydramine), older (tricyclic or tetracyclic) antidepressants (eg, imipramine), some of the centrally acting antimuscarinics that are used for parkinsonism (eg, benztropine and trihexyphenidyl), scopolamine (used for motion sickness), and most of the phenothiazine antipsychotics (eg, chlorpromazine). Owing to the often strong antimuscarinic side effects of these drugs, treating overdoses of any of them probably will involve managing what amounts to "atropine poisoning"—and many other problems too.

(You may not know this, but perhaps it will have some meaning or help jog your memory: the trade name for physostigmine is Antilirium. Recall that one of the hallmark CNS signs of atropine/antimuscarinic poisoning is delirium. Hence, "*anti-lirium*" makes sense.)

89. The answer is d. *(Brunton, pp 238, 240t-241t, 250-251. Katzung, pp 140, 216-217.)* Dobutamine behaves, for all practical purposes, as a selective

β_1 agonist. Norepinephrine is a β_1 agonist that also activates α-adrenergic receptors effectively. However, when it is administered with phentolamine (prototype α-blocker) its spectrum of activity is, qualitatively, identical to that of dobutamine.

High doses of dopamine (a) cause positive inotropic and chronotropic effects, but also release neuronal norepinephrine and probably activate α-adrenergic receptors directly (causing unwanted vasoconstriction). These vasoconstrictor effects would negate vasodilator effects due to stimulation of dopamine D_1 receptors found in some arterioles; and of D_2 receptors found on some ganglia, and in the cardiovascular control center of the CNS.

Ephedrine (b) weakly activates all adrenergic receptors and also leads to norepinephrine release. Overall, its effects are quite similar to those produced by norepinephrine itself. Regardless, if one administers ephedrine with propranolol (c), the prototypic nonselective (β_1 and β_2) blocker, ephedrine's remaining actions amount to selective α-adrenergic activation (ie, phenylephrine-like)—not at all like dobutamine, and not at all what we want in this situation.

Phenylephrine (α agonist) plus atropine (muscarinic antagonist) (e) causes effects that in no way resemble those of dobutamine or the norepinephrine-phentolamine combination. From a cardiovascular perspective, this combination would give us a rise of blood pressure due to peripheral vasoconstriction. The vasoconstriction would elicit a baroreceptor reflex tantamount to withdrawing sympathetic tone and increasing opposing parasympathetic tone. However, the presence of atropine would blunt parasympathetic-mediated cardiac slowing. The overall and combined effect on heart rate of reduced sympathetic tone to the SA node, and concomitant blockade of ACh-mediated cardiac slowing (also an effect on the SA node) can vary. However, it would be reasonable to predict a slight increase of rate over predrug rates. Nonetheless, there would not be a positive inotropic response, which is what would occur with either dobutamine or a norepinephrine-phentolamine combination.

90. The answer is a. *(Brunton, pp 143t, 243-246. Katzung, p 78.)* With only two major exceptions (eccrine sweat glands and the arrectores pilorum), the neurotransmitter released by postganglionic sympathetic nerves (adrenergic nerves) to activate their targets is norepinephrine (NE). NE is a "good" agonist for only α- and β_1-adrenergic receptors, but not β_2. In contrast, epinephrine (EPI; from the adrenal medulla) is a very efficacious agonist for both classes of adrenergic receptors and their main subtypes, including β_2. Of the responses listed in the question, only airway smooth-muscle relaxation is a process that involves (depends on) autonomic activation of β_2-adrenergic receptors. There is no innervation of these muscles, and so no NE to be released. Even if NE were injected, its lack of β_2-agonist activity would render it ineffective as a bronchodilator.

Atrioventricular nodal automaticity and conduction (b) are increased, in terms of sympathetic influences, by β_1 receptors, which can be activated by either or both NE and EPI. The same applies to the coronary vasculature, which constricts in response to α-adrenergic receptor activation by either or both NE or EPI. (If the answer choice were coronary vasodilation involving sympathetic influences, then only EPI would be a correct answer, since sympathetic coronary vasodilation involves β_2 receptors.) Either NE or EPI will cause mydriasis (d), which is an α-mediated response. Finally, sympathetically influenced renin release from the juxtaglomerular apparatus involves β_1 activation, which can be caused by either NE or EPI.

Note: You may have learned something like "if it's a sympathetic response involving the heart, the receptor involved is β_1." Well, that's usually true, but now you see that sympathetic mediated coronary vascular smooth muscle relaxation—a response that occurs "in the heart"—involves β_2 receptors. You may have also learned "if a β_1 receptor is involved, the response is occurring (only) in the heart." Again, the statement is usually true, but juxtaglomerular cell renin release is obviously occurring outside the heart, but it is a β_1-mediated response nonetheless.

91. The answer is b. *(Brunton, 143t-145t, 234t. Katzung, pp 88t-89t, 131t, 136-137.)* To me, the tip-off that helps get to the correct answer, isoproterenol, is to focus (no pun intended) on the fact that the unknown drug did not change the size of the pupil of the eye. Of all the main autonomic receptor types, adrenergic and cholinergic, only the β-receptors play no role in regulating the size of the pupil. That narrows things down to isoproterenol or propranolol. Propranolol might lower BP (particularly in a hypertensive patient), but it would not raise heart rate or dilate the bronchi. Only isoproterenol fits the bill.

And the other answers? Atropine (a) might raise heart rate, it is not likely to lower BP, and it will relax airway smooth muscle cells and increase bronchiolar diameter, but it would cause mydriasis, which we don't see in the results presented in the diagram. Neostigmine (c) would slow heart rate, perhaps lower BP (probably not), and constrict the airways and pupils. Phenylephrine (d) would raise BP, and if the BP rise is sufficiently high and quick, reflexly lower heart rate (baroreceptors). It would do nothing to airway diameter, but would cause mydriasis.

92. The answer is e. *(Brunton, pp 163-164. Katzung, pp 82-84, 89, 92t, 133f.)* In short, the answer is "reuptake." A norepinephrine transporter plays the main role in terminating the activity of neuronally (physiologically) released NE. This transporter is blocked by cocaine and tricyclic antidepressants (eg, imipramine). Diffusion of released NE from the synaptic space, leading to metabolism by such enzymes as COMT (d), is overall a minor process in terms of the physiologic inactivation of the effects of NE. Metabolic inactivation by MAO (c) requires reuptake of the catecholamines into the neuron, since the MAO that degrades catecholamines is located intraneuronally (and intramitochondrially).

93. The answer is c. *(Brunton, pp 263-270. Katzung, pp 129-130, 150f, 152-154.)* Tamsulosin is a selective α_1-adrenergic blocker, and presumably its affinity is greater for α-receptors on smooth muscles in the prostate (hence, its use for BPH, due to relaxation of smooth muscles there) than for those in the peripheral vasculature. Nonetheless, its pharmacologic profile is most similar to that of prazosin, which can be considered the prototypic α_1-selective adrenergic blocker that is mainly used to treat hypertension because it competitively blocks vasoconstriction caused by α agonists such as epinephrine and norepinephrine. (Remember: drugs with a generic name that ends in "-osin" or "-zosin" are selective α_1-adrenergic blockers: eg, tamsulosin, prazosin, terazosin, doxazosin.)

So, of the answers listed above, orthostatic hypotension is the most likely side effect. Among the many classes of adrenergic drugs, bradycardia (a) would most likely be caused by a β-blocker (or lesser prescribed drugs such as reserpine, a catecholamine depletor), or a muscarinic agonist or cholinesterase inhibitor, and certainly not by a drug that has no direct cardiac effects and is more likely to elicit reflex cardiac stimulation secondary to reduced blood pressure. There are no known interactions between α-blockers and atorvastatin or related drugs, whether involving skeletal muscle pathology and dysfunction (b) or other adverse responses that a statin might cause. Photophobia (d) is an exceedingly unlikely problem: it is usually caused by drugs that cause mydriasis (eg, α-adrenergic agonists or antimuscarinics), and if anything tamsulosin is likely to prevent the mydriasis that is a common cause of photophobia. Exacerbations of emphysema (e), whether due to bronchoconstriction or other causes, is unlikely too. From an autonomic perspective, epinephrine is the main bronchodilator substance (via β_2 activation), ACh is the main autonomic bronchoconstrictor (via muscarinic activation). Tamsulosin affects neither.

94. The answer is c. *(Brunton, pp 186-188, 1712, 1720-1722. Katzung, pp 88t, 89t, 93f, 116, 119.)* There are a couple of ways you could have arrived at this answer, even if you did not learn specifically about homatropine being a shorter-acting, semisynthetic derivative of atropine, the prototypic antimuscarinic drug.

First off, consider major autonomic innervation of the eye. The sympathetic nervous system, via α-adrenergic receptors, controls mainly the size of the pupil of the eye; there is very little influence on the ciliary muscle or other structures that control accommodation. (β-Adrenergic influences play no role in controlling pupil size or tone of the ciliary muscle.) The parasympathetic branch of the ANS, and its influences on muscarinic receptors, can alter both pupil size and accommodation—precisely what we have here. So, we can rule-out any "sympathetic" drug, agonist or antagonist, as a correct answer. Thus, we reject epinephrine (b), an α and β agonist that would cause mydriasis; isoproterenol (d), the $\beta_{1/2}$ agonist and propranolol (f), the $\beta_{1/2}$-blocker, that affect neither pupil size nor accommodation. We reject ACh (A); this muscarinic agonist would cause miosis and facilitates accommodation. The same applies to pilocarpine (e). This leaves us with homatropine (c). So you could arrive at this correct answer either by the process of elimination, or by making an educated guess (correctly, of course) that homatropine is an atropine-like (antimuscarinic) drug.

95. The answer is d. *(Brunton, pp 30, 177, 184-187, 395-396. Katzung, pp 100-102.)* ACh, in vivo or in vitro, causes its vasodilator response via an action on the endothelium, where the muscarinic receptors are located. The vasodilator response ultimately depends on endothelial cell formation of nitric oxide (NO), which in the case of ACh is a process that emanates from and involves endothelial cell integrity. When the endothelium is damaged or removed (d; the most likely case described here), the direct effect of ACh on vascular smooth muscle is contraction (constriction of arterioles). Atropine, the prototype muscarinic antagonist, will prevent ACh-mediated vasodilation of intact arterioles (b), with intact endothelium, by blocking the interaction between ACh and endothelial cell muscarinic receptors, but it will not cause vasoconstriction when the endothelium is intact (it is important here to distinguish between preventing vasodilation and causing vasoconstriction). Botulinum toxin (c) prevents ACh release from cholinergic nerves, but in our experimental set-up that is irrelevant because the in vitro preparation is devoid of innervation, and ACh is added directly to the tissue bath. Moreover, even if the smooth muscle preparation were innervated, botulinum toxin would not convert the usual vasodilator response to ACh into a vasoconstrictor one.

96. The answer is b. *(Brunton, pp 151-152. 171, 224, 229. Katzung, 81, 82t, 465.)* Botulinum toxin, the cause of botulism, inhibits release of ACh from all cholinergic nerves, particularly those in the autonomic and somatic/motor nervous systems. (Take a look at the schematic of the peripheral nervous systems in the answers to Questions 36-42 to refresh your memory about where these sites are.) It has no agonist (a) activity on any cholinergic receptors, nor an ability to block nicotinic (e) or muscarinic receptors. The toxin has no direct effects on adrenergic nerves (other than preventing their physiologic activation by ACh, normally released by preganglionic sympathetic nerves. Thus, NE reuptake is not affected (c; recall that cocaine and tricyclic antidepressants do inhibit NE reuptake); nor is NE released (d) as occurs with, say, amphetamines.

97. The answer is c. *(Brunton, pp 197-198, 634t, 637-640, 642, 1002. Katzung, pp 116, 275-279.)* The peripheral autonomic actions of diphenhydramine (an ethanolamine-class "first-generation" histamine H_1 antagonist) are very similar to those of atropine, the prototypic competitive muscarinic receptor antagonist. These effects are seen with both therapeutic doses (eg, dry mouth, blurred vision, and occasionally urinary retention or constipation) and with toxicity. In life-threatening cases physostigmine, the "antidote for atropine poisoning" may be a valuable adjunct.

Diphenhydramine, and other H_1 blockers for that matter, have no direct effects either as agonist (a) or antagonist (b) on adrenergic receptors; and no nicotinic receptor-activating activity, whether in autonomic ganglia (d) or at the adrenal medulla (suprarenal gland; e).

98. The answer is d. *(Brunton, pp 210-211. Katzung, pp 103, 117, 989t.)* Pralidoxime is classified as a "cholinesterase reactivator" and is used specifically, and adjunctively, for managing poisoning with the long-acting ("irreversible") organophosphate cholinesterase inhibitors that are found in some insecticides and "nerve gases" such as soman, sarin, and VX. Pralidoxime, an oxime, has very high affinity for phosphorus in the organophosphates. If given early enough in the poisoning it will prevent or reverse the binding of the organophosphate to, and longterm inhibition of, the active binding site on the cholinesterase. The need for early pralidoxime administration is critical: if it is delayed too long the enzyme will "age," yielding a largely permanent and irreversible enzyme configuration.

Methylphenidate (a) is an indirect-acting (norepinephrine-releasing or amphetamine-like) sympathomimetic; pralidoxime has no effect on its actions, nor on the actions of epinephrine (b) or prazosin (e), a selective α_1-adrenergic blocker. Although neostigmine (d) is a cholinesterase inhibitor it is not an organophosphate (it is a carbamate), and it is spontaneously and relatively quickly hydrolyzed leading to loss of cholinesterase-inhibitory activity. Thus, use of pralidoxime for excesses of neostigmine (or other carbamate) doses would be both ineffective (mechanistically) and unnecessary.

99. The answer is b. *(Brunton, pp 143t, 1720-1722. Katzung, pp 88t, 89t, 93.)* Start off with a fundamental review of autonomic innervation of the eye insofar as control of pupil size, and effects on the ciliary muscle (which affects accommodation—the ability of the lens of the eye to thicken so we can see close-up). The sympathetic nervous system, via α-adrenergic receptor activation, has the ability to cause mydriasis. Activate those receptors and the pupil dilates; or block the opposing parasympathetic influences (via muscarinic receptor blockade) and the same thing happens, since there's a relatively comparable influence of both branches of the autonomic nervous system on pupil size. However, there is little resting influence of the sympathetic nervous system (or adrenergic receptors) on the tone of the ciliary muscle. That is mainly a parasympathetic-dependent phenomenon that indirectly affects the shape of the lens of the eyes and, so, the point of sharp focus. And, for all practical purposes, β-receptor activation has no influence on pupil size or accommodation.

Now, classify the drugs by their sites and mechanisms of action.

Eliminate atropine (a) as a possible answer choice. By blocking all ocular effects of normal parasympathetic innervation (muscarinic blockade), it will both dilate the pupil and impair accommodation. The same applies to homatropine (c), a drug that is, for all practical purposes, atropine-like.

Pilocarpine (e), a muscarinic agonist, will constrict the pupil of the eye and impair cholinergic mechanisms involved in focusing of the lens. Isoproterenol (d) activates all β-adrenergic receptors, timolol (f) blocks them all; and as I said, β-receptors are not relevant in terms of pupil size or accommodation. This leaves us with epinephrine: it has both α-adrenergic and β-adrenergic activating activity, and no cholinergic/muscarinic activity. It will dilate the pupil and not significantly affect accommodation.

100. The answer is e. *(Brunton, pp 631-632, 640-641. Katzung, pp 275-278.)* You may have chosen d (histamine H_2 receptor blocker) as your answer to this question. However, H_2 receptors are mainly involved in regulating gastric acid secretion, not typical responses to seasonal allergies. What if I had given "Histamine H_1 receptor blockade" as an answer choice? Although diphenhydramine blocks H_1 receptors quite well, histamine plays a relatively minor role in the symptoms of rhinovirus infections (in contrast with a much more important role in, say, seasonal allergies). As a result, blocking the effects of histamine on H_1 receptors per se does not account for most of the symptom relief in the common cold. The drying up of nasal secretions afforded by diphenhydramine in this instance is due to the drug's rather intense muscarinic receptor-blocking (atropine-like) actions.

The antihistamines (first-generation drugs like diphenhydramine or second-generation ones such as loratadine) lack any antagonist or agonist activity on α-adrenergic receptors (a) or on β-adrenergic receptors (b); and have no direct or major effect on calcium channels (d).

101. The answer is c. *(Brunton, pp 254, 260, 263-267, 269-271. Katzung, pp 137-139.)* Phenylephrine raises blood pressure by activating α-adrenergic receptors on vascular smooth-muscle cells. Prazosin competitively blocks those receptors, and when present at sufficiently high doses (as might occur with an acute, severe overdose) may eliminate the vasopressor response to even higher than usual doses of phenylephrine. β-Blockers (atenolol, propranolol) have no α-blocking activity and so won't reduce the vasopressor response to phenylephrine. Nor will bethanechol, which causes vasodilation by activating muscarinic receptors for ACh. And reserpine? See the answer to question 102.

102. The answer is e. *(Brunton, pp 161-162, 171t, 173-174, 856. Katzung, p 89.)* Reserpine treatment of sufficient duration (because its effects develop slowly) depletes neuronal norepinephrine. This accounts for the lowered blood pressure with therapeutic doses or frank hypotension with overdoses. One consequence of this, long-term, is development of adrenergic receptor supersensitivity because the receptors just aren't being activated as they should. And a consequence of that, in turn, there will be heightened (and sometimes extreme) responses to a given dose of adrenergic agonists that can activate their receptors (α or β) directly, including the phenylephrine you administered. (That is, the dose-response curve for direct-acting adrenergic agonists is "shifted to the left" after long-term reserpine treatment.)

Atenolol (a) and propranolol (d) are β-blockers. Although atenolol preferentially blocks β_1 receptors, while propranolol (and most other β-blockers) affects both β_1 and β_2, neither drug will alter the expected vascular responses to an α-agonist such as phenylephrine. Prazosin (c) competitively antagonizes the effects of an α-agonist. Bethanechol (b) is a muscarinic agonist; if effective concentrations of the drug were in the circulation at the same time as phenylephrine was given, its effects would physiologically antagonize the pressor responses to the vasoconstrictor.

103. The answer is e. *(Brunton, pp 205-207, 212-214. Katzung, pp 103-104, 106-107.)* Edrophonium is fast- and short-acting parenteral acetylcholinesterase inhibitor—one of the relatively few therapeutic AChE inhibitors with a generic name that doesn't end in "-stigmine."

The question states that we are dealing with a patient experiencing a cholinergic crisis. That means, of course, that she has received either relatively or absolutely excessive doses of the oral cholinesterase inhibitor (eg, pyridostigmine, neostigmine, several others) used to manage her myasthenia gravis. Because of the dosage excess, and the excess ACh accumulating at the skeletal neuromuscular junctions (owing to reduced metabolic inactivation of the neurotransmitter), her skeletal muscles are weakened and fatigued from what amounts to overstimulation of nicotinic receptors by the ACh. This skeletal muscle hypofunction involves not only muscles in the extremities, but also the diaphragm and intercostals that must function normally for adequate ventilation. So, when we give a cholinesterase inhibitor to patients like the one described above, who is already experiencing excessive cholinergic effects, further (over) activation of the diaphragm and intercostals may be sufficient to cause ventilatory distress or total ventilatory failure. This is a main reason why the "edrophonium test" is so dangerous should the underlying problem actually be the cholinergic crisis, and why edrophonium is preferred to other ACh esterase inhibitors because it has a very short duration of action (highly desirable should adverse effects occur).

Edrophonium is not at all likely to trigger a hypertensive crisis (a) in response to the edrophonium. It and other drugs in its class, or direct muscarinic agonists (eg, bethanechol) for that matter, have no vasoconstrictor activity (when vascular endothelial cells are intact). Cholinesterase inhibitors are far more likely to lower heart rate (via indirect muscarinic receptor activation secondary to inhibited ACh hydrolysis at the SA node) than stimulate it (b); and just as the drug causes no peripheral vasoconstriction, it causes no coronary vasoconstriction. Ventricular automaticity is likely to decrease further, not increase (c), in response to increased muscarinic activation. Edrophonium will not improve skeletal muscle tone and function (d) if the problem is a cholinergic crisis; that is the expected response, however, if the patient has a myasthenic crisis (reflecting inadequate dosages of the cholinesterase inhibitor used for maintenance therapy).

Note: For many patients with myasthenia gravis, and who are being treated with an oral cholinesterase inhibitor, you should be able to differentiate between a myasthenic and a cholinergic crisis without resorting to the "edrophonium test." You simply need to assess your patient carefully, and apply some basic autonomic pharmacology knowledge. In either crisis, the main common features are skeletal muscle fatigability, weakness, or paralysis due to inadequate (myasthenic crisis) or excessive (cholinergic crisis) activation of nicotinic receptors on skeletal muscle. With a myasthenic crisis the primary problems are confined to skeletal muscle function (and secondary consequences of that, such as inadequate ventilation).

Things usually present quite differently, however, if the underlying problem is a cholinergic crisis. Remember that cholinesterase inhibitors do not act only at skeletal neuromuscular junctions. They also act at all cholinergic synapses in the peripheral nervous systems: at all the postganglionic parasympathetic nerve "endings" and at the synapses between postganglionic sympathetic fibers and sweat glands and the arrectores pilorum—inhibiting ACh metabolism there, and leading to signs and symptoms of muscarinic activation in addition to nicotinic/skeletal muscle effects.

Thus, in patients who are experiencing a cholinergic crisis many or most of the signs and symptoms typically associated with parasympathetic (muscarinic) activation will occur, and they will be useful to you in making the differential diagnosis if you look and listen carefully: miosis and excessive lacrimation; salivation; bradycardia (and possibly AV block determined by an ECG); wheezing or other manifestations of bronchoconstriction and/or increased airway mucus secretions; gut and bladder hypermotility (eg, defecation, urinary frequency or incontinence, increased bowel sounds); and diaphoresis. See some of these in addition to skeletal muscle dysfunction and you should be thinking cholinergic crisis and placing myasthenic crisis further down on your list of possible diagnoses.

104. The answer is c. *(Brunton, 189-194, 198, 636-641. Katzung, 275-278, 1099t.)* First off, I think you should know that the main active ingredient in OTC sleep aids (other than those advertised as "natural" supplements such as melatonin, vitamins, etc) is a sedating antihistamine: doxylamine or, more likely, diphenhydramine. Doxylamine is extremely similar to diphenhydramine, the prototype first-generation (older) "antihistamine"—a competitive H_1-receptor antagonist. Chemically, they are in the ethanolamine class and are used not only for allergy relief, but also for sedation and sleep. If one wanted to stay awake and alert (e) these certainly would not be drugs that achieve that goal; moreover, they don't have any amphetamine-like catecholamine-releasing activity. These drugs also block muscarinic receptors—and quite effectively to boot. So the answer to this question boils-down to "What best describes the actions or effects of atropine?" As you should know, atropine or drugs with similar antimuscarinic actions should not be used by patients with prostatism or angle-closure (narrow-angle) glaucoma.

Given the antimuscarinic effects, if therapeutic doses do anything to heart rate it will be an increase, not a decrease (a) since chronotropic effects of ACh on the SA node are inhibited. ACh normally increases gut motility, facilitates micturition by stimulating the bladder's trigone and detrusor, and relaxes sphincters in the GI and urinary tracts. Blocking those influences on the gut would tend to cause constipation, not diarrhea (b). Blood pressure will not rise because of catecholamine-like vasoconstriction; these drugs have no α-adrenergic (or any other) agonist activity.

Note: Once again I wrote a question about an ostensibly "miscellaneous" drug, so why did I ask about doxylamine? I did so not to be picky, but because doxylamine (and more so diphenhydramine) is widely used; can cause problems for certain people; and is available OTC, which means your patient can take them without your advice, consent, or knowledge.

Central Nervous System Pharmacology

Alzheimer drugs
Antidepressants and other mood-stabilizing drugs
Antiepileptics/anticonvulsants
Antiparkinson drugs
Antipsychotics
Anxiolytics
Central nervous system stimulants and anorexigenic agents
Ethanol
General anesthetics
Intravenous anesthetics and anesthesia adjuncts
Opioid analgesics and antagonists
Psychotomimetics
Sedatives, hypnotics

Questions

Questions 105 to 109

The next five questions refer to the table below. It's the same one shown earlier for Questions 76 to 82 in the previous chapter the anesthesia record from a patient undergoing two procedures during laparoscopic abdominal surgery. Here I ask you about some drugs not addressed before. Remember: this medication administration plan is typical of what you'll see with many similar surgical procedures.

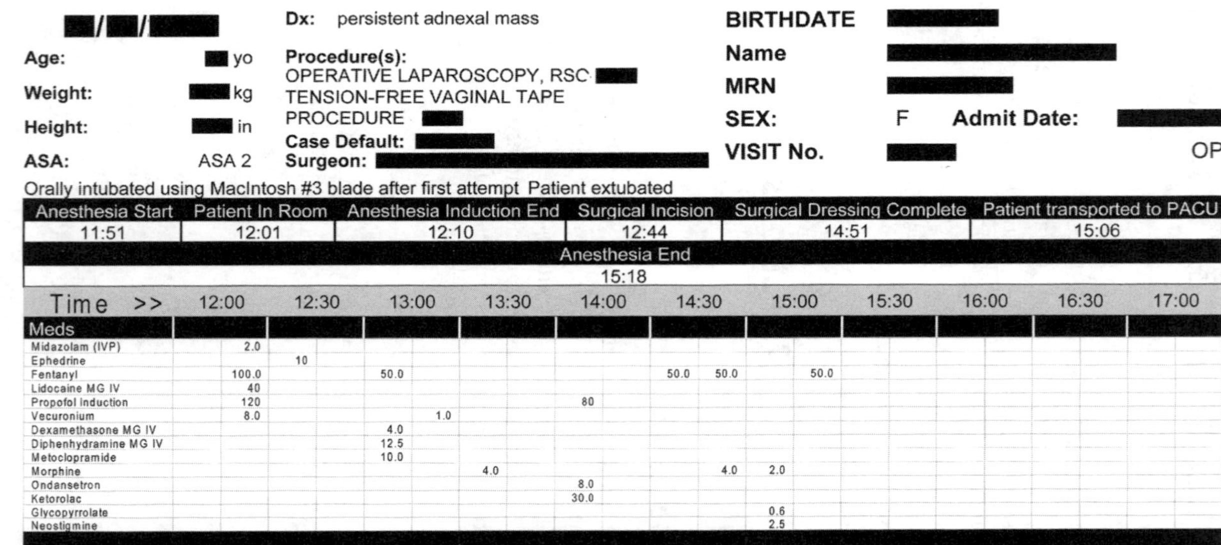

■■/■■/■■■■		Dx: persistent adnexal mass	BIRTHDATE ■■■■
Age:	■ yo	Procedure(s):	Name ■■■■
Weight:	■ kg	OPERATIVE LAPAROSCOPY, RSC ■■	MRN ■■■■
Height:	■ in	TENSION-FREE VAGINAL TAPE PROCEDURE ■■	SEX: F Admit Date: ■■■■
ASA:	ASA 2	Case Default: ■■■■ Surgeon: ■■■■	VISIT No. ■■■■ OP

Orally intubated using MacIntosh #3 blade after first attempt Patient extubated

Anesthesia Start	Patient In Room	Anesthesia Induction End	Surgical Incision	Surgical Dressing Complete	Patient transported to PACU
11:51	12:01	12:10	12:44	14:51	15:06

Anesthesia End
15:18

Time >>	12:00		12:30		13:00		13:30		14:00		14:30		15:00		15:30		16:00		16:30		17:00	
Meds																						
Midazolam (IVP)		2.0																				
Ephedrine			10																			
Fentanyl		100.0			50.0						50.0	50.0		50.0								
Lidocaine MG IV		40																				
Propofol induction		120							80													
Vecuronium		8.0				1.0																
Dexamethasone MG IV					4.0																	
Diphenhydramine MG IV					12.5																	
Metoclopramide					10.0																	
Morphine							4.0					4.0	2.0									
Ondansetron									8.0													
Ketorolac									30.0													
Glycopyrrolate													0.6									
Neostigmine													2.5									

105. You see that midazolam was the first drug given to the patient—actually right before she was transported into the OR. (The notation IVP next to midazolam means "IV push," ie, a rapid bolus injection.) In addition to causing sedation, anxiety relief, and generally "smoothing" the induction of anesthesia, what is the most likely other effect you would expect to occur as a result of premedicating with midazolam?

a. Potentiating the analgesic effects of the morphine
b. Preventing an intraoperative fall of blood pressure
c. Preventing seizures likely to be caused by the propofol
d. Prophylaxis of cardiac arrhythmias
e. Providing amnestic effects (suppressing recall of perioperative events)

106. The record shows that propofol was given for induction. What would be the most likely adverse response(s) associated with the administration of this widely used drug?

a. Hypotension and respiratory (ventilatory) depression
b. Laryngospasm
c. Long-term memory loss
d. Malignant hyperthermia
e. Seizures
f. Unintended or excessively prolonged skeletal muscle paralysis

107. Assume that instead of inducing anesthesia with propofol, the nurse anesthetist used a parenteral barbiturate (eg, methohexital, thiamylal, thiopental) with an extremely fast onset of action and short duration (sometimes called "ultrashort"). These barbiturate induction agents are effective, but are associated with a fairly high incidence of a certain and rather unique adverse effect. What best describes what that adverse effect is?

a. Hyperalgesia (heightened perception of pain)
b. Hypertensive crisis
c. Laryngospasm
d. Malignant hyperthermia
e. Seizures, typically monoclinic

108. The patient received an intravenous dose of ketorolac shortly before the wounds were closed and surgery was done. What is the most likely purpose for which it was given?

a. Control of anticipated postoperative nausea and vomiting
b. Postoperative pain control
c. Reversal of CNS depression caused by multiple depressant drugs
d. Reversal of drug-induced neuromuscular blockade (paralysis)
e. Suppression of wound inflammation

109. Ondansetron was administered about an hour before the anticipated end of surgery (because it has a relatively slow onset of action). What is the most likely reason for giving it to the patient?

a. Hasten recovery of consciousness while effects of anesthetics wear off
b. Intensify pain-relieving effects of other analgesics given to the patient
c. Lessen risks of postop urinary retention through effects on bladder musculature
d. Prevent or reduce the risk of postoperative paralytic ileus
e. Reduce the risk of postoperative nausea and vomiting

110. A 42-year-old woman develops akathisias, parkinsonian-like dyskinesias, galactorrhea, and amenorrhea, during drug therapy. What drug-receptor-based mechanism, occurring in the central nervous system, most likely caused these responses?

a. Blockade of α-adrenergic receptors
b. Blockade of dopamine receptors
c. Blockade of muscarinic receptors
d. Supersensitivity of dopamine receptors
e. Stimulation of nicotinic receptors

111. A patient on the trauma-burn unit received a drug to ease the pain of debridement and dressing changes for several severe burns. They experience good, prompt analgesia, but despite the near absence of pain their heart rate and blood pressure rise considerably, consistent with sympathetic nervous system activation. As the effects of the drug develop, their skeletal muscle tone progressively increases. They appear awake at times because their eyes periodically open. As drug effects wear off, they hallucinate and behave in a very agitated fashion. Hallucinations, "bad dreams," and periods of delirium recur over several days after receiving the drug. What drug was most likely given?

a. Fentanyl
b. Ketamine
c. Midazolam
d. Succinylcholine
e. Thiopental

112. A patient who has been treated with levodopa is switched to a regimen with a product that contains levodopa plus carbidopa. What is the main action of carbidopa that provides the rationale for using it in this dual-drug approach?

a. Blocks ACh release in the CNS, thereby facilitating levodopa's ability to restore a dopamine-ACh balance
b. Helps activate dietary vitamin B_6, a deficiency of which occurs during levodopa therapy
c. Increases permeability of the blood-brain barrier to levodopa, giving levodopa better access to the CNS
d. Inhibits metabolic conversion of levodopa to dopamine outside the CNS
e. Reduces levodopa-induced hypotension by blocking vascular dopamine receptors

113. A physician considers placing a patient on long-term (months, years) phenobarbital for control of a relatively common medical condition. For most of these indications, newer and arguably more efficacious drugs that participate in fewer drug interactions are available and preferred. For which one of the following uses, nonetheless, is this barbiturate still considered reasonable and appropriate?

a. Alcohol withdrawal signs/symptoms
b. Anxiety management
c. Certain epilepsies
d. Endogenous depression (adjunct to SSRIs)
e. Sleep disorders such as insomnia

114. One reason for the declining use of tricyclic antidepressants such as imipramine, and the growing use of newer classes, is the prevalence of common tricyclic-induced side effects or adverse responses. What side effect or adverse response is most likely to occur with usual therapeutic doses of a tricyclic?

a. Anticholinergic (antimuscarinic) effects
b. Arrhythmias
c. Hepatotoxicity
d. Nephrotoxicity
e. Seizures

115. A 17-year-old male was diagnosed with epilepsy after developing repeated episodes of generalized tonic-clonic seizures following a motor vehicle accident in which he received a head injury. After treating acute seizures with the proper injectable drugs, he is started on a regimen of oral phenytoin, with the daily dose titrated upward until symptom control and a therapeutic plasma concentration are reached. The overall elimination half-life of the drug during initial treatment was measured to be 24 hours, a value that is quite for otherwise healthy adolescents and adults taking no other drugs.

Today he presents in the neurology clinic with nystagmus, ataxia, diplopia, cognitive impairment, and other signs and symptoms consistent with phenytoin toxicity. A blood sample, drawn at noon, has a plasma phenytoin concentration of 30 mcg/mL. That value is 50% higher than typical peak therapeutic plasma concentrations, and twice the usual minimum effective blood level. These values are summarized in the figure on the next page.

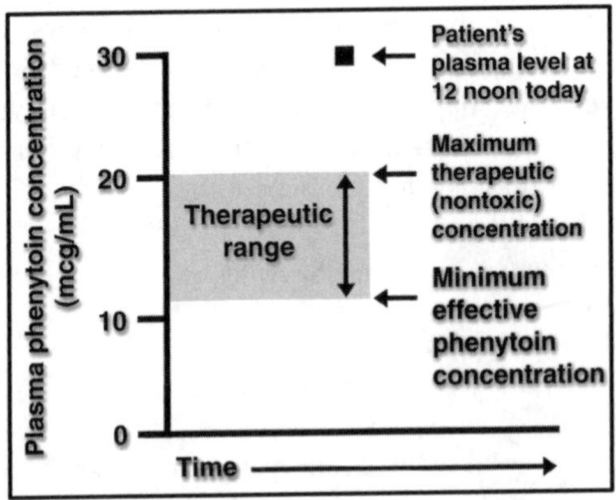

We will withhold further doses of phenytoin until plasma levels fall into the therapeutic range, and the patient is largely free of signs and symptoms of phenytoin toxicity. In the interim, what would you do or expect to occur next?

a. Administer flumazenil, which will quickly reverse signs and symptoms of phenytoin toxicity but may cause seizures to recur
b. Elimination of phenytoin from the plasma will follow zero-order kinetics for several days
c. Give an amphetamine or other CNS stimulant to reverse generalized CNS depression due to the phenytoin excess
d. Give phenobarbital to induce the P450 system, thereby hastening phenytoin's metabolic elimination
e. Plasma phenytoin concentrations will fall to 15 mcg/mL, in the middle of the therapeutic range, by noon tomorrow (24 h later, per the usual half-life)

116. A patient with Parkinson disease has signs and symptoms that can be considered "moderate" now, but they are worsening and not responding well to current drug therapy. The physician decides to empirically assess an antiparkinson drug that is a selective inhibitor of monoamine oxidase type B (MAO-B). Which of the following drugs would that be?

a. Bromocriptine
b. Carbidopa
c. Phenelzine
d. Selegiline
e. Tranylcypromine

117. Meperidine is similar to morphine in many ways, but has some decided differences that are clinically relevant: with very high blood levels or with true overdoses, meperidine can cause significant adverse responses that simply aren't seen with morphine or most other opioid analgesics. What is that rather unique effect of meperidine?

a. Constipation leading to paralytic ileus
b. Heightened response to pain (paradoxical hyperalgesia)
c. Intense biliary tract spasm
d. Psychosis-like state, possibly seizures
e. Respiratory depression, apnea, ventilatory arrest

118. A patient has mild to moderate pain that is expected to last for at least a month. The physician appropriately decides that a strong opioid analgesic is not indicated, and so prescribes another analgesic drug at usual recommended doses. Seeking greater pain relief, the patient promptly doubles the daily prescribed dose. Within a couple of days, they manifest rather strong symptoms of psychosis and some ventilatory depression. Administration of usually effective doses of naloxone fails to reverse the initial drug's adverse effects. What drug was the patient probably taking?

a. Acetaminophen
b. Aspirin
c. Codeine
d. Hydrocodone
e. Propoxyphene

119. Chlorpromazine and haloperidol can be considered prototypes of two relatively old but still-used antipsychotic drugs—the phenothiazines and the butyrophenones—respectively. While many of the actions and side effects of these drugs are qualitatively similar, they are different quantitatively: that is, in terms of incidence and severity. Which of the following effect or side effect typically occurs more frequently, is usually more severe, and has a relatively rapid onset, with haloperidol?

a. Extrapyramidal reactions
b. Intense atropine-like side effects
c. Lethal blood dyscrasias
d. Orthostatic hypotension
e. Urinary retention necessitating bladder catheterization

120. A patient is transported to the emergency department. A friend who accompanies the patient says he was experimenting with "angel dust." What best describes the actions or other characteristics of this recreational drug?

a. Causes peripheral and central effects via antimuscarinic properties
b. Causes significant withdrawal symptoms
c. Has strong opioid receptor-activating activity
d. Has amphetamine-like properties and is an hallucinogen
e. Overdoses should be treated with flumazenil

121. Package inserts for a drug caution against administering it concurrent with any other drug that can raise or lower sodium concentrations. The risks are inadequate or excessive effects of the drug, depending on the direction in which sodium concentrations change. This, of course, requires cautious use or avoidance (if possible) of the common diuretics. To which drug does this caution or warning apply?

a. Cholestyramine
b. Lithium
c. Nifedipine
d. Phenylephrine
e. Statin-type cholesterol-lowering drugs

122. A 12-year-old boy has been treated with methylphenidate for the last three years. His younger sister finds the bottle of pills and consumes enough to cause significant toxicity. Which of the following findings would you most likely expect?

a. Hypertension, tachycardia, seizures
b. Hypotension, bronchospasm
c. Drowsiness, obtunded reflexes, diarrhea
d. Miosis, bradycardia, profuse salivation, sweating
e. Hypothermia, skeletal muscle weakness or paralysis, pupils that are not responsive to light

123. Two inhaled general anesthetics, A and B, have the following MAC values:

$$X: MAC \approx 2\%$$
$$Y: MAC \approx 100\%$$

Based only on this information (note that we have not named any drugs), which statement is true?

a. Drug X has a longer duration of action than drug Y
b. Drug X is more soluble in the blood than drug Y
c. Drug Y causes greater analgesia and skeletal muscle relaxation than drug X
d. The concentration of drug in inspired air that is needed to cause adequate surgical anesthesia is higher for drug Y than for drug X
e. The time to onset of adequate general anesthesia is 50 times longer for drug Y than for drug X

124. A 31-year-old woman has been treated with fluoxetine for 5 months. She is diagnosed with another medical problem and receives one or more drugs that would otherwise be suitable and probably problem-free. She is rushed to the ED with unstable vital signs, muscle rigidity, myoclonus, CNS irritability, altered consciousness, and shivering. What add-on drug(s) most likely caused these responses?

a. Codeine for cough
b. Loratadine for seasonal allergies
c. Midazolam and fentanyl, used to ease discomfort from endoscopy
d. Sumatriptan for migraine
e. Zolpidem for short-term insomnia

125. A 42-year-old woman with a long history of anxiety that has been treated with diazepam decides to triple her daily dose because of increasing fearfulness about global warming. Two days after her attempt at self-prescribing, she is found extremely lethargic and nonresponsive, with markedly obtunded reflexes and reactions to painful stimuli. Respirations are 8/min and shallow. What drug would you give to manage these drug-induced signs and symptoms?

a. Dextroamphetamine
b. Flumazenil
c. Naltrexone
d. Physostigmine
e. Pralidoxime

126. A patient who has been treated for Parkinson disease for about a year presents with purplish, mottled changes to her skin. What drug is the most likely cause of this cutaneous response?

a. Amantadine
b. Bromocriptine
c. Levodopa (alone)
d. Levodopa combined with carbidopa
e. Pramipexole

127. A young boy who has been treated for epilepsy for a year is referred to a periodontist for evaluation and treatment of massive overgrowth of his gingival tissues. Some teeth are almost completely covered with hyperplastic tissue. Which drug is the most likely cause of the oral pathology?

a. Carbamazepine
b. Lorazepam
c. Phenobarbital
d. Phenytoin
e. Valproic acid

128. A patient with undiagnosed coronary artery disease is given a medication. Shortly thereafter she develops intense tightness and "crushing discomfort" of her chest. An ECG reveals ST-segment changes indicative of acute myocardial ischemia in tissues supplied by the left anterior descending coronary artery and distal vessels. Which drug most likely caused this reaction?

a. Clozapine
b. Pentazocine
c. Phenytoin
d. Sumatriptan
e. Zolpidem

129. Nitrous oxide is a common component in the technique of balanced anesthesia. It is used in conjunction with such other drugs as a halogenated hydrocarbon volatile liquid anesthetic, and usually included as 80% of the total inspired gas mixture. Which phrase best summarizes why nitrous oxide cannot be used alone for general anesthesia?

a. Almost total lack of analgesic activity, regardless of concentration.
b. Inspired concentrations greater than 10% or so tend to profound cardiac negative inotropic effects.
c. MAC (minimum alveolar concentration) is greater than 100%.
d. Methemoglobinemia occurs even with low inspired concentrations.
e. Such great solubility in blood that its effects take an extraordinarily long time to develop.
f. Very high frequency of bronchospasm.

130. A patient develops a severe and rapidly worsening adverse response to a drug. The physician orders prompt administration of antipyretics, IV hydration, and bromocriptine or dantrolene to manage symptoms and hopefully to prevent a fatal outcome. Which drug or drug group most likely caused these adverse responses?

a. Benzodiazepines, especially those used as hypnotics
b. Chlorpromazine
c. Levodopa
d. Phenytoin
e. SSRIs

131. Ropinirole is a relatively new drug that is approved to treat what's commonly called restless leg syndrome (also known as Ekbom syndrome). The drug works as a dopamine receptor agonist in certain parts of the brain. Given this mechanism of action, what other disorder is, most likely, another indication for this drug?

a. Daytime anxiety
b. Hypersomnia (excessive sleepiness)
c. Parkinson disease
d. Schizophrenia
e. Status epilepticus
f. Treatment of severe pain

132. A 34-year-old man with mild anxiety and depression symptoms has heard about buspirone on TV and asks whether it might be suitable for him. According to recent diagnostic and treatment criteria the drug would be appropriate, particularly for short-term symptom control. Which phrase correctly describes an important property of buspirone?

a. Associated with a withdrawal syndrome that, if unsupervised or controlled, may be fatal
b. Has a significant potential for abuse
c. Is likely to potentiate the CNS-depressant effects of alcohol, benzodiazepines, and sedative antihistamines (eg, diphenhydramine), so such interactants must be avoided at all cost
d. Requires almost daily dosage titrations in order to optimize the response
e. Seldom causes drowsiness

133. A patient in the neurology unit at your hospital develops status epilepticus, and at the time there is no good information about the etiology. What drug should be given first for the fastest suppression of the seizures?

a. Carbamazepine
b. Lorazepam
c. Phenobarbital
d. Phenytoin
e. Valproic acid

134. A patient has had a documented severe allergic reaction to ester-type local anesthetics. What other drug is a member of the ester class, and so would be the most likely to provoke an allergic or anaphylactic reaction if this patient received it?

a. Bupivacaine
b. Lidocaine
c. Mepivacaine
d. Prilocaine
e. Tetracaine

135. A 66-year-old woman is diagnosed with Alzheimer disease, with symptoms being described as mild-to-moderate. What pharmacologic approach is generally considered the most fruitful in terms of alleviating symptoms of early Alzheimer and probably slowing the course of her underlying brain pathology?

a. Activate a population of serotonin receptors
b. Block dopamine release or receptor activation
c. Inhibit acetylcholinesterase
d. Inhibit MAO
e. Dissolve cerebral vascular thrombi

136. Trihexyphenidyl is prescribed as an adjunct to other drugs being used to manage a patient with Parkinson disease. What is the most likely purpose or action of this drug as part of the overall drug treatment plan?

a. To counteract sedation that is likely to be caused by the other medications
b. To help correct further the dopamine-ACh imbalance that accounts for parkinsonian signs and symptoms
c. To manage cutaneous allergic responses that are so common with typical antiparkinson drugs
d. To prevent the development of manic/hypomanic responses to other antiparkinson drugs
e. To reverse tardive dyskinesias if the parkinsonism was induced by an antipsychotic drug

137. In early 2006, the FDA granted approval to market a new prescription drug (drug X) that will be administered in the form of a dermal patch (apply the patch to intact skin; the drug is absorbed from there).

Drug X belongs to a very old class of drugs that, when given by its usual route, orally, can interact with foods such as cheese and processed meats (certain breads, other foods, and alcoholic beverages) leading to an interaction that can elevate blood pressure to severe and sometimes fatal levels. After more than a decade of testing, the FDA approved its use for adults. In its lowest dose, no dietary restriction(s) are required.

Based on this information, how is drug X most likely classified and what is its most likely clinical use?

a. Amphetamine-like agent for ADD/ADHD
b. Barbiturates used for daytime anxiety
c. Benzodiazepine for anxiety and sleep
d. MAO inhibitor for depression
e. Morphine-like analgesic for severe/chronic pain

138. The pediatrician writes a prescription for a combination (of several drugs) product that contains dextromethorphan, which is an isomer of a codeine analog. The patient is a 12-year-old boy. What is the most likely purpose for which the drug is prescribed?

a. Control mild-moderate pain after the lad broke his wrist playing soccer
b. Manage diarrhea caused by food-borne bacteria
c. Provide sedation because the child has ADD/ADHD
d. Suppress severe cough associated with a bout of influenza
e. Treat nocturnal bed-wetting

139. We administer a "usually effective" and otherwise therapeutic dose of thiopental to a patient. It is given by IV bolus injection. Within a matter of seconds the patient is asleep. We will give no other drug. What is most likely to occur thereafter, assuming the patient has no unusual genetic traits that might alter the thiopental's pharmacodynamics or pharmacokinetics?

a. Significant and clinically useful analgesia will persist for an hour or so
b. Significant increase in cerebral oxygen consumption
c. The drug will be promptly metabolized by the hepatic P450 system
d. The patient develops acute seizures (eg, status epilepticus)
e. The patient will awake in about 3 to 5 minutes

140. Many legal jurisdictions have imposed various restrictions on over-the-counter sale of products that contain pseudoephedrine, for example in various oral decongestant products. That is because pseudoephedrine can be rather easily used to synthesize which of the following highly psychoactive and abuse-prone drugs?

a. Methamphetamine
b. Morphine
c. Oxycodone
d. Pentazocine
e. Phencyclidine (PCP)

141. The anesthesiologist prepares to administer several drugs to a patient as part of normal pre- and intraoperative care. What drug lacks the ability to cause generalized CNS depression, to reduce or impair the patient's level of consciousness, or to prevent or reduce pain?

a. Droperidol
b. Midazolam
c. Pancuronium
d. Propofol
e. Thiopental

142. A 26-year-old woman has been on antidepressant therapy for several months. Today she complains of missing her period and having what is eventually determined to be galactorrhea. Your careful assessment reveals that she has developed some dyskinesias not unlike those you would typically associate with a phenothiazine or butyrophenone (eg, haloperidol) antipsychotic drug. Pregnancy tests are negative. What drug is most likely to have caused these findings?

a. Amoxapine
b. Citalopram
c. Fluoxetine
d. Sertraline
e. Tranylcypromine

143. A patient has been taking an oral monoamine oxidase inhibitor (MAOI), but that fact is unknown to the health team who is now taking care of her, for unrelated medical conditions, in the hospital. The patient receives a drug that leads to a fatal response characterized by profound fever, delirium, psychotic behavior, and status epilepticus. It was found to have occurred because of an interaction with the MAOI. Which of the following is this second drug or the drug class to which it belongs?

a. Barbiturate
b. Diazepam
c. Meperidine
e. Morphine
e. Phenytoin

144. A young woman is taken to the emergency department by some friends. It seems they were out on "bar night" and someone slipped something into her alcoholic beverage, the first and only one she consumed that night. She is now extraordinarily drowsy and has little recall of what happened between the time she sipped her drink and now. Someone overheard another bar patron talking about "roofies." You suspect her drink was spiked with Rohypnol, the lesser-known generic name of which is flunitrazepam. A positive response (ie, symptom improvement) to administering what drug below would confirm your suspicion?

a. Diazepam
b. Flumazenil
c. Ketamine
d. Naltrexone
e. Triazolam

145. In deciding on pharmacotherapy for many patients you've diagnosed with depression, you've usually considered starting with an SSRI or, in some cases, a tricyclic. Today you assess a patient and suspect endogenous depression. While discussing treatment options they refer to a drug by name and ask you about it; they've seen many advertisements for it in magazines and on TV. The drug (generic name) is bupropion. In what main way does bupropion differ from the SSRIs and the tricyclics?

a. Higher incidence of CNS depression, drowsiness
b. Higher incidence of weight gain
c. Less drug-induced sexual dysfunction
d. Much more common and severe falls of resting blood pressure and orthostatic hypotension
e. More severe and more frequent peripheral anticholinergic (atropine-like) side effects
f. Stronger inhibition of monoamine oxidase

146. A 33-year-old woman patient who has been treated with haloperidol is seen in the emergency department. Her husband reports that she has complained of rapidly worsening fever and muscle stiffness, and she has "the shakes" (tremor). Her level of consciousness is diminishing. Her temperature is 104°F, and her blood creatine kinase level is elevated. What is the most likely explanation for these findings?

a. Allergic response to her medication
b. Neuroleptic malignant syndrome (NMS)
c. Overdose
d. Parkinsonism
e. Tardive dyskinesia

147. Nearly all the drugs used as primary therapy, or as adjuncts, for the treatment of Parkinson disease or drug-induced parkinsonism exert their desired effects directly in the brain's striatum. Which one exerts its main effects in the gut, not in the brain?

a. Amantadine
b. Benztropine
c. Bromocriptine
d. Carbidopa
e. Selegiline

148. You have a patient with severe postoperative pain who is not getting adequate analgesia from usually effective doses of morphine. The physician orders an immediate switch to pentazocine (at usually effective analgesic doses). What is the most likely outcome of stopping the morphine and immediately starting the pentazocine?

a. Abrupt, added respiratory depression
b. Acute development of physical dependence
c. Coma
d. Seizures
e. Worsening of pain

149. Our chosen pharmacologic approach to managing a patient with mild and recently diagnosed parkinsonism will be to enhance the activity of endogenous brain dopamine by inhibiting its metabolic inactivation. What drug works primarily by that mechanism?

a. Benztropine
b. Selegiline
c. Trihexyphenidyl
d. Bromocriptine
e. Chlorpromazine

150. Chlorpromazine has been prescribed for a patient with schizophrenia, and the patient has been taking the drug, at usually effective doses, for about 6 months. Today he comes to the hospital with other medical conditions that require surgery and the administration of other drugs, and we decide it is unwise to stop the chlorpromazine and run the risk of psychotic behavior while we perform other interventions. What other signs/symptoms that the patient may also have, or acquire as the result of surgery and drug therapy, are most likely to be affected beneficially by the continued use of chlorpromazine?

a. Epilepsy and the risk of seizures
b. Hypotension
c. Nausea and vomiting
d. Urinary retention caused by abdominal surgery
e. Xerostomia (dry mouth) caused by antimuscarinic drugs used to prevent intraoperative bradycardia

151. There are, rightfully, concerns about cocaine abuse, and too many deaths have occurred from smoking "crack" cocaine or injecting or nasally inhaling the drug. What statement best describes the main mechanism by which cocaine exerts its deleterious effects in the central nervous system or in the periphery?

a. Directly activates, as an agonist, both α- and β_1-adrenergic receptors
b. Enhances neuronally mediated adrenergic receptor activation by inhibiting neuronal norepinephrine (NE) reuptake
c. Inhibits catecholamine inactivation by inhibiting MAO and catechol *O*-methyltransferase.
d. Produces bradycardia and vasodilation, leading to hypotension and acute heart failure, by blocking neuronal NE release
e. Stimulates autonomic nerve conduction effectively, leading to increased neuronal NE release

152. One approach to managing hyperprolactinemia is to administer a drug that has relative selectivity, as an agonist, for central dopamine D_2 receptors. What drug works in that manner?

a. Bromocriptine
b. Chlorpromazine
c. Fluphenazine
d. Haloperidol
e. Promethazine

153. We perform a meta-analysis on the ability of various antipsychotic drugs to cause constipation, urinary retention, blurred vision, and dry mouth—all of which reflect significant blockade of muscarinic receptors in the peripheral nervous systems. Which of the following drugs most likely caused these unwanted effects?

a. Chlorpromazine
b. Clozapine
c. Haloperidol
d. Olanzapine
e. Sertraline

154. A 66-year-old woman has terminal cancer and is in a hospice. She is receiving round-the-clock opioids, at rather high doses, but still reports what she describes as significant burning, shooting pain. The physician believes it is neuropathic pain, which is often difficult to manage. Increasing the dose of opioids may be helpful, but that option is ruled out at this time because doing so is likely to suppress ventilation excessively. In addition, the patient does not want the excessive grogginess that is apt to occur with more opioid on board. Although the patient is not at all hypertensive, the physician prescribes an opioid analgesic adjunct that is far more widely used as an antihypertensive agent. What is the most likely adjunctive drug she prescribed?

a. Captopril
b. Clonidine
c. Hydrochlorothiazide
d. Labetalol
e. Prazosin

155. A patient is on long-term methadone therapy as part of a holistic plan to curb their opioid addiction and abuse. Which of the following phrases best describes a characteristic of this drug?

a. Causes pentazocine-like activation of κ receptors and blockade of μ receptors
b. Has greater oral bioavailability than morphine, especially when oral administration is started
c. Remarkably devoid of such typical opioid analgesic side effects as constipation and respiratory depression
d. Useful for maintenance therapy in opioid- (eg, heroin-) dependent individuals, but lacks clinically useful analgesic effects
e. When abruptly stopped after long-term administration, causes a withdrawal syndrome that is more intense, but briefer, than that associated with morphine or heroin withdrawal

156. An 8-year-old girl is brought to the ED by her mother, who has observed that her daughter experiences frequent impairments of consciousness associated with episodes of staring into space lasting approximately 30 seconds. Further neurologic evaluation indicates signs and symptoms consistent with absence seizures. Which of the following drugs is generally considered the preferred starting agent for this type of epilepsy?

a. Alprazolam
b. Diazepam
c. Ethosuximide
d. Midazolam
e. Phenytoin

157. A 43-year-old woman becomes hypertensive and suffers a fatal acute coronary syndrome shortly after starting therapy on a drug. Autopsy shows little in the way of coronary atherosclerosis, but ECG changes noted just before her death revealed significant myocardial ischemia in the myocardium served by the left anterior descending and circumflex coronary arteries. The cause of death is thought to involve coronary vasospasm. Which of the following drugs most likely precipitated this event?

a. Bromocriptine used for Parkinson disease
b. Ergotamine given to abort a migraine attack
c. Morphine given for post-trauma analgesia
d. Phenoxybenzamine used for carcinoid syndrome
e. Phenytoin administered to manage generalized tonic-clonic seizures

158. Promethazine, a phenothiazine derivative with substantial antiemetic, antitussive, and H_1-histamine receptor blocking activity, has a clinical profile quite similar to diphenhydramine. Recently the FDA mandated a "black box warning" against use of the drug, in all doses and forms, for children aged 2 years or younger. Fatalities have occurred in these young patients, even in response to dosages that previously were considered therapeutic and safe. What is the most likely cause of death from promethazine in these patients?

a. Complete heart block followed by asystole
b. Hypertensive crisis, intracranial hemorrhage
c. Parkinsonian-like dyskinesias, including tardive dyskinesias
d. Severe and refractory diarrhea leading to fluid and electrolyte loss
e. Ventilatory depression, apnea, excessive CNS depression

159. A 55-year-old woman undergoes surgery. She receives several drugs for preanesthesia care, intubation, and intraoperative skeletal muscle paralysis; and a mixture of inhaled agents to provide balanced anesthesia. Toward the end of the procedure she develops a rapidly progressing fever, hypertension, hyperkalemia, tachycardia, muscle rigidity, and metabolic acidosis. What drug combination most likely interacted and elicited this reaction?

a. Fentanyl and midazolam
b. Midazolam and morphine
c. Nitrous oxide and etomidate
d. Propofol and midazolam
e. Succinylcholine and isoflurane

160. A 30-year-old woman with partial seizures is treated with vigabatrin. What is the principal mechanism of action of this anticonvulsant?

a. Sodium channel blockade
b. Increase in frequency of chloride channel opening
c. Increase in GABA
d. Calcium channel blockade
e. Increased potassium channel permeability
f. NMDA receptor blockade

161. A 24-year-old woman has a history of epilepsy that is being treated with phenytoin. She becomes pregnant. What would you do throughout the remainder of her pregnancy, in addition to providing otherwise proper perinatal care, with regard to her seizure disorder?

a. Add valproic acid.
b. Discontinue all anticonvulsant medication.
c. Increase daily dietary iron intake.
d. Prescribe daily folic acid supplements.
e. Switch from the phenytoin to phenobarbital.

162. A patient is transported to the emergency department by ambulance after repeated syncopal episodes. The cause was attributed to severe drug-induced orthostatic hypotension due to α-adrenergic blockade from one of the drug's main side effects. What drug most likely caused this problem?

a. Buspirone
b. Chlorpromazine
c. Diphenhydramine
d. Haloperidol
e. Zolpidem

163. Clozapine, as an example of the "atypical antipsychotics," seldom is used as first-line (initial) therapy of schizophrenia. Compared with the older antipsychotics, it is associated with a much higher risk of a serious adverse response. What is that greater risk?

a. Agranulocytosis
b. Extrapyramidal side effects (parkinsonian)
c. Hypoglycemia
d. Hypotension, severe
e. Ventilatory depression or arrest

164. You're at the end of the first week of your M3 ob-gyn clerkship. You are about to go into the delivery room to see your first childbirth. You've reviewed the mother's chart and see that she was taking, before and throughout pregnancy, a certain drug. You also note that starting about 1 month before her due date (today) she was prescribed daily oral vitamin K supplements. These supplements were given specifically because of the other drug she was taking. The baby is born and promptly gets an injection of vitamin K. Knowing what you do about vitamin K, you correctly reason that these measures were taken to reduce the risks of excessive or abnormal bleeding caused by drug-induced impairments of hepatic vitamin K-dependent clotting factors in the newborn. What drug did the mother most likely receive during pregnancy that necessitated the vitamin K administration?

a. Bupropion
b. Diazepam
c. Methadone
d. Phenytoin
e. Warfarin

165. When carbidopa is administered along with levodopa for Parkinson disease, it increases the bioavailability of levodopa by inhibiting the formation of dopamine in the gut. However, the carbidopa-induced inhibition of dopa decarboxylase favors the peripheral metabolism of levodopa to another metabolite (3-*O*-methyldopa) that competes with levodopa for transport across the blood-brain barrier. This is catalyzed by catechol *O*-methyltransferase (COMT). If your goal is to inhibit COMT, and so further increase the central bioavailability and effects of levodopa, which of the following drugs would you choose?

a. Donepezil
b. Entacapone
c. Selegiline
d. Tacrine
e. Trihexyphenidyl

166. A patient has a long history of excessive alcohol consumption. He was arrested yet again for drunk driving and referred to a substance abuse program for therapy. The physician there prescribed a drug to stifle further alcohol ingestion, to be used along with other nondrug interventions. The doctor properly instructed the patient not to consume any alcohol, not to use alcohol-containing mouthwashes, nor even apply alcohol-based toiletries, because alcohol may cause a disturbing, if not dangerous, interaction with his medication. The patient ignored the advice and decided to have a shot of whiskey. Within minutes he develops flushing, a throbbing headache, nausea, and vomiting. Which drug was he most likely taking to curb his alcohol use?

a. Naltrexone
b. Diazepam
c. Disulfiram
d. Phenobarbital
e. Tranylcypromine

167. We start a patient with endogenous depression on a drug that selectively inhibits neuronal serotonin (5-HT) reuptake and has minimal effect on the reuptake of NE or dopamine. Which drug best fits this description?

a. Amitriptyline
b. Bupropion
c. Fluoxetine
d. Imipramine
e. Venlafaxine

168. A 29-year-old man uses an oral barbiturate and alcohol to help satisfy his addiction to CNS depressants. During the past week he has been incarcerated and is not able to obtain the drugs. He is brought to the medical ward because of the onset of severe anxiety, increased sensitivity to light, dizziness, and generalized tremors due to drug withdrawal. On physical examination, he is hyperreflexic. Which drug would be the best choice to help diminish his withdrawal symptoms?

a. Buspirone
b. Chloral hydrate
c. Chlorpromazine
d. Lorazepam
e. Trazodone

169. A 50-year-old man has been consuming large amounts of ethanol on an almost daily basis for many years. One day, unable to find any ethanol, he ingests a large amount of methanol (wood alcohol) that he had bought for his camp lantern. What drug would be administered to best treat underlying biochemical consequences of the methanol poisoning?

a. Diazepam
b. Ethanol
c. Flumazenil
d. Phenobarbital
e. Phenytoin

170. Many news reports have told of a large number of deaths of opioid abusers who purchased and self-administered illicit drugs that contained lethal amounts of fentanyl. One patient who received a fentanyl-laced drug presents in your emergency department, barely alive. Which of the following drugs would you administer first, with the best hope that it can promptly reverse the potentially lethal effects of the fentanyl?

a. Diazepam
b. Flumazenil
c. Naloxone
d. Naltrexone
e. Phenytoin

171. A 10-year-old boy has nocturnal enuresis. His parents take him to a clinic that specializes in management of this condition. The physician writes an order for a low dose of imipramine. After a couple of weeks on the drug, the episodes of bed-wetting decrease dramatically. What is the most likely mechanism by which the imipramine provided benefit?

a. Alleviated depression signs and symptoms by increasing neuronal catecholamine reuptake
b. Blocked muscarinic receptors in the bladder musculature
c. Caused sedation such that the boy sleeps through the night without voiding
d. Reduced renal blood flow, glomerular filtration, and urine output
e. Released antidiuretic hormone (ADH)

172. A patient is transported to your emergency department because of a seizure. A review of his history reveals that he has been treated by different physicians for different medical conditions, and there has been no dialogue between them in terms of what they've prescribed. One physician prescribed a drug for short-term management of depression. Another prescribed the very same drug, marketed under a different trade name, to help the patient quit smoking cigarettes. What drug was most likely prescribed by both doctors, and was the most likely cause of the seizures?

a. Bupropion
b. Chlordiazepoxide
c. Fluoxetine
d. Imipramine
e. Lithium

173. About one year ago you diagnosed schizophrenia in a 23-year-old otherwise healthy man. As a result of intensive psychotherapy, careful titration of chlorpromazine dosages, and remarkably good compliance with drug and other therapies, he is well enough to return to work. Several months later, at a scheduled visit, you observe numerous signs and symptoms of drug-induced parkinsonism, and the patient reports rather distressing symptoms of akathisias (inner restlessness, jitteriness, etc). However, typical manifestations of schizophrenia seem to be well controlled. Which approach is most likely to alleviate the motor and subjective parkinsonian responses, and pose the lowest risk of causing schizophrenia signs and symptoms to reappear?

a. Add a catechol *O*-methyltransferase inhibitor (eg, tolcapone).
b. Add a centrally acting cholinesterase inhibitor (eg, donepezil or tacrine).
c. Add benztropine.
d. Add levodopa or levodopa plus carbidopa.
e. Switch from chlorpromazine to haloperidol.

174. Consider isoflurane and halothane as somewhat representative examples of volatile liquid general anesthetics. Which statement best compares or contrasts their actions?

a. Both typically raise blood pressure via direct vasoconstrictor effects in the peripheral vasculature
b. Halothane is associated with a higher risk of renal and hepatic toxicity, especially in patients who have been anesthetized with this drug before
c. Isoflurane prolongs the QT interval and is associated with a much higher risk of causing potentially fatal ventricular tachyarrhythmias, including torsades de pointes, than halothane
d. Isoflurane sensitizes the myocardium to the arrhythmogenic effects of catecholamines much more than halothane does
e. Use of isoflurane for balanced anesthesia requires adjunctive use of nitrous oxide and neuromuscular blockers, use of halothane does not

175. A patient with Parkinson disease starts therapy with a drug that acts in the CNS as an agonist for dopamine receptors. It has no direct effects on dopamine synthesis, neuronal reuptake, or metabolic inactivation. Which drug fits this description the best?

a. Amantadine
b. Apomorphine
c. Belladonna
d. Bromocriptine
e. Selegiline

176. A patient develops profound fever, skeletal muscle rigidity, autonomic hyperactivity, and systemic electrolyte imbalances as part of a severe adverse response to a psychoactive drug. The working diagnosis is neuroleptic malignant syndrome. In addition to administering dantrolene in an attempt to restore some semblance of normal skeletal muscle function, which other drug is most likely to be given to help provide additional symptom relief?

a. Benztropine
b. Bromocriptine
c. Diazepam
d. Flumazenil
e. Naloxone
f. Propranolol

177. It is obvious that morphine should always be administered with care. However, one of its expected effects makes giving it particularly dangerous for certain patients unless "special measures" can be taken to prevent it. Which comorbidity weighs against using morphine unless we first take precautions to prevent adverse consequences from occurring?

a. Acute pulmonary edema
b. Closed-head injury
c. History of epilepsy
d. Hypertension
e. Recent/evolving myocardial infarction

Central Nervous System Pharmacology

Answers

105. The answer is e. *(Brunton, pp 361-362, 402-404, 410-412, 446, 452. Katzung, pp 375t, 378-379, 382.)* Benzodiazepines as a class tend to cause short-term memory loss following administration. The intensity of the effect depends on the unique drug, its pharmacokinetics, and its administration route. For example, the amnestic effect is common and intense (and clinically useful) with midazolam, which has a fast onset and short half-life; and flunitrazepam (Rohypnol, better known as roofies on the street).

The memory loss does not affect recall of prior events but rather events occurring shortly after the drug is given. This *antegrade* amnesia is valuable in settings such as described in the scenario, where many unpleasant or anxiety-provoking events may occur between preop medication, the trip to the operating room, and other unpleasantries that might occur before the patient is anesthetized. (The patient here had absolutely no recall of events occurring within about 30 s after the midazolam was given, up to about an hour after she regained consciousness postop. Many patients who receive midazolam for short endoscopic procedures such as colonoscopy or bronchoscopy also lack recall.)

Midazolam intensifies the overall sedative and mental clouding effects of opioids, but does not potentiate analgesia (a). It does not prevent or reverse hypotension (b), and if the dose is too large or it is administered too quickly the drug may actually lower blood pressure in its own right. Midazolam has some anticonvulsant effects but it is seldom used for that purpose (lorazepam is one benzodiazepine that is routinely used for certain seizures, particularly status epilepticus, for which it is the first drug that should be injected). More importantly the question stated "seizures likely to be caused by propofol," but propofol rarely causes seizures (c). Benzodiazepines are not arrhythmogenic nor do they have antiarrhythmic activity (d).

106. The answer is a. *(Brunton, pp 343-345, 350-353, 422. Katzung, pp 423-424, 434-437.)* Hypotension and respiratory/ventilatory depression are common side effects of propofol and, indeed, of most other classes of CNS depressants injected for preanesthetic sedation, anesthesia induction, or anesthesia maintenance. Laryngospasm (b) sometimes and rather uniquely applies to injection of rapidly acting barbiturate induction agents (see Question 107). Memory loss (c)—specifically short-term antegrade amnesia—is associated with certain benzodiazepines (here, the midazolam, previous question).

Propofol does not cause malignant hyperthermia (d), or interact with other medications (those listed in the MAR, or others) to cause it. Malignant hyperthermia is mainly linked, in the surgical setting, to the combined use of a halogenated hydrocarbon inhaled anesthetic (particularly halothane, the use of which is declining) and a neuromuscular blocker (typically succinylcholine more so than a curare-like nondepolarizing agent). Propofol does not cause seizures (e); of the injectable induction agents, seizures are mainly a problem with etomidate. Finally, aside from generalized suppression of the CNS, propofol causes no significant or clinically relevant effects on skeletal muscle, and tends not to cause nausea or emesis (when used alone) that is common with other reasonable alternatives.

107. The answer is c. *(Brunton, pp 347-350, 417, 419. Katzung, pp 372-380, 434-435.)* Laryngospasm is associated with the barbiturate induction agents, whether the drug is an oxybarbiturate (methohexital) or a thiobarbiturate (thiamylal, thiopental, others; "thio" refers to a sulfur atom replacing an oxygen atom at a certain point in the molecule). The mechanism is not known for sure, but the phenomenon is, and the laryngospasm may be sufficient in a small number of cases to make airway intubation difficult. Barbiturates also cause ventilatory depressant effects (centrally mediated), but in the situation described here that is not worrisome because the patient is receiving mechanical ventilation—assuming there were no difficulties with intubation.

Barbiturates lack analgesic effects at blood levels not far lower than lethal. They can actually increase the sensation of pain (hyperalgesic effect; a) when therapeutic doses of oral agents (mainly phenobarbital nowadays) are given (inappropriately) to patients with pain and who are not being treated with true analgesic drugs suitable for the degree of pain the patient has. This is one of the reasons why barbiturates or benzodiazepines should never be used as analgesics, even though they may cause generalized CNS depression. Note, however, that when the fast-acting injectable barbiturates are given at usual induction/anesthetic doses the hyperalgesic effect does not occur because it is obscured by true analgesic drugs that are also administered (eg, the morphine this patient got).

Barbiturates as a class, whether given parenterally or orally, and regardless of the pharmacokinetics of a specific drug, tend to lower blood pressure (not raise it, answer b; the probable sites of action are both central and directly on the heart and resistance vessels). Barbiturate IV induction agents tend to lower blood pressure significantly and sometimes excessively. Malignant hyperthermia (d) is a serious adverse perioperative response that is associated with the combined administration of skeletal neuromuscular blockers and inhaled halogenated hydrocarbon anesthetics (Question 106). Barbiturates do not interact or cause malignant hyperthermia in their own right. All the barbiturates have some anticonvulsant activity (dose-dependent and also dependent on which barbiturate is being used), and they do not cause myoclonus or other types of seizures (e). A higher risk of myoclonic seizures is mainly associated with etomidate, which is another IV induction agent. The seizure risk can be reduced, apparently, by premedication with an opioid or a benzodiazepine.

108. The answer is b. *(Brunton, 677t, 682, 697-698. Katzung, pp 624t, 628.)* Ketorolac is usually presented in a text book chapter on NSAIDs. It is presented here because it provides excellent analgesia that has been described as equivalent to that provided by usual doses of an opioid (eg, codeine, hydrocodone, oxycodone, or even relatively low doses of morphine) when pain is "mild to moderate" and relatively short-lived, and an opioid might otherwise be used. The mechanism probably involves inhibited prostaglandin synthesis (as with all NSAIDs) and does not involve activation of any opioid receptors. The drug has no antiemetic effects (a); does not affect ventilatory rate or depth (c); and has no effect on skeletal neuromuscular transmission or the effects of neuromuscular blockers (d). Unlike most opioids, with meperidine being a notable exception, ketorolac also lacks adverse effects on the biliary tract, usually making it a good choice for patients with cholecystitis or other conditions that trigger gallbladder/bile duct spasm and pain.

Ketorolac is not suitable, alone, for severe pain (when an opioid truly is indicated) nor for chronic pain. In surgical settings such as the one described here it is used as a supplement to an opioid. What are the advantages of ketorolac, whether used alone or as a supplement, compared with an opioid? Because, as noted above, it has excellent analgesic activity with none of the common and sometimes unwanted effects of drugs like codeine or morphine. It is often used as an opioid supplement precisely because the main alternative approach—simply giving a higher dose of an opioid—could lead to excessive ventilatory depression and hypotension.

The main adverse responses to ketorolac are similar to those of traditional NSAIDs on the GI tract: the potential for gastric ulceration, potentially with GI bleeding or hemorrhage; for renal impairment; and for prolonged bleeding due to antiplatelet effects (weak and not therapeutically useful). These adverse effects are most likely to occur with long-term use, which is why ketorolac should be used only for short-term pain control (no more than 5 days). Most of the contraindications that apply to traditional NSAIDs apply to ketorolac, for example, peptic ulcer disease (active or a risk thereof); renal dysfunction; active bleeding (especially intracranial); pregnancy; and prior hypersensitivity.

Notes: You should know about ketorolac because it is used widely in general surgical settings such as described in the question; in orthopedics; and in oral surgery and other settings where "good" short-term analgesia is needed and it is best to minimize or avoid unwanted effects of opioids.

When ketorolac was first approved, many practitioners used it frequently and prescribed it for chronic pain control. (Some described prescribing the drug "like candy." After all, it provided excellent pain control with no opioid-like problems.) Not long thereafter prescribers realized the strong ulcerogenic actions of the drug, and so new guidelines and warnings were made to restrict its use to no more than several days in a row.

109. The answer is e. *(Brunton, pp 300t, 604, 999-1003, 1701. Katzung, pp 285, 1084-1087.)* Ondansetron, like a related drug, dronabinol, is used to manage drug-induced nausea and vomiting that can occur postoperatively or in response to emetogenic drugs (eg, many anticancer drugs). It is a serotonin receptor (5-HT_3) blocker that acts mainly in the CTZ and inhibits vagal control of parts of the upper GI tract smooth muscles.

Ondansetron has no general CNS or cortical stimulating effects that would help restore consciousness, alertness, or awareness of time and place (a); no analgesic-intensifying effects (b); no significant effects on the bladder (c); and does not reduce the risk of paralytic ileus (d) because vagal tone to intestinal smooth muscles is suppressed.

110. The answer is b. *(Brunton, pp 477-481. Katzung, pp 472-475.)* Unwanted extrapyramidal side effects produced by antipsychotic drugs (eg, chlorpromazine, as the exemplar of the phenothiazines; and, more so, haloperidol, the butyrophenone) include a parkinsonian syndrome, akathisia, dystonias, galactorrhea, amenorrhea, and infertility. These side effects are due to the ability of these agents to block dopamine receptors. The phenothiazines also block muscarinic and α-adrenergic receptors, which are responsible for other effects in both the CNS and (especially) in the periphery. The incidence and severity of these autonomic side effects is much greater with low-potency antipsychotics (eg, chlorpromazine and other phenothiazines) than with haloperidol.

111. The answer is b. *(Brunton, pp 351-353. Katzung, pp 437, 538, 563.)* The scenario describes most of the classic responses to ketamine, a "dissociative anesthetic": analgesia; an ostensibly light sleep-like state; a trance-like or cataplectic state (with increased muscle tone); and activation of most cardiovascular/hemodynamic parameters. Various psychosis-like emergence reactions are the main disadvantages of using a drug that, otherwise, causes many of the desired elements of balanced anesthesia, usually without the need for complicated and expensive anesthesia administration devices or personnel. The only other drug listed that provides adequate analgesia is fentanyl (a). Midazolam (c; benzodiazepine), succinylcholine (d; depolarizing neuromuscular blocker), and thiopental (e; thiobarbiturate) lack analgesic activity. Moreover, if any cardiovascular or autonomic changes were to occur in response to any of those drugs, they would be better characterized as depression, not activation.

112. The answer is d. *(Brunton, pp 533-534. Katzung, pp 142, 471-474, 484.)* When levodopa is administered orally, the vast majority of the administered dose (about 90%) is metabolized in the gut to dopamine by DOPA decarboxylase. However, dopamine cannot cross the blood-brain barrier, and so only a fraction of the parent drug gets into the CNS to be metabolized and cause its desired effects there. Carbidopa inhibits DOPA decarboxylase in the periphery (it cannot cross the blood-brain barrier), reducing peripheral metabolism of levodopa to dopamine and "sparing" a bigger fraction of the levodopa dose so it can be metabolized in the nigrostriatum. By reducing peripheral conversion of levodopa to dopamine, the adjunctive use of carbidopa may also allow management of parkinsonian signs and symptoms with lower doses of levodopa. One additional benefit of that is a reduction in the number and severity of peripheral side effects of the levodopa (or, more precisely, its metabolite, dopamine). Adding carbidopa to a regimen involving levodopa only may also help (at least transiently) combat such problems as dopamine's "on-off" phenomenon and "end-of-dose" failure.

Carbidopa, whether considered in its own right or in the context of coadministration with levodopa, has no effects on ACh release (a). Vitamin B_6 deficiencies do not occur in response to therapy with either or both drugs (b); and it is important to note that ingesting large amounts of that vitamin, whether as part of the diet or in the form of supplements, will antagonize the desired effects of levodopa with or without added carbidopa. Carbidopa does give "better access" of levodopa to the CNS, but that effect has nothing to do with increasing blood-brain barrier permeability to dopamine (c). It is due, as noted, to increased concentrations of levodopa in the circulation due to inhibited peripheral conversion to dopamine. Carbidopa has no beneficial effects on dopamine-induced blood pressure changes, and has no ability to block dopamine receptors in the vasculature (e) or anywhere else.

Note: DOPA decarboxylase is an aromatic L-amino acid decarboxylase. The enzyme is also responsible for the metabolism of L-tryptophan to serotonin, and carbidopa inhibits that metabolic conversion too.

113. The answer is c. *(Brunton, pp 126, 416t, 418, 510-511, 522-523. Katzung, pp 381-382, 407.)* Phenobarbital's role in the primary management of all of the named conditions has waned dramatically, and appropriately, as newer drugs have been developed. The only use in the list given in Question 113, for which phenobarbital is still considered reasonable for long-term therapy in some patients, is for managing certain epilepsies (mainly as an alternative to phenytoin). Benzodiazepines are almost always preferred for managing alcohol withdrawal (a) and anxiety (b). Benzodiazepines, or the benzodiazepine-like agents zalpelon or zolpidem, are almost always turned to for insomnia (e). Phenobarbital—and other barbiturates for that matter—have no beneficial effects on depression signs and symptoms (d), and they are not properly used alone or in combination with an SSRI, a tricyclic, or an atypical antidepressant.

Major reasons for selecting a benzodiazepine over a barbiturate include fewer drug-drug interactions (phenobarbital is a classic P450 inducer); a lower risk of dependence; withdrawal syndromes that are typically less severe or dangerous; lower risk of fatal ventilatory depression with oral overdoses (and the availability of flumazenil, the specific benzodiazepine antagonist, to treat them); and less narrowing between lethal and effective doses (better therapeutic index or margin of safety) as use continues and tolerance develops.

Note that even though benzodiazepines may be preferred, treatment for such problems as anxiety and insomnia should be kept as short as possible.

114. The answer is a. *(Brunton, pp 433-434, 447-448. Katzung, pp 514, 518-519, 524.)* The most common side effects associated with tricyclic antidepressants are their antimuscarinic effects, which may occur and be prominent in over 50% of patients. Clinically, these effects may manifest as dry mouth, blurred vision, constipation, tachycardia, dizziness, and urinary retention. These are, of course, some of the typical and common side effects associated with atropine or any other drug with substantial antimuscarinic effects. At therapeutic plasma concentrations these drugs usually do not cause changes in the ECG (b)—but with severe overdoses lethal arrhythmias often do occur. These drugs are not particularly hepatotoxic or nephrotoxic (c, d). Seizures are not likely to occur unless the patient has a history of seizure disorders or massive overdoses have been taken.

Note: in terms of tricyclic toxicity, that is, with overdoses, you might want to recall what some students learn as the "three Cs"—Coma, Cardiotoxicity (mainly arrhythmias that are often difficult to treat), and Convulsions. In addition, all the other manifestations of "atropine poisoning" will develop and usually be severe.

115. The correct answer is b. *(Brunton, pp 509-510, 1860t. Katzung, pp 40t, 403-405, 1031t.)* The hepatic enzymes responsible for phenytoin metabolism (mainly CYP2C9) become saturated at plasma drug concentrations above approximately 10 to 15 mcg/mL, which are clearly within the typical therapeutic range yet well below maximum or peak therapeutic levels. At daily dosages associated with or below those 10 to 15 mcg/mL concentrations, dose increases give relatively proportional increases in plasma drug concentrations, and phenytoin elimination follows usual first-order kinetics (a constant fraction of drug is eliminated with the passing of each half-life). Once the metabolic capacity for the drug is exceeded (as it has in our patient, which may arise with intentional or inadvertent increases in the daily dose), small increases in dosage lead to disproportionately large increases of plasma concentrations (and effects) because, in essence, "drug in greatly exceeds drug out." Zero-order kinetics now describes the drug's elimination, such that a constant amount (not fraction) of drug is eliminated per unit time. Therefore, the first-order half-life no longer applies; elimination is slower, and the plasma concentration will be much greater than 15 mcg/mL (half of 30 mcg/mL; answer e) 24 hours after the initial blood sample is taken.

The figure below shows an approximation of the relationship between plasma phenytoin levels and daily doses (the placement of the curve along the x-axis can vary from patient to patient). From the rapid rise in the curve at dosages above about 300 mg/d, you can deduce a significant reduction of clearance rates owing to slowed metabolism (since metabolism is the main pathway for phenytoin's elimination).

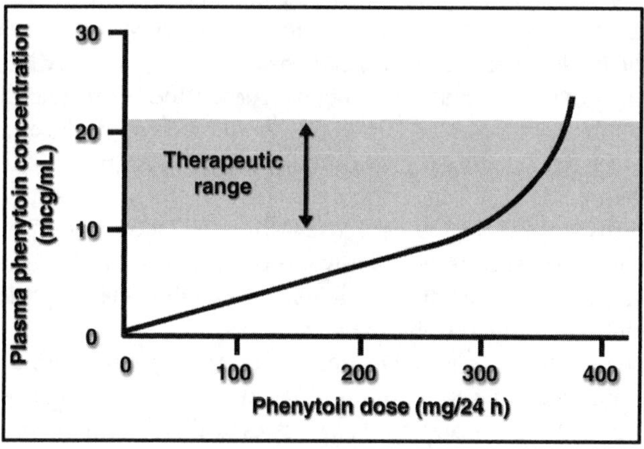

Answer a is incorrect; flumazenil is a benzodiazepine receptor antagonist (competitive blocker) that has no effects on the elimination or effects of phenytoin. It would be inappropriate—and dangerous—to give an amphetamine or any other CNS stimulant to counteract the excess CNS depression. Titrating upward the dose of a CNS stimulant to combat CNS depression (whether caused by a drug or from another cause) is a risky endeavor due to the chance of inducing seizures from excessive CNS stimulation, and the risks are far greater in a person with a history of seizure disorders.

Phenobarbital (d) is a classic example of a P450 inducer, and indeed it is metabolized mainly by CYP2C9, on which phenytoin's elimination mainly depends. In theory, giving phenobarbital might increase phenytoin's metabolism via P450 induction. In reality, the pharmacokinetic outcomes of a phenobarbital-phenytoin interaction are quite variable (and dependent on blood levels of each drug), but the more likely consequence is inhibited phenytoin elimination as the barbiturate competes with it for conversion by the same cytochromes. Regardless, adding phenobarbital is likely to add to the generalized CNS depression caused by the phenytoin, and complicate both the clinical picture and its management. Therefore, this approach, too, would be inappropriate.

116. The answer is d. *(Brunton, pp 174, 299, 443, 529-533, 535, 537. Katzung, pp 84, 786f, 519-520.)* Two of the important types of MAO are: (1) MAO-A, which metabolizes NE and serotonin and other biogenic amines, and is the predominant hepatic form of the enzyme; and (2) MAO-B, which metabolizes dopamine and other monoamines in the brain. Selegiline is a selective inhibitor of MAO-B. It inhibits the breakdown of dopamine and prolongs the therapeutic effectiveness of levodopa (endogenous or that provided pharmacologically) in parkinsonism. The risks of serious drug interactions in patients taking nonselective MAO inhibitors (eg, phenelzine, tranylcypromine), such as hypertensive crisis in response to mixed- and indirect-acting sympathomimetics (tyramine, pseudoephedrine, amphetamines) are much less, but still possible, with selegiline.

Bromocriptine (a) is a dopamine receptor agonist. Carbidopa (b) inhibits the peripheral metabolism of levodopa by DOPA decarboxylase. Both are useful in the treatment of some cases of idiopathic (but not antipsychotic drug-induced) parkinsonism. Phenelzine (c) and tranylcypromine (e) are nonselective MAOIs. Combining them with L-dopa may lead to a potentially fatal hypertensive crisis, and thus they are not used in the therapy of parkinsonism. A similar interaction may occur with tyramine-rich foods and beverages; and with catecholamine-releasing sympathomimetics (ephedrine, pseudoephedrine, amphetamines, and amphetamine-like drugs such as methylphenidate). As a result of these common and potentially lethal interactions, nonselective MAO inhibitors are rarely used for anything unless no other usually effective therapies work adequately or are otherwise contraindicated.

117. The answer is d. *(Brunton, pp 568-571. Katzung, pp 546, 560.)* High or frankly toxic plasma levels of meperidine can cause seizures, hypertension, and a psychosis-like state, in addition to typical morphine-like effects (eg, analgesia and ventilatory depression). Interestingly, it appears that administration of naloxone to combat excessive effects of meperidine may increase the risk of seizures. This is something that is extraordinarily rare when naloxone is administered to counteract excessive effects of morphine and most other opioids in patients who otherwise are not at an increased risk of seizures.

The rather unique adverse effects associated with meperidine are probably due to a major metabolite, normeperidine. A weak opioid analgesic, propoxyphene (structurally related to methadone), can produce toxic reactions similar to those of meperidine. One of its metabolites, norpropoxyphene, is thought to be the cause. The risks account for why meperidine doses should be kept as low as possible, and the duration of treatment with it should be kept short (usually no more than a day or two).

Meperidine, like other opioids, can cause constipation (a) through its actions on longitudinal muscles and sphincters in the GI tract. Hyperalgesia (b), an increased perception of pain, does not occur. Biliary tract/ sphincter of Oddi spasm (c) is much less likely to occur with meperidine than with most other opioids (say, the prototype, morphine). Indeed, meperidine can be considered a preferred opioid (for short-term) use for patients with moderate-to-severe pain and gallbladder disease.

Respiratory depression (e), possibly leading to ventilatory arrest, is a property shared by all the opioid analgesics, but of course to varying degrees based on their efficacy and dose.

Note: Before the unusual risks of meperidine were fully appreciated, the drug was often prescribed for days or weeks on end. That should never be done anymore.

118. The answer is e. *(Brunton, pp 513, 573-574, 580t. Katzung, p 546.)* Propoxyphene is a methadone analog that has been on the market for decades. It has much lower analgesic efficacy and potency than methadone, other strong-moderate opioids, and even codeine, oxycodone, hydrocodone, and other similar drugs. Indeed, its analgesic effects are comparable to those afforded by acetaminophen (not all that great), and the two drugs are often administered together (combination products are available).

Compared with other opioids, the risks of dependency are quite low with propoxyphene. While that may seem advantageous, propoxyphene has a very low margin of safety (or therapeutic index), and only slight increases above the recommended dose can cause psychosis. These are not characteristics of acetaminophen (a), aspirin (b), codeine (c), or hydrocodone (d). In addition, while the toxic effects of codeine or hydrocodone (and other opioids or opioid-like drugs) can be reversed by a narcotic antagonist (naloxone, naltrexone, etc), the blockers have no effects on propoxyphene.

Notes: Your course or text may pay little attention to propoxyphene. Why address it here? Despite the low efficacy and high risk of serious problems with propoxyphene—and despite the fact that it has been banned in such countries as the United Kingdom because of them—propoxyphene still (as of early 2010) is a widely prescribed (misprescribed?) drug in the United States; indeed, for years it has been one of the "Top 25" drugs in terms of the number of prescriptions written for it. Soon after you pass Step 1 and hit the wards, you'll likely encounter patients taking it unless the FDA bans it first. In July 2009, the FDA notified healthcare professionals that it is taking several actions to reduce the risk of overdose in patients using pain medications that contain propoxyphene because of data linking the drug to fatal outcomes. FDA will also require stronger label warnings (black box) emphasizing the potential for overdose, and will provide a medication guide to patients stressing the importance of using the drug as directed.

FDA is also requiring a new safety study to address unanswered questions about the effects of propoxyphene at higher than recommended doses.

119. The answer is a. *(Brunton, pp 474, 477-481, 572t. Katzung, pp 487-507.)* It is common to classify chlorpromazine and other phenothiazine antipsychotics as "low-potency" agents, in comparison with haloperidol (butyrophenone class), which has been called a "high-potency" antipsychotic. Potency, of course, usually and more properly refers to the dose needed to cause a stated effect of a certain intensity, and does not necessarily give good insight into a particular drug's absolute or relative efficacy or its side effects profile. Nonetheless, haloperidol is more potent than phenothiazines and is more selective for blocking dopamine D_2 receptors. But another implied and arguably more practical meaning of (mis)using the "low potency-high potency" terminology is that haloperidol, compared with chlorpromazine and other phenothiazines, tends to cause a higher incidence of extrapyramidal reactions that can be severe and of sudden onset (hours or days in some cases, particularly when haloperidol is given parenterally for acute psychosis). In contrast, haloperidol tends to cause much milder and less frequent peripheral autonomic side effects—α-adrenergic blockade leading to blood pressure falls (d) and antimuscarinic effects (b, e) than a typical phenothiazine. Haloperidol also seems to be associated with a lower risk of blood dyscrasias (c) than with a phenothiazine.

120. The answer is d. *(Brunton, pp 332, 624-625. Katzung, pp 563, 577t, 1029t.)* "Angel dust" is phencyclidine (PCP), a hallucinogen with an amphetamine-like mechanism of action. Thus, the problems that arise are due to blockade of neuronal reuptake of such monoamines as dopamine, NE, and serotonin. The drug does not have central or peripheral muscarinic receptor antagonist activity (a), nor opioid agonist actions (c). A phencyclidine withdrawal syndrome (b) has not been documented consistently in humans, largely because it is used episodically and is not chronically present in the circulation. In overdose, the treatment of choice for manifestations of drug-induced psychosis is haloperidol, although rapidly acting and highly sedating benzodiazepines may be used instead. Flumazenil (e) is a benzodiazepine receptor antagonist with no use or efficacy in phencyclidine toxicity.

121. The answer is b. *(Brunton, pp 429, 485-490, 753. Katzung, pp 40t, 500-504.)* In essence, the intensity of effects from any given plasma concentration of lithium are inversely related to sodium concentrations. When sodium concentration falls, the effects of lithium can be intensified to the point of causing toxicity. By way of their actions to increase renal sodium loss, virtually all the common diuretics also reduce renal lithium excretion. It is probably of greatest concern with thiazides or thiazide-like diuretics, which have the greatest potential of all the common diuretics to cause hyponatremia. Cholestyramine (a) is a cholesterol-binding resin (bile acid sequestrant) that also has the ability to bind (adsorb) a variety of other drugs present in the GI tract at the same time, thereby reducing their bioavailability. Given concomitantly with an oral diuretic, the most likely outcome of cholestyramine administration would be reduced bioavailability of the diuretic, not increased or decreased effects of the resin. Nifedipine (c), a dihydropyridine calcium channel blocker, may cause excessive antihypertensive effects when administered with any diuretic, although combined administration is common and usually problem-free if due diligence is given. If excessive effects of nifedipine occur in conjunction with a diuretic, they are not specifically due to changes of sodium concentrations. Phenylephrine's (d) vasoconstrictor effects are not likely to be altered appreciably in the presence of a diuretic. The same lack of a clinically significant interaction applies to the statins (e; HMG Co-A reductase inhibitors, eg, atorvastatin).

122. The answer is a. *(Brunton, pp 259, 263. Katzung, pp 134f, 141, 145, 1020.)* Methylphenidate, which is widely used to manage ADD-ADHD, has amphetamine-like sympathetic and CNS-stimulating effects. Indeed, amphetamine itself (and derivatives or mixtures of amphetamines) is used for treatment of ADHD.

Peripheral sympathetic (adrenergic) effects arise from the drug's ability to release neuronal NE. Related findings would include increased vasoconstriction (greater α_1-receptor activation of vascular smooth muscle), and therefore increased blood pressure; and tachycardia, increased cardiac contractility, and electrical impulse conduction rates, probably accompanied by tachyarrhythmias, from β_1 activation.

At toxic doses, the CNS effect of the drug is likely to cause seizures.

There is no mechanism by which direct effects of methylphenidate or amphetamine (whether at normal or toxic doses) would cause bronchospasm, bronchoconstriction, or even bronchodilation (because NE that is released has no ability to activate or block β_2 receptors on airway smooth muscle). Miosis (which occurs with either muscarinic activation or α-blockade) would be the opposite of what you would predict in terms of ocular effects.

In terms of autonomic effects, skeletal muscle weakness or paralysis are findings you would expect from drugs that either blocked nicotinic cholinergic receptors (eg, tubocurarine or another similar nondepolarizing neuromuscular blocker) or caused depolarizing block (succinylcholine).

123. The answer is d. *(Brunton, p 344. Katzung, pp 430-431.)* MAC (minimum alveolar concentration) is an expression of inhaled anesthetic potency. It is defined as the minimum inspired concentration needed to abolish a specified painful response in 50% of treated patients. (Thus, it is much like the ED_{50}, measured in a population dose-response curve, for most other drugs.) Obviously, giving a drug at a dose that suppresses a response in only half the treated patients is not desirable, so inhaled anesthetics are typically given at a dose more than the MAC. (Recall, too, that MAC is not absolute: it can change depending on the use of other anesthesia adjuncts and such other factors as body temperature, ventilatory rate, presence of other diseases, etc.)

A drug's MAC gives us no useful and invariable information about onsets or durations of action (a, e). You cannot state correctly that drug Y (MAC ≈ 100%) causes greater analgesia and/or skeletal muscle relaxation than another drug any more than we can say that a drug with an ED_{50} of 5 mg causes a greater response than one with an ED_{50} of 1 mg. It all depends on the dose given, not the MAC or ED_{50}.

124. The answer is d. *(Brunton, pp 305-306, 441-442, 446-447, 450. Katzung, pp 282-284, 525-526, 1021.)* This patient probably has the serotonin syndrome. Serotonin is already present in increased amounts in synapses because of blockade of its reuptake by the SSRIs. When sumatriptan (or other triptans used for migraine therapy; they are $5\text{-HT}_{1B/2D}$ agonists) is added, rapid accumulation of serotonin and/or the triptan in serotoninergic synapses of the brain can occur.

The risk of the serotonin syndrome in SSRI-treated patients is much higher when MAO inhibitors are used concomitantly. Nonetheless, such severe reactions from an SSRI-triptan interaction have been reported. In addition, do not forget that MAO inhibitors can also cause an acute and potentially fatal hypertensive crisis when coadministered with tricyclic/tetracyclic antidepressants (eg, imipramine); such combined use should be avoided.

None of the other drugs listed (codeine, a; loratadine or another second-generation antihistamine, b; midazolam or fentanyl—or other benzodiazepines or opioids—c; or zolpidem or the related drug zalpelon, e) interact with fluoxetine or other SSRIs in terms of specifically raising systemic or synaptic serotonin levels.

125. The answer is b. *(Brunton, pp 402-406, 413-414, 615. Katzung, pp 378, 380-382.)* Flumazenil is a competitive antagonist of benzodiazepines at the GABA receptor. Repeated administration is necessary because of its short half-life relative to that of most benzodiazepines—especially diazepam, which forms many long-lasting active metabolites.

Dextroamphetamine (a) is a CNS stimulant that will increase the patient's level of consciousness, but it is not indicated for this use. High doses will probably be needed to overcome the intense benzodiazepine effects, and they may cause dangerous CNS and cardiovascular responses rather than simply "normalizing" variables depressed by the diazepam. Naltrexone (c) specifically antagonizes the effects of opioid agonists on μ and κ receptors and is used to diagnose or treat opioid overdoses; it has no benzodiazepine receptor-blocking activity. Physostigmine (d) is a lipophilic acetylcholinesterase inhibitor that may be a lifesaving intervention for severe poisoning with many drugs having significant antimuscarinic (atropine-like) actions. Pralidoxime (e) is a cholinesterase reactivator used in the adjunctive management of poisoning with such "irreversible" cholinesterase inhibitors as the organophosphate insecticides and many "nerve gases" (soman, sarin, VX).

126. The answer is a. *(Brunton, pp 538, 1256-1258. Katzung, pp 477, 871-872.)* This cutaneous response, called livedo reticularis, is characteristically associated with amantadine. Recall that this seldom-used antiparkinson drug probably works by releasing endogenous dopamine and blocking its neuronal reuptake. Livedo reticularis is not associated with levodopa (used alone or with carbidopa; c or d), nor with the dopamine agonists bromocriptine (d) or pramipexole (e; a newer and generally preferred drug for starting treatment of mild parkinsonian signs and symptoms). You might also recall that amantadine is also used for prophylaxis of some strains of influenza virus infections. The mechanism of action in this setting is not well understood.

127. The answer is d. *(Brunton, pp 509-510. Katzung, pp 403-405.)* For many years, phenytoin has been cited as a classic example of a drug that can cause gingival hyperplasia. (It is often referred to as Dilantin® hyperplasia, in recognition of phenytoin's common proprietary name.) The mechanism is unknown, but we suspect the drug alters collagen metabolism in the gingival tissues. Although phenytoin isn't the only drug associated with potential gingival hyperplasia (verapamil is another common one), it is the only one listed as a choice. Note that phenobarbital, which is still used as an alternative to phenytoin for seizures, does not cause gingival hyperplasia. It is precisely because of the low gingival hyperplasia risk that phenobarbital is sometimes prescribed for children with responsive seizure disorders in lieu of phenytoin.

128. The answer is d. *(Brunton, pp 308, 447, 450, 570. Katzung, pp 279-284.)* The serotonin receptor agonist actions of the "triptans," including the prototype, sumatriptan, can trigger intense vasoconstriction in various vascular beds. The cerebral vasoconstrictor effects of these drugs contribute importantly to the relief they afford in migraine headaches. However, coronary vasospasm can occur also; it may be particularly intense and potentially life-threatening in patients with coronary vasospastic disease (ie, "variant" or Prinzmetal angina), for whom the triptans are contraindicated.

None of the other drugs listed have any significant coronary (or other) vasoconstrictor effects. Indeed, some such as phenytoin and zolpidem (a benzodiazepine-like hypnotic) may cause slight cardiovascular changes (eg, afterload reduction) that would actually reduce the degree of myocardial ischemia and the risk of angina.

129. The answer is c. *(Brunton, pp 344, 353f, 360-361. Katzung, pp 426t, 430-431.)* Recall that nitrous oxide has a MAC (minimum alveolar concentration) of about 105%. Achieving that concentration in an inspired gas mixture is physically impossible at normal atmospheric pressure. Even if we could safely give pure nitrous oxide (we obviously cannot), and we rounded-off the MAC to 100%, the drug would (1) cause abolition of a painful response in only 50% of subjects (this is one element of the definition of MAC) and (2) be lethal, since 100% nitrous oxide means no (0%) oxygen at normal atmospheric pressures. This very effective analgesic gas is poorly soluble in the blood, so equilibration between alveolar and blood concentrations and the onset of its central effects are quite rapid.

Even at the usual concentrations (typically 80% of the inspired gas mixture), and whether used only with air (as in many aspects of dental practice) or with other inhaled agents (common in surgery), nitrous oxide causes little or no bronchospasm nor significant cardiac depression.

130. The answer is b. *(Brunton, pp 464, 474-479, 535. Katzung, pp 283t, 284, 482, 499.)* The question describes common and necessary interventions for managing neuroleptic malignant syndrome, which is characteristically associated with older antipsychotics—chlorpromazine and other "low potency" antipsychotics to a degree, but more so with haloperidol (butyrophenone). Signs and symptoms include muscle tetany/rigidity, profound fever, rapid swings of heart rate, rhythm, blood pressure (autonomic instability), electrolyte abnormalities, and dehydration. None of the other agents listed are associated with this syndrome, whether acutely or with long-term therapy or at therapeutic or toxic plasma levels, nor would the interventions described be indicated.

131. The answer is c. *(Brunton, pp 535-536. Katzung, pp 474-475, 482.)* This is a question about a drug you may not have learned about explicitly, but given the description of its mechanism, which should be quite familiar, you should have no problem arriving at the right answer. Ropinirole (a related drug is pramipexole) directly activates striatal dopamine receptors. It is one of several dopaminergic drugs that can be used to initiate therapy of early Parkinson disease. Dyskinesias and hypotension are relatively common side effects, as also applies to alternatives such as levodopa and bromocriptine. (A similar ergot-derived direct-acting dopamine agonist, pergolide, was withdrawn from the US market in 2007 because it was linked to cardiac valve damage). Ropinirole also causes drowsiness or sleepiness; either would render the drug not ideal for managing daytime anxiety (a), but anxiety management is not an indication for the drug, nor is hypersomnia (b). Ropinirole's dopaminergic action may exacerbate signs and symptoms of schizophrenia (d). Like many other antiparkinson drugs it may lower the seizure threshold in patients with epilepsy, and so would be irrational for managing status epilepticus (e). It has no clinically useful analgesic activity (f).

Note: Ropinirole stimulates the brain's "dopamine reward system" and has been linked to compulsive behaviors including gambling and hypersexuality. Both of these effects have been widely publicized.

132. The answer is e. *(Brunton, pp 436t, 447-451. Katzung, pp 283, 373, 381t.)* Buspirone is an attractive drug for managing mild short-term anxiety. Among the reasons (and especially when compared with more traditional anxiolytics, such as benzodiazepines) are a lack of sedation (buspirone is not a CNS depressant); very little (if any) potentiation of the effects of other CNS depressants, including alcohol; no known abuse potential (it is not regulated by the Controlled Substances Act) or tendency for development of tolerance; and no major withdrawal syndrome. One major drawback is a slow onset of symptom relief (a week or two), and typically it takes about a month from the onset of therapy for antianxiety effects to stabilize. (Knowing this slow onset, one should resist the temptation to titrate the dosage upward, to hasten or increase the drug's effects, prematurely.)

You should recall that long-term benzodiazepine administration is associated with withdrawal phenomena (and, depending on the use, dose, exact drug, and other patient-related factors, the syndrome can be severe). Thus, one can envisage a switch from a benzodiazepine to buspirone. Because buspirone lacks CNS-depressant effects and its effects take some time to develop, one should start the buspirone several weeks before stopping the benzodiazepine and then taper the benzodiazepine dose once it's time to stop the drug.

133. The answer is b. *(Brunton, pp 403t, 504, 523. Katzung, pp 381t, 382, 415, 418-419.)* Intravenous lorazepam is generally regarded as the drug of choice for initial treatment of status epilepticus. (It has surpassed diazepam because of a faster onset of action and less venous irritation, among other things.) Lorazepam, like the benzodiazepines in general, increases the apparent affinity of the inhibitory neurotransmitter GABA for binding sites on brain cell membranes. Lorazepam's anticonvulsant effects are relatively short-lived. If lorazepam was the only drug given for status epilepticus seizures would stop quickly but could return quickly too as the drug is eliminated and blood concentrations fall. Therefore, immediately after giving the lorazepam either phenytoin or fosphenytoin should be given to provide longer seizure suppression and "coverage" because lorazepam's effect wanes so quickly.

Why not just give phenytoin or fosphenytoin and skip the lorazepam? Recall that the longer status epilepticus persists, the greater the risk of brain damage or death. The goal is to terminate the seizures as fast as possible. While phenytoin or fosphenytoin have relatively long-lasting effects, their onsets of action are not fast enough to achieve prompt seizure suppression. Lorazepam works quickly, and that's why we give it first.

None of the other drugs listed in the question are appropriate for initial therapy of status epilepticus, despite their widespread use for oral therapy of seizure disorders long-term. Phenobarbital might be used for seizures refractory to any of the preferred initial drugs, however.

134. The answer is e. *(Brunton, pp 369-371f, 376. Katzung, pp 440-442, 447-449.)* This may seem like a picky question, or perhaps a tricky one, if you've been taught the main properties of only one or two prototypic local anesthetics. For example, you may have learned about lidocaine as the prototype amide and prototype local anesthetic overall; procaine as the prototype of the ester class; and perhaps a third drug, benzocaine, which is suitable only for topical administration because it is largely insoluble and can't be given safely or effectively by other routes. Nonetheless, there are a couple of important points here, and they revolve around a fundamental difference between amides and esters, and you need to know the class to which a particular local anesthetic belongs for several reasons. (1) Allergic reactions of various severities are more common with esters than with amides; (2) there is class-based cross-reactivity, meaning that if a patient has had a true immunologic reaction to any ester, he or she is at risk for a similar reaction from subsequent exposure to any ester; and (3) there is no cross-reactivity between esters and amides, such that use of an amide in an "ester-sensitive" patient is not likely to pose problems of allergenicity.

Now, some learning "tricks," if you haven't learned them before: how to tell whether a local anesthetic (one you've learned about, or not) is an ester or amide. Look at the drug's generic name; if there are two occurrences of the letter "i" in it, it's an amide; if not, it's an ester. Thus, we have such esters as cocaine, chlor(o)procaine, procaine itself, and tetracaine, which is the correct answer for this question. The others I listed are amides.

135. The answer is c. *(Brunton, 188, 201, 204, 211-214, 538-540. Katzung, pp 108, 1040-1042.)* Initial recommended therapy includes use of acetylcholinesterase inhibitors (donepezil, tacrine, galantamine, rivastigmine; all are reversible cholinesterase inhibitors). These drugs are not cures, but they appear to slow symptoms of brain neurodegeneration in some patients. None appears to be invariably superior to any other. Their actions almost certainly involve activation of central muscarinic receptors—indirectly, by inhibiting metabolism of ACh released from viable nerves, of course—in part because drugs with central antimuscarinic actions reduce their efficacy. Tacrine is noteworthy, compared with the other drugs noted in the answer, because it causes more cholinesterase inhibition in the periphery: more and more disturbing symptoms typical characteristic of increased (and indirect, due to cholinesterase inhibition) muscarinic effects on the gut, bladder, airways, etc.

Activating serotonin receptors (a) or blocking dopaminergic effects (b) are not suitable or effective therapies for Alzheimer disease. Selegiline (MAO-B inhibitor, d) and high doses of vitamin E (antioxidant) apparently slow neurodegenerative processes, but so far there are no convincing data that they slow cognitive decline and they are not first-line therapies. Thrombolytic drugs (e) are not indicated, as the signs and symptoms of idiopathic Alzheimer disease are not due to clots or other vaso-obstructive causes.

136. The answer is b. *(Brunton, pp 533t, 537. Katzung, p 477, 484.)* Trihexyphenidyl (and the related drug benztropine) causes significant antimuscarinic (atropine-like) actions in the CNS—hence, these drugs have been classified as "centrally acting antimuscarinics." These drugs are quite lipophilic and enter the CNS well (this accounts for the drug's marked sedative effects, too) to block muscarinic receptors there. That helps adjust the dopamine-ACh imbalance that appears to be a main biochemical underpinning of parkinsonism. Diphenhydramine can be used instead of trihexyphenidyl or benztropine, but it causes more drowsiness in most patients. Nonetheless, none of these drugs is used to counteract CNS depression caused by other antiparkinson drugs.

Diphenhydramine does help alleviate cutaneous allergy symptoms (eg, urticaria; d), but those are rare with any of the common antiparkinson drugs (and I did not specify which "other" drug was given). None of these drugs affect manic/hypomanic episodes that might occur with, say, high doses of levodopa. They do not reverse antipsychotic-induced tardive dyskinesias (e); no drug does that effectively.

137. The answer is d. *(Brunton, pp 173, 239, 240t, 449, 537. Katzung, pp 476, 519-520, 524, 526, 544t, 1147t.)* Many drugs (but not amphetamines, a; barbiturates, b; benzodiazepines, c; or morphine or related opioid analgesics, e) participate in significant interactions with certain foods or beverages. However, when you read phrases along the lines of those noted in the question—"severe and sometimes fatal hypertension from consuming such foods as cheeses and processed meats"—you should automatically be thinking of the older, nonselective (MAO-A/B) monoamine oxidase inhibitors. These drugs have been used for severe hypertension or depression, but due to the potentially lethal interactions with tyramine-containing foods or beverages, their use has dwindled because the risks were too great. (Nonetheless, you need to know your pharmacology for such drugs as pargyline, phenelzine, and tranylcypromine.) Recall that tyramine is a catecholamine-releasing drug with sympathomimetic actions in its own right. When we consume tyramine-rich foods or beverages much of that sympathomimetic is metabolized by hepatic MAO before it reaches the systemic circulation (first-pass metabolism), and so its effects are slight. In the presence of a nonselective MAO inhibitor, however, the metabolic inactivation does not occur and significant amounts of the drug reach the circulation to cause more intense and potentially very intense effects that involve adrenergic receptor activation. In addition, catecholaminergic (eg, adrenergic) nerves in the MAO-treated patient can be considered "loaded" with an abundance of NE due to inhibited intraneuronal metabolism of the neurotransmitter.

Although the NE may not be released physiologically, in response to an action potential (at least in the peripheral sympathetic nervous system), it can be released by such drugs as tyramine or by pseudoephedrine and ephedrine (mixed-acting sympathomimetics) or amphetamines (indirect-acting sympathomimetics). This can then trigger possibly fatal hypertensive crisis, profound cardiac stimulation, and the consequences thereof. These problems led to the development of MAO inhibitors (eg, selegiline) that have preferential effects on MAO in the brain (MAO-B) and far less an effect on MAO forms in the liver and peripheral nervous system (MAO-A). Nonetheless, as stated in the question, there is a new nonselective MAO inhibitor that has just been approved for use, for depression, in the form of a transdermal delivery system (skin patch).

138. The answer is d. *(Brunton, pp 578-579. Katzung, pp 547, 1008t.)* Dextromethorphan is, indeed, chemically related to codeine, but it lacks many effects you probably associate with codeine or other opioids, except one: it has excellent antitussive activity. This cough-suppressant effect presumably occurs via some ill-defined central mechanism, but does not involve agonist actions on opioid receptors. (Some have speculated that the mechanism involves suppression of the afferent limb of the 10th cranial nerve.)

Dextromethorphan does not have analgesic effects (a); alter gut motility (b); or have effects on the bladder musculature that might relieve nocturia. Very high doses of dextromethorphan can cause CNS depression, but regardless of the dose it is not used therapeutically as a sedative or other agent for controlling symptoms of ADD/ADHD. Finally, unlike codeine and most other opioids, dextromethorphan lacks significant addictive properties or potential, although clearly cough syrups that contain dextromethorphan (and alcohol) and abused.

139. The answer is e. *(Brunton, pp 347-349, 416t. Katzung, pp 426t, 434-435.)* Thiopental can be considered the prototype of the thiobarbiturates (in contrast with oxybarbiturates such as phenobarbital). It is often used as an IV preanesthetic induction adjunct because of its ability to cause unconsciousness in a matter of seconds. This occurs because the drug is very lipophilic, quickly concentrating in the brain and spinal cord. However, the drug also has a very short duration of action, with patients awaking within minutes unless repeated doses or other CNS depressants are administered afterward. This is because thiobarbiturates rapidly distribute out of the CNS to other tissues following their rapid CNS uptake. The brief duration is not due to prompt hepatic metabolism (c). Actually the plasma half-life of thiopental is on the order of 10 to 12 hours—a value that not only reflects further redistribution from tissues, but rather slow metabolism. None of the barbiturates cause clinically useful analgesia (a) at dosages that could be considered safe. Thiopental and other barbiturates (at sufficiently high CNS levels) routinely decrease, not increase (b), cerebral metabolic rates. This effect is often beneficial. Seizures are rare with any of the barbiturates; indeed phenobarbital (and some related drugs as metharbital and mephobarbital) is used long-term as anticonvulsants; and induction of a "barbiturate coma" with thiopental or other barbiturates might be used to manage seizures refractory to more first-line anticonvulsants.

140. The answer is a. *(Brunton, pp 240t, 242, 258-260, 622. Katzung, p 141.)* Whether you have learned or read about restrictions on pseudoephedrine sales specifically in a pharmacology class or text, for medicolegal and societal (and board-related?) reasons you should be aware of the growing problem of illicit "meth labs" that use pseudoephedrine (pseudo) as the starting point for a rather easy chemical synthesis of this highly addictive and dangerous CNS stimulant. None of the other drugs listed can be synthesized using this common indirect-acting sympathomimetic as a starting point.

141. The answer is c. *(Brunton, pp 220-222. Katzung, pp 458-460.)* Pancuronium is a curare-like nondepolarizing neuromuscular blocker that is commonly used to induce or maintain skeletal muscle paralysis for surgery. It has no effects on brain functions such as levels of consciousness or sensations such as of pain. The drug prevents activation of nicotinic receptors on skeletal muscle (it is a competitive antagonist), thereby preventing myocyte depolarization and other elements of normal skeletal muscle activation and ultimately causing flaccid paralysis. The onset and duration of this effect depends on the actual drug being administered.

Droperidol (a) is a haloperidol-like neuroleptic drug. It causes drowsiness and sedation in its own right. In some instances it is administered with fentanyl to cause neurolept analgesia (a calming effect, indifference to pain and surroundings); or with fentanyl and nitrous oxide for greater pain control (neurolept anesthesia). However, droperidol does not have any clinically useful intrinsic analgesic effects. A limitation to using droperidol for any purpose is its tendency to prolong ventricular repolarization, which renders patients with long QT syndrome at risk of serious arrhythmias (especially torsades).

Intravenous administration of midazolam (b), propofol (d), or thiopental (e) causes prompt sedation or loss of consciousness (dose-dependent) and can be used for such purposes as induction of anesthesia or sedation. Some are used for other purposes, for example patients on ventilators, and those undergoing endoscopy or other noninvasive procedures. These drugs lack intrinsic analgesic effects at the dosages in which they are usually given, and should not be used alone for pain control.

142. The answer is a. *(Brunton, pp 432t-436t, 438-440. Katzung p 519-520, 524, 526.)* The mention of menstrual irregularities, galactorrhea, and what appears to be extrapyramidal side effects, should be a tip-off that we are dealing with a drug that interacts with dopamine receptors—specifically D_2, by blocking them. Amoxapine, the correct answer, is a tricyclic antidepressant (secondary amine). It is rather unique among all the tricyclics (other secondary amines, and tertiary amines such as the more familiar amitriptyline and imipramine) in several respects. For one thing it inhibits neuronal dopamine and NE reuptake (the others affect mainly NE and serotonin). That, however, does not readily explain the amenorrhea-galactorrhea and extrapyramidal side effects. What provides the explanation or mechanism relates to another rather unique property of amoxapine: one of its metabolites is a strong dopamine receptor antagonist, an action not shared by any of the other tricyclics; by the SSRIs (eg, citalopram, fluoxetine, sertraline; answers b, c, and d); or by the monoamine oxidase inhibitors (eg, tranylcypromine, e; or phenelzine).

You should recall that such antipsychotic drugs as the phenothiazines and haloperidol may also cause amenorrhea-galactorrhea and extrapyramidal side effects, by the same dopaminergic receptor-blocking mechanism. Conversely, drugs that activate dopamine receptors in one way or another (eg, bromocriptine) can be used to manage these endocrine dysfunctions. Amoxapine's dopamine receptor blockade also seems to account for why the drug exerts some antipsychotic properties, theoretically making it useful for patients with both psychosis and depression.

143. The answer is c. *(Brunton, pp 450, 570. Katzung, pp 533t, 537-542, 545-546.)* Meperidine appears to be rather unusual among the common opioid analgesics in terms of its ability to inhibit neuronal reuptake of serotonin. The MAO inhibitor causes increased synaptic levels of serotonin (and other endogenous monoamines) in the central synapses, and so the presence of the opioid has enabled massive overstimulation of serotonin receptors. We have caused the "serotonin syndrome." None of the other drugs listed participate in such an interaction. However, other important drugs not listed in the question certainly do. They include, especially, both tricyclic and SSRI-type antidepressants; and the serotonin agonists commonly referred to as "triptans" (eg, sumatriptan.)

Note: Compared with other opioid analgesics, meperidine causes strong antimuscarinic side effects, which may be problematic or dangerous for some patients. The concerns over interactions with MAOIs, the strong antimuscarinic activity, and the general prevalence of toxicity owing to ready accumulation of the drug's toxic metabolite (normeperidine; especially when the drug is used for long-term pain management) has led some to state that its use as a "first-line analgesic is (becoming) increasingly rare." That may be true for long-term pain control, but for single dose or other short-term management of moderate-to-severe pain, meperidine is still used often. See the explanation for the answer to Question 117 for more information.

144. The answer is b. *(Brunton, pp 403-412, 424, 516. Katzung, pp 376-379, 567.)* The generic name for Rohypnol ("roofies" on the street) is flunitrazepam, a very lipophilic and potent benzodiazepine that manifests a typical but unusually strong benzodiazepine-ethanol interaction. Given the unfortunate frequency with which this drug is used illegally (there are some legal uses outside the United States), you need to know about it, and I suspect you know that flumazenil is a competitive benzodiazepine receptor antagonist used to reverse (or diagnose) benzodiazepine overdoses. If you said that flumazenil has no effect on ethanol-induced CNS depression you would be correct, but our patient has consumed little alcohol; her problems are due to the excessive benzodiazepine effects and the interaction with the alcohol. Diazepam (a) and triazolam (e), being in the same class as the offending drug in this situation, are likely to exacerbate the clinical problems. Ketamine, a dissociative anesthetic (b; see Question 111 for more) would be inappropriate. Naltrexone (d) is an opioid antagonist, much like naloxone, but is used orally for uses somewhat different than those for naloxone. Naloxone's specificity is for opioid receptors, and so it would have no good or bad impact on our patient's symptoms or vital signs.

145. The answer is c. *(Brunton, pp 450-451, 616, 731. Katzung, pp 519-522, 526, 562, 1021.)* One of the most noteworthy actions of bupropion, compared with tricyclics or other common antidepressants, is the lowest incidence of sexual dysfunction. In males there is no antimuscarinic action (e) that might interfere with erection, and no peripheral α-adrenergic blockade (d) that might interfere with ejaculation or cause orthostatic hypotension. In fact, the drug seems to enhance sexual drive and performance. This has been clinically useful when the drug has been used to counteract the suppressed sexual desire caused by many of the SSRI antidepressants, and most of the tricyclics. Women with depression who report a decreased interest in intercourse also seem to benefit from this drug more than others. Bupropion has structural similarities with amphetamine and so is largely nonsedating (and so a is incorrect); and tends to suppress, rather than increase, appetite (b). The drug lacks any effects on monoamine oxidase (f). However, bupropion's metabolism is dependent on MAO, and it should not be given within about 2 to 3 weeks of stopping MAO inhibitor therapy to minimize risks of toxicity—the main and most serious of which is a predisposition to seizures.

You may also remember that bupropion is marketed as a smoking cessation aid, under a different trade name than the one labeled for use for depression. It is in situations such as this, where the same active ingredient is sold under two different trade names for decidedly different uses, that accidental overdoses can occur if both products are inadvertently prescribed for the same patient.

146. The answer is b. *(Brunton, pp 474-479, 535. Katzung, pp 283-284, 482, 499.)* Neuroleptic malignant syndrome (NMS) is thought to be a severe form of an extrapyramidal syndrome that can occur at any time with any dose of a neuroleptic agent. However, the risk is higher when a so-called "high-potency antipsychotic" (eg, haloperidol) is used in high doses, especially if given parenterally. Mortality from NMS is greater than 10%. Allergic reactions (a) to haloperidol are rare. While haloperidol overdoses (c) may trigger NMS, that is not a prerequisite for the development of the syndrome. Haloperidol clearly causes extrapyramidal side effects (d) and tardive dyskinesias (e), but the fever, elevations of CK, and diminishing level of consciousness would be consistent with a diagnosis of NMS.

147. The answer is d. *(Brunton, p 534. Katzung, pp 447-472, 474.)* Carbidopa is used as an adjunct to levodopa. It works by inhibiting dopamine decarboxylation, and subsequent metabolism of levodopa to dopamine, in the gut. This is important because the majority of an orally administered dose of levodopa is metabolized to dopamine in the gut, and dopamine in the systemic circulation does not cross the blood-brain barrier (and so never reaches the striatum to cause desired antiparkinson effects). Amantadine (a) works in the CNS to promote dopamine release from functional dopaminergic nerves. Benztropine (b) works centrally to block muscarinic receptors, thereby helping to normalize a dopamine-ACh imbalance that seems to be important in parkinsonism. Bromocriptine (c) works centrally as a direct dopamine receptor agonist. Selegiline (e) is a centrally acting MAO-B inhibitor that works by reducing metabolic inactivation of dopamine.

148. The answer is e. *(Brunton, pp 574-575. Katzung, p 547.)* Pentazocine is a partial agonist: it acts as an agonist on κ receptors, and blocks μ receptors. Adding it to an analgesic regimen involving morphine or another "pure" opioid agonist will counteract key effects of morphine. In this case, the patient's pain will grow worse, not become less; and such other effects as ventilatory depression will be counteracted also. Under the circumstances described in the question, the worsening of pain is far more likely to occur than seizures, which have been reported "occasionally."

To answer this question you need to remember that morphine causes the following effects by acting as an agonist on μ receptors: analgesia, respiratory depression, euphoria, sedation, physical dependence, and decreased gut motility. Pentazocine, given alone, causes analgesia, sedation, and decreased gut motility by acting as an agonist on κ receptors. However, although pentazocine is a weak agonist it is fully capable of antagonizing the actions of morphine on μ receptors in a concentration-dependent fashion, and so pain returns in this patient.

Concomitant with antagonism of a strong opioid agonist's analgesic effects, administration of pentazocine will antagonize (not intensify, a) respiratory depression. It will not promote, accelerate, or intensify strong opioid-related physical dependence (b); induce coma (c), nor induce seizures (d).

149. The answer is b. *(Brunton, pp 174, 299, 443, 529, 533-537. Katzung, p 476.)* Selegiline inhibits MAO-B, thus inhibiting the metabolic breakdown of dopamine and making more neuronally released dopamine available for its postsynaptic receptor activation. It increases the effectiveness of both endogenous and pharmacologically administered L-dopa. Benztropine (a) and trihexyphenidyl (c) are cholinergic muscarinic antagonists that mainly act in the CNS. They have no effect on dopamine metabolism, release, or direct receptor-mediated agonist actions. Bromocriptine (d) is a dopamine receptor agonist. Chlorpromazine (e) is an antipsychotic drug with antiadrenergic properties, and it also competitively blocks dopamine receptors in both the CNS and in the periphery.

150. The answer is c. *(Brunton, pp 474, 641, 1004. Katzung, pp 153, 487, 489-499, 1024t.)* Chlorpromazine, the prototype phenothiazine antipsychotic drug, is also indicated for managing nausea and vomiting, in both adults and children, from a number of causes. The drug can be administered orally, rectally, or intramuscularly for this very purpose. (Some phenothiazines with better antiemetic activity, such as prochlorperazine or promethazine, are usually used instead.) Regardless, the antiemetic mechanism appears to involve blockade of dopaminergic receptors in the chemoreceptor trigger zone of the brain's medulla.

Chlorpromazine (and most other antipsychotics) can lower the brain's "seizure threshold," thereby increasing the risk of seizures (a) in susceptible patients. (Consider the seizure threshold to be the point at which further CNS stimulation leads to seizures; the lower it is, the greater the likelihood that a drug such as a phenothiazine, a dopaminergic drug, etc, can cause epileptiform brain changes.) Chlorpromazine, and most phenothiazines, tend to lower blood pressure (b) by blocking α-adrenergic receptors in the vasculature, and so probably would aggravate preexisting hypotension. Most of the phenothiazines also cause significant antimuscarinic effects, which would aggravate bladder hypomotility (d) and xerostomia (e; and other conditions involving reduced exocrine gland secretions). The antimuscarinic effects would inhibit activation of the bladder's detrusor muscle and inhibit relaxation of the sphincter, thereby aggravating problems with micturition in such patients as elderly men with an enlarged prostate.

Note: In general, phenothiazines are not used often for managing emesis or nausea. That is, in part, because of the risk of excessive sedation, extrapyramidal reactions, orthostatic hypotension, and occasional cholestatic jaundice or blood dyscrasias. Nowadays we tend to turn to other dopamine antagonists (eg, metoclopramide), a cannabinoid (dronabinol), or a serotonin receptor blocker (ondansetron; a 5-HT_3-selective blocker).

151. The answer is b. *(Brunton, pp 66, 161, 239, 377, 620-621. Katzung, pp 142-143, 439, 448.)* Cocaine, an ester of benzoic acid, has local anesthetic properties; it can block the initiation or conduction of a nerve impulse. It is metabolized by plasma esterases to inactive products. Most important, cocaine (and tricyclic antidepressants) blocks the neuronal reuptake of NE and other monoamines (eg, dopamine). This action produces CNS-stimulant effects including euphoria, excitement, and restlessness. Peripherally, the blocked NE reuptake causes sympathomimetic effects including tachycardia and vasoconstriction. Death from acute overdose can be from cardiac failure, stroke (hypertensive crisis), seizures, or apnea during the seizures. Cocaine does not directly activate adrenergic (a) or cholinergic receptors; it has no effect on catecholamine metabolism (c); tachycardia and vasoconstriction, not the opposite (d), are expected responses; and cocaine has local anesthetic activity and so actually suppresses the conduction of a variety of neuron types.

152. The answer is a. *(Brunton, pp 479, 535, 1500. Katzung, pp 474, 492-493.)* The main subclasses of dopamine receptors in the CNS are D_1 and D_2 receptors. Bromocriptine is a selective D_2 agonist, and is useful to treat parkinsonism or hyperprolactinemia. Chlorpromazine (b), fluphenazine (c), haloperidol (d), and promethazine (e) are competitive D_2 receptor antagonists, and are used mainly as antipsychotic drugs.

153. The answer is a. *(Brunton, pp 472t, 474, 477. Katzung, pp 287-288, 474, 656.)* Of all the antipsychotics the incidence and severity of these adverse responses are highest with the phenothiazines, of which chlorpromazine can be considered the prototype. Clozapine (b) blocks α-adrenergic, histamine (H_1), and ACh (muscarinic) receptors, but the affinity for those receptors is very low in comparison with dopamine and serotonin receptor blockade. Haloperidol has considerable dopamine receptor-blocking activity, and little effect on muscarinic receptors that might account for the side effects described here. (See Question 119 for more on fundamental differences between "high-potency" and "low-potency" antipsychotics, especially as they predict the relative incidence of peripheral autonomic and central [extrapyramidal] side effects.) Olanzapine (d) is pharmacologically most similar to clozapine, except for the fact that the risk of agranulocytosis is quite low. Sertraline (e) is an SSRI, and you should recall that SSRIs (eg, the prototype, fluoxetine) lack clinically significant antimuscarinic effects.

154. The answer is b. *(Brunton, pp 255-256, 450, 854-855. Katzung, pp 145, 173-174.)* In addition to being approved (and widely used) as an antihypertensive drug, clonidine is also approved for managing severe pain in situations such as the one described in the question. For analgesia it is mainly used as an adjunct to an opioid, and it seems to provide significant added relief from pain or other unpleasant sensations that are neuropathic in origin. The drug is given by continuous epidural infusion at rates and dosages lower than those reached when the drug is given orally or transdermally for blood pressure control. The receptor-based analgesic mechanism of this very lipophilic drug is probably similar to its central antihypertensive effects. Whereas antihypertensive doses act as an agonist for a population of α_2-adrenergic receptors in the cardiovascular control center of the brain (medulla), analgesic doses of clonidine primarily act in parts of the spinal cord. Once those adrenergic receptors are activated neurotransmission by afferent sensory nerves is inhibited. (The drug acts only in those parts of the spinal cord that have sensory afferent pain pathways from peripheral structures.) Clonidine-mediated analgesia is not suppressed or abolished by traditional opioid receptor antagonists (naloxone, naltrexone). Nonetheless, when clonidine is used for pain (or to manage drug withdrawal signs and symptoms), you still should anticipate all the drug's expected side effects, including a fall of blood pressure (reduced sympathetic vasoconstriction) and of heart rate and stroke volume (reduced β_1-activation). Also, even when used as an analgesic, when the drug is to be stopped the daily doses need to be tapered gradually to reduce the risk of rebound hypertensive episodes.

None of the other drugs listed as possible answers, or members of their class—ACE inhibitors, diuretics, β-blockers (of any sort or selectivity), or peripherally acting α-blockers—share clonidine's analgesic actions or use. Indeed, of all the antihypertensive drugs clonidine is the only one with this approved analgesic use.

155. The answer is b. *(Brunton, pp 552t, 566, 572-573, 1848t. Katzung, pp 545, 560.)* Methadone is a slow-onset, long-acting, opioid receptor (μ and κ) agonist. It is used as an analgesic for long-term pain control when an opioid is indicated, and for maintenance therapy of individuals dependent on opioids. It has greater oral bioavailability than morphine, especially when oral therapy is started. (Recall that morphine is subject to extensive first-pass hepatic metabolism, and only with repeated oral administration can we saturate its drug-metabolizing enzymes such that bioavailability is improved enough to get good analgesia. That's why, if our analgesic of choice is morphine, we start treatment with parenteral administration.) Methadone's long biologic half-life accounts for the milder but more protracted abstinence syndrome when the drug is stopped. Methadone does not possess opioid antagonist properties (whether μ or κ) and, thus, would not precipitate withdrawal symptoms in a heroin addict, as would naloxone or naltrexone, so long as we administer sufficient doses of the methadone, and that is precisely what we do with methadone maintenance therapy or when we switch a patient to it from another opioid. Excessive doses of methadone can cause typical opioid-related ventilatory depression.

156. The answer is c. *(Brunton, pp 506, 513-514, 523. Katzung, pp 412-413.)* The symptoms describe absence seizures, for which ethosuximide is very effective (and, according to many, the drug of choice). Phenytoin (e) may aggravate absence seizures. None of the other drugs are effective or indicated for long-term therapy of epilepsy: alprazolam (a); diazepam (b); or midazolam (d).

157. The answer is b. *(Brunton, pp 308-311. Katzung, pp 285-290.)* For years ergotamine has been considered a mainstay of aborting migraine headaches. Its likely mechanism involves antagonizing cerebral vasodilation. It activates 5-HT_3 receptors, which in turn causes cerebral vasoconstriction. This ergot alkaloid also can cause significant and long-lasting systemic vasoconstriction via α-adrenergic receptor activation. While normal coronary vessels aren't uniquely sensitive to this effect, those of patients who are prone to developing coronary vasospasm (Prinzmetal or variant angina) are at greater risk, and that is likely what this patient had. (Perhaps you've heard of "St. Anthony's Fire"—what we now call ergotism—that occurred in the Middle Ages. It was characterized by gangrene and "bloodless" loss of the fingers and toes [among other problems], and was due to intense vasoconstriction caused by eating spoiled grains laden with a fungus that produced large amounts of ergot alkaloids.)

Bromocriptine (a), another ergot alkaloid, has little effect on 5-HT or adrenergic receptors. However, it is an efficacious dopamine D_2 agonist, and that provides the basis for its use for parkinsonism, hyperprolactinemia, and treatment of some prolactin-secreting pituitary tumors. Morphine (c) is not likely to cause hypertension, and would produce myocardial ischemia (of a global nature) only when such high doses are given that hypotension and ventilatory depression ensue.

Phenoxybenzamine (d) blocks 5-HT receptors (and ACh and histamine receptors too), which explains its rather infrequent use for carcinoid syndrome—a tumor that secretes large amounts of serotonin and peptides that stimulate smooth muscles (primarily in the airways and GI tract). However, its main pharmacologic effect is long-lasting and noncompetitive blockade of α-adrenergic receptors, and the related use is adjunctive management of catecholamine-secreting tumors (ie, pheochromocytoma). Thus, it lowers blood pressure and also would block coronary vasoconstriction or spasm mediated by α-adrenergic activation. Dosages needed to block 5-HT receptors are much higher than those needed to block serotonin receptors.

Phenytoin (e), an important anticonvulsant, has no ability to cause hypertension (nor any other significant increase of blood pressure), nor to cause or exacerbate coronary vasospasm.

158. The answer is e. *(Brunton, p 462. Katzung, pp 276-279, 489-490, 494-495.)* Promethazine, like most other phenothiazines, tends to cause dose-dependent CNS depression. Of the answers given here, the most likely outcome of that effect is ventilatory depression and apnea, and that is precisely the reason why the FDA bolstered the warnings for children. Like most other phenothiazines, promethazine has significant antimuscarinic activity, and that would not cause heart block (a) or diarrhea (d). It has α-adrenergic blocking activity, which would lower, rather than raise, blood pressure (b). Promethazine may, indeed, cause parkinsonian side effects (c), but they are not likely to be a cause of death unless the patient develops neuroleptic malignant syndrome that goes undiagnosed and improperly treated until it is too late.

159. The answer is e. *(Brunton, pp 227-228, 356. Katzung, pp 283-284, 433, 465.)* The syndrome described is that of malignant hyperthermia (MH). (Some folks like to use the mnemonic FEVER—**f**ever, **e**ncephalopathy, **v**itals unstable, **e**levated enzymes such as creatine kinase, and **r**igidity of muscles.) For decades it has been attributed to an interaction between halogenated hydrocarbon volatile liquid anesthetics—primarily halothane (the use of which is declining owing to the relatively high MH risk, coupled with a host of other adverse responses such as sensitizing the myocardium to catecholamine-induced arrhythmias), but still a possibility with others, including isoflurane; and skeletal neuromuscular blockers, particularly succinylcholine. It can occur intraoperatively or in the immediate postoperative period. The overall incidence is about 1 in 50,000 anesthesias, and 1 in about 15,000 pediatric anesthesias. Worldwide, MH is fatal about 80% of the time, but only about 10% to 15% of the time in the United States. There is almost certainly a genetic basis for MH, involving an autosomal dominant trait that accounts for about half of all MH cases. On a molecular basis it is characterized by aberrant function of the so-called ryanodine-sensitive calcium channel in the sarcoplasmic reticulum. In essence, it impairs the ability of the scarcoplasmic reticulum to take up (via an ATPase) and retain Ca^{2+} as is necessary for skeletal muscle to relax, albeit briefly, between contractions. The resulting rise of free intracellular Ca^{2+} leads to tonic skeletal muscle activation (hence, rigidity). The heightened ATP consumption that occurs to maintain cross-bridge formation uses an abundant amount of oxygen, and heat is generated (the fever). As muscle function deteriorates and ATP is depleted, metabolism switches to glycolysis and lactic acid accumulation (acidosis). Damaged muscle cells leak K^+ that in turn causes hyperkalemia, tachycardia, and cardiac arrhythmias. Myoglobin and large intracellular enzymes such as creatine kinase also leak out of damaged myocytes. Unless treated promptly (dantrolene, physical means to cool the body, attempts to correct blood pH and electrolyte profiles), the consequences can be fatal.

None of the other drugs, individually or in the combinations given, are associated with malignant hyperthermia.

160. The answer is c. *(Brunton, pp 503-506, 523. Katzung, pp 408-409.)* Vigabatrin (γ-vinyl GABA) is useful in partial seizures. It is an irreversible inhibitor of GABA aminotransferase, an enzyme responsible for the termination of GABA action. This results in accumulation of GABA at synaptic sites, thereby enhancing its effect.

161. The answer is d. *(Brunton, pp 509-510. Katzung, pp 419, 575.)* Folic acid supplementation is recommended during normal uncomplicated pregnancy, and it is critical when the mother is receiving anticonvulsant drugs (AEDs) during gestation. The purpose is to reduce the risk of spina bifida and other neural tube defects (and some other teratogenic consequences). The condition is known as the "fetal hydantoin syndrome." The question's scenario describes no reason to add valproic acid (or add or switch to any other AED, including phenobarbital) if the mother is kept seizure-free during pregnancy and gets proper perinatal care. Valproic acid is in pregnancy class D; most others are C), and so it appears to carry the highest risk of teratogenic effects of all the common AEDs. Discontinuing any or all AEDs during pregnancy (b) is risky in this and most circumstances, as it carries the risk of seizure recurrence that can be more dangerous to the mother and the fetus than continuing effective therapy and providing good prenatal care—and folic acid supplementation.

Notes: Current recommendations (Folic acid for the prevention of neural tube defects: U.S. Preventive Services Task Force recommendation statement. Ann. Intern. Med. 150:626, 2009) are that women "(even) planning or capable of pregnancy should take a daily supplement (in addition to any folate in the diet) containing between 0.4 and 0.8 mg of folic acid." These recommendations apply even to women who are otherwise healthy and taking no teratogenic drugs, AEDs, or any others. As an aside, the overall risk of having a child born with neural tube defects or other anomalies is about 1%. With single-dose AED therapy throughout pregnancy, and with proper perinatal care, the risk (overall) rises to about 2%. The risk goes up considerably, however, when the mother is taking more than one AED during pregnancy, whether that drug is valproic acid (a) or any other agent.

Finally, judicious supplementation of the mother's diet with iron (c) is often recommended. That is to reduce the risk or severity of hematologic abnormalities, and has nothing to do with prevention of teratogenesis or other similar AED-related problems.

162. The answer is b. *(Brunton, pp 463t, 474. Katzung, pp 492-495, 497-499.)* Chlorpromazine, of all the drugs listed, has strong α-adrenergic receptor-blocking activity. This accounts for a relatively high incidence of orthostatic hypotension and explains why measuring the patient's blood pressure in both the supine and standing positions is important. At clinically relevant dosages, buspirone (a) has no significant autonomic or cardiovascular effects. Diphenhydramine strongly blocks both muscarinic and H_1-histamine receptors, and neither action would likely cause hypotension. Haloperidol (d), a butyrophenone antipsychotic, causes few peripheral autonomic side effects, including those noted in the question. Zolpidem (e) is a benzodiazepine-like hypnotic that lacks appreciable peripheral autonomic side effects.

163. The answer is a. *(Brunton, pp 194, 313, 462-466. Katzung pp 487, 491t, 493.)* Clozapine causes agranulocytosis in 1% to 2% of treated patients—perhaps a small number in an absolute sense, but far more common and potentially serious with other drugs that might be used in lieu of this unusual antipsychotic. It is generally reversible on discontinuation of the drug but this, of course, depends on frequent blood tests to detect the problem early on. Monitoring for this adverse response is so critical that the initial prescription for the drug, and refills for continued therapy, cannot be filled without proof of blood counts that are within "acceptable" levels. Other concerns with clozapine, for which monitoring is important, include the development of seizures; weight gain (it is common and the patient may put on an extra 10 or 20 lb); rises of blood glucose levels (perhaps with the development of new-onset diabetes, and so answer c is incorrect); and myocarditis. Extrapyramidal side effects (b) are rare, in contrast with typical antipsychotics, because of clozapine's low affinity for dopamine D_2 receptors. Hypotension (d) and ventilatory depression (e) are not at all common with this drug.

164. The answer is d. *(Brunton, pp 510, 523-524. Katzung, pp 403-405, 1025-1029.)* Phenytoin, given throughout pregnancy, can inhibit hepatic synthesis (activation) of vitamin K-dependent clotting factors in utero. Phenobarbital and several other anticonvulsants can do the same, and so vitamin K prophylaxis applies to their use as well. None of the other drugs listed is associated with such an effect. Warfarin (e), arguably the most widely used oral anticoagulant in the world, is absolutely contraindicated (FDA pregnancy category X) during pregnancy because of the risks of so-called "warfarin embryopathy." See the explanation for answers to Question 195 in Chapter 4 on Cardiovascular Pharmacology, for more information.

Notes: Bupropion is pregnancy category B (low risk in humans). Most of the benzodiazepines, including diazepam, are in pregnancy category D (definite risks, not absolutely contraindicated). Estazolam, flurazepam, quazepam, temazepam, and triazolam are category X. Opioids, including methadone (c) are generally category B or C agents.

165. The answer is b. *(Brunton, pp 174, 536-537. Katzung, p 476.)* Entacapone is a COMT inhibitor. COMT normally is a minor player in the metabolism of levodopa, but when the major pathway for levodopa metabolism to dopamine (via dopa decarboxylase) is inhibited, as it is with administration of carbidopa, COMT plays a more important role. It helps form 3-*O*-methyldopa, which competes with levodopa for uptake into the brain. So, when we have poor responses to levodopa (alone or in combination with carbidopa), or when levodopa therapy has been ongoing for so long that the patient develops acute or chronic refractoriness to its effects (eg, the "on-off" or the "wearing-off" phenomena), adding entacapone (or a similar drug, tolcapone) might be reasonable. Donepezil (a) and tacrine (d) are centrally acting cholinesterase inhibitors with no effect on dopamine metabolism. Selegiline (c) is a selective inhibitor of dopamine metabolism by MAO in the brain (MAO-B). Trihexyphenidyl (e) is a centrally acting muscarinic receptor blocking drug. Related drugs are benztropine and diphenhydramine (the latter of which also exerts strong peripheral muscarinic-blocking effects.

166. The answer is c. *(Brunton, pp 593, 602-603, 613. Katzung, pp 65t, 388, 395, 596t, 1145t.)* This is a classic description of an alcohol-disulfiram interaction. Disulfiram is sometimes used in controlling alcohol abuse. It acts by inhibiting aldehyde dehydrogenase, resulting in the accumulation of acetaldehyde. This "acetaldehyde syndrome" is characterized by the signs and symptoms described in the question. The onset of symptoms is almost immediately following ingestion of alcohol and may last for several hours in some patients. None of the other drugs listed in the answers can cause these outcomes. Naltrexone (a), an opioid antagonist, would have no effect on the responses to ethanol. Diazepam (b) and phenobarbital (d), both CNS depressants that clearly have their depressant effects potentiated by alcohol, would not lead to the described effects. Tranylcypromine (e) is an older nonselective MAO inhibitor. MAO plays no role in the metabolism or responses to alcohol.

Note: Several other drugs or drug classes can cause clinically significant disulfiram-like reactions. They include the older sulfonylureas (tolbutamide, chlorpropamide) used for oral therapy of Type 2 diabetes mellitus; and some of the cephalosporin antibiotics.

167. The answer is c. *(Brunton, pp 447-448, 450-451, 616, 731. Katzung, pp 513-514, 516-525, 527t.)* Fluoxetine—and related SSRI antidepressants such as sertraline, fluvoxamine, citalopram, and escitalopram—selectively inhibit neuronal serotonin uptake, with minimal effects on other monoamines. The tricyclics (amitriptyline and imipramine, a, d) and venlafaxine (e) inhibit serotonin and NE reuptake (and, apparently to a small degree, dopamine). Bupropion (b) affects reuptake of both NE and dopamine.

168. The answer is d. *(Brunton, pp 410t-411t, 601. Katzung, pp 394, 563.)* Benzodiazepines (particularly those with prompt and significant sedating activity) are considered good choices for alleviating barbiturate and alcohol withdrawal symptoms. The anxiolytic effects of buspirone (a) take several days to develop, rendering it unsuitable for acute, severe withdrawal signs and symptoms. In addition, it causes little or no CNS depression in most patients. Chloral hydrate (b) and ethanol interact by inhibiting the metabolism of each other, with the main result being profound CNS depression. That is, each drug potentiates the effects of the other. We would not want to give chloral hydrate to any patient who still may have alcohol in the circulation. Chlorpromazine (c) is used mainly for psychosis, and is not likely to beneficially affect the signs and symptoms that our patient has. Trazodone (e) is an atypical antidepressant with a fair amount of generalized CNS-depressant effects, which makes it often prescribed for patients who have insomnia as a major depression symptom. It weakly inhibits neuronal serotonin reuptake and seems to increase serotonin release from serotoninergic nerves. It would not be suitable for the immediate management of this patient.

169. The answer is b. *(Brunton, pp 593, 600. Katzung, pp 396-397, 1024.)* Methanol is metabolized by the same enzymes that metabolize ethanol, but the products are different: formaldehyde and formic acid in the case of methanol. Headache, vertigo, vomiting, abdominal pain, dyspnea, and blurred vision can occur from accumulation of these metabolic intermediates. However, the most dangerous (or at least permanently disabling) consequence in severe cases is hyperemia of the optic disc, which can lead to blindness. The rationale for administering ethanol to treat methanol poisoning is fairly simple. Ethanol has a high affinity for alcohol and aldehyde dehydrogenases and competes with methanol as a substrate for those enzymes, reducing metabolism of methanol to its more toxic products. Important adjunctive treatments include hemodialysis to enhance removal of methanol and its products; and administration of systemic alkalinizing salts (eg, sodium bicarbonate) to counteract metabolic acidosis. None of the other drugs listed would be appropriate. They may alleviate some of the signs and symptoms resulting from methanol poisoning, but they would have no beneficial effects on the crux of the problem—the metabolism of the methanol.

170. The answer is c. *(Brunton, pp 560, 571-574, 577-578. Katzung, pp 547-549, 560.)* Naloxone is given parenterally. It specifically blocks opioid receptors that are activated by such agonists as morphine, heroin, and fentanyl (among many others). Diazepam (a) and other benzodiazepines (eg, lorazepam) have no effects on opioid receptors. Flumazenil (b) is a specific benzodiazepine antagonist. It may be lifesaving in cases of benzodiazepine overdoses, but has no effects on the responses to opioids. Naltrexone (d) is an opioid receptor antagonist (as is naloxone), but it is given orally, has a slow onset of action, and so will be of little benefit in this acute, life-threatening situation. Fentanyl is unlikely to cause seizures. Phenytoin (e) is, of course, an anticonvulsant; it would be inappropriate to administer, and if the administered dose was sufficiently high it could contribute to the CNS and ventilatory depression caused by the fentanyl.

171. The answer is b. *(Brunton, pp 432t, 446-447, 450-451. Katzung, pp 83f, 512, 514-519, 522-527.)* Imipramine, a tricyclic antidepressant, causes strong peripheral antimuscarinic effects. In the context of our patient, recall that muscarinic receptor activation contracts the detrusor muscle of the bladder, and relaxes the bladder sphincter. Imipramine blocks those effects, and that seems to explain its effects in managing nocturnal enuresis—especially in children. The drug, and other members of its class, does relieve depression signs and symptoms. However, they are due to inhibition, not increases of (a) monoamine neurotransmitter reuptake via the so-called norepinephrine transporter at the "endings" of catecholaminergic neurons. Imipramine and its group members tend to cause sedation (c), but that is not likely to reduce the frequency of enuresis. These drugs also have α-adrenergic blocking activity, and one consequence of that would most likely be an increase, not a decrease, of renal blood flow and GFR. Tricyclic antidepressants, nor other major classes of antidepressants, have any important effects on the release of antidiuretic hormone or the responses of the renal tubules to ADH.

172. The answer is a. *(Brunton, pp 436t, 447-448, 453, 616, 731. Katzung, pp 520-522, 562, 1021.)* Bupropion is marketed, under different trade names, for two main purposes: anxiety relief, and suppression of the cravings for nicotine. Since too many physicians prescribe by brand-name, and ignore the active generic drug, such problems as the one I described in the scenario, due to accidental duplication and overdoses of a drug, are more common than you'd like to believe. One of the main consequences of bupropion overdose is seizures. Chlordiazepoxide (b) is a benzodiazepine that is not indicated for depression or as a stop-smoking aid. If anything, the drug will suppress, rather than cause, seizures. Fluoxetine (c) and imipramine (d) are antidepressants, but they are not normally prescribed as smoking-cessation aids, nor are they marketed in products approved for that use. Lithium (e) is a mood-stabilizing drug used in bipolar illness. It is not at all likely to have been approved for managing depression or for smoking cessation.

173. The answer is c. *(Brunton, 537-538. Katzung, 447-448.)* At first blush it would seem that choosing any antiparkinson drug would be appropriate for this man. However, if you think about the etiology of schizophrenia and of parkinsonism (especially drug-induced), and the mechanisms of action of the drugs listed, you would select benztropine (or a related drug, trihexyphenidyl)—or diphenhydramine, a β-blocker, or a benzodiazepine, none of which was listed as a choice).

Phenothiazines (chlorpromazine), and especially butyrophenones (haloperidol, e), relieve schizophrenia signs and symptoms largely by blockade of central dopamine (D_2) receptors, particularly in the mesolimbic-mesocortical system. Simultaneously, D_2 blockade in the nigrostriatum, and concomitant unmasking of opposing muscarinic-cholinergic effects, seems to account for the extrapyramidal/parkinsonian side effects that have surfaced in patients like the one I describe. Recall that despite the imprecision of the terminology, "high-potency" antipsychotics such as haloperidol are associated with a much higher incidence of extrapyramidal side effects than are the "low-potency" antipsychotics (ie, the phenothiazines), due to their stronger central D_2 blockade, and so switching from chlorpromazine to haloperidol would not at all alleviate this patient's parkinsonian side effects: it would likely worsen them.

In idiopathic Parkinson disease there is deterioration of dopaminergic neurons and, inferentially, a decrease of central dopamine content or release. That pathophysiology provides a rationale for pharmacologically boosting dopaminergic influences: increasing central dopamine synthesis (levodopa, alone or with carbidopa; d); inhibiting dopamine's metabolic inactivation with either a COMT inhibitor (tolcapone, a; or entacapone) or an MAO inhibitor (eg, selegiline, not listed); or using such other strategies as dopamine-releasing or -mimetic agents (amantadine, bromocriptine).

In this situation of drug-induced parkinsonism, however, dopamine receptors are blocked by the antipsychotic. While we could try to overcome that blockade (since it is surmountable and competitive antagonism we are dealing with), that approach is not likely to be effective nor tolerable to the patient, since we would have to try very large doses of a dopaminergic drug—doses sufficient to cause, in all likelihood, significant side effects.

So what we do, therefore, is attack the dopamine-ACh imbalance from the "other side"—administer a centrally acting antimuscarinic drug. Note that since we are dealing with symptoms arising from a relative excess of cholinergic influences, a centrally acting cholinesterase inhibitor (donepezil or tacrine, b) would worsen the problems by making even more ACh available at central muscarinic synapses.

174. The answer is b. *(Brunton, pp 354-358. Katzung, pp 424f, 426t, 429, 431-433.)* One of the main reasons why halothane is used infrequently in adult anesthesia is because of the risk of renal and hepatic toxicity. Such halothane-related problems are uncommon in children, and rare in either children or adults anesthetized with the more commonly used drug, isoflurane. Neither halothane nor isoflurane tends to raise blood pressure (a). Isoflurane seems to lower blood pressure mainly as a result of vasodilation; with halothane, both cardiac depression and vasodilation seem to cause hypotension. Another limitation to the use of halothane is its arrhythmogenic effects, which occur by two main mechanisms. (1) It sensitizes the myocardium to catecholamines; (2) prolongs ventricular repolarization (prolongs the QT interval), thus predisposing susceptible patients to ventricular tachycardia, torsades de pointes, or other potentially lethal ventricular arrhythmias. The risks are far lower with isoflurane. Finally, while both halothane and isoflurane are potent anesthetics (they have MACs <2%), these drugs lack sufficient analgesic and skeletal muscle-relaxing effects to be used routinely without other appropriate adjuncts (eg, nitrous oxide, neuromuscular blocking drugs).

175. The answer is d. *(Brunton, pp 479, 535, 1500. Katzung, pp 474, 492-493.)* Bromocriptine mimics the action of dopamine in the brain but is not as readily metabolized and inactivated as the endogenous neurotransmitter. It is especially useful in parkinsonism that is unresponsive to L-dopa. Apomorphine (b) is also a dopamine receptor agonist, but its side effects (mainly emesis) preclude its use for parkinsonism. Selegiline (e) is an MAO-B inhibitor. Belladonna preparations (c) are atropine and atropine-like antimuscarinics. Centrally acting antimuscarinics such as benztropine and trihexyphenidyl are important drugs for managing some patients with parkinsonism, but they work not by enhancing the effects of dopamine but rather by blocking the central effects of ACh. Amantadine (a) is an antiviral agent that also is useful in some cases of parkinsonism. It either (or both) enhances the synthesis or inhibits neuronal reuptake of dopamine. It is not a dopamine receptor agonist.

176. The answer is b. *(Brunton, p 479. Katzung, p 474.)* Bromocriptine, an ergot derivative, is a direct-acting dopamine receptor agonist. Its main uses are for adjunctive management of Parkinson disease, and for management of amenorrhea and infertility (and, if present, galactorrhea) due to hyperprolactinemia. It is also used, long-term, for management of some pituitary adenomas. However, it has gained acceptance as an important adjunct (usually along with dantrolene, as noted in the question) for management of neuroleptic malignant syndrome (NMS). Recall that NMS is a rare but potentially fatal response to traditional neuroleptic/antipsychotic drugs (phenothiazines such as chlorpromazine, and butyrophenones such as haloperidol). The newer, atypical antipsychotics (clozapine, olanzapine, and risperidone) may also cause NMS, but the clinical presentation seems not to include muscle rigidity that is usually an accompaniment of NMS caused by phenothiazines or butyrophenones.

177. The answer is b. *(Brunton, pp 547, 552t, 560, 563-568, 574. Katzung, pp 534, 537-540, 544.)* Morphine, and other strong opioids, cause ventilatory depression. That, in turn, raises blood P_{CO_2} and lowers P_{O_2}. Cerebral blood vessels respond to the rise of P_{CO_2} by autoregulating (dilating) to increase cerebral perfusion. This, in turn, increases intracranial pressure (ICP)—which is already likely to be high with a closed-head injury. If ICP rises sufficiently high from brain swelling (the combined effects of drug-induced cerebral vasodilation and trauma-induced edema), then cerebral blood flow can be reduced to dangerous or even fatal levels (ie, ischemic stroke).

Now let's consider a scenario that's germane to the question. Assume the patient suffered the closed head injury, along with numerous and severe lacerations, fractures, and internal injuries, in a motor vehicle accident. They hurt. Will we let them hurt by avoiding use of morphine or any other strong opioid analgesic that also suppresses ventilation and raises ICP? Of course not, so what can we do? (1) Mechanically ventilate the patient to control and maintain reasonably normal blood gases; (2) administer mannitol, the osmotic diuretic, to help counteract brain swelling; (3) perhaps give a corticosteroid with strong anti-inflammatory activity, such as dexamethasone; (4) drill a burr hole in the skull to help reduce intracranial pressure; and so on.

And the other answer choices? Morphine is indicated as adjunctive therapy for acute pulmonary edema (a; improves pulmonary hemodynamics, helps normalize ventilation, helps allay anxiety); and also does similar things for a recent or evolving MI or acute coronary syndrome (e). A history of epilepsy (c) or hypertension (d) does not pose any clinically relevant problems in terms of morphine administration.

Cardiovascular Pharmacology

Antianginals
Antiarrhythmics
Anticoagulants
Antihyperlipidemics
Antihypertensives
Antiplatelet drugs
Heart failure therapy
Thrombolytics (fibrinolytics)
Vasodilators

Questions

178. A patient with chronic-stable ("effort-induced") angina is on prophylactic β-blocker therapy, with sublingual nitroglycerin (NTG) used PRN (as needed) for managing acute angina. One day he experiences particularly severe angina and takes the usually recommended dose of sublingual NTG. His discomfort is not reduced at all. Seeking relief, he repeats the usual recommended NTG dose 6 times over a period of about 10 minutes, and now has taken far too much of the nitrovasodilator. An electrocardiogram taken by the paramedics, who were called for the patient's emergency, shows changes consistent with severe myocardial ischemia. The patient incurs a massive infarction, goes into cardiac arrest, and cannot be resuscitated. Which of the following is the most likely cause of or contributing factor to the patient's ultimately fatal response to the excessive dosage of NTG? Assume the patient was taking no other drug(s) except the NTG and a β-blocker.

a. Cyanide, a toxic metabolite of NTG, accumulated.
b. The NTG directly induced coronary vasoconstriction.
c. The NTG lowered arterial (coronary perfusion) pressure excessively.
d. The patient had vasospastic (variant or Prinzmetal) angina, the original diagnosis of chronic-stable angina was incorrect.
e. The β-blocker counteracted the effects of the NTG and increased the risk and severity of myocardial ischemia.

179. A 65-year-old man with heart failure is unable to climb a flight of stairs without experiencing dyspnea. After several years of therapy with carvedilol, captopril, and furosemide, the therapeutic plan probably needs to change now. You empirically add digoxin to improve cardiac muscle contractility. Within 4 weeks, he has a marked improvement in his symptoms. Which of the following best describes the main cellular action of digoxin that accounts for its ability to improve his cardiovascular function and overall hemodynamic status?

a. Activates β_1-adrenergic receptors
b. Facilitates GTP binding to specific G proteins
c. Increases mitochondrial calcium (Ca^{2+}) release
d. Inhibits sarcolemmal Na^+,K^+-ATPase
e. Stimulates cyclic adenosine 5′-monophosphate (cAMP) synthesis

180. A patient has frequent episodes of paroxysmal supraventricular tachycardia (PSVT). Which of the following drugs would be most suitable for outpatient prophylaxis of these worrisome electrophysiologic events?

a. Adenosine
b. Lidocaine
c. Nifedipine
d. Nitroglycerin
e. Verapamil

181. A patient with chronic-stable angina begins taking metoprolol, and once blood levels reach the therapeutic range the frequency and severity of anginal attacks and the need for sublingual nitroglycerin were reduced. Which of the following states the direct pharmacologic action by which the β-blocker produced the desired effects?

a. Decreased myocardial oxygen demand
b. Dilated the coronary vasculature
c. Directly inhibited angiotensin II synthesis
d. Reduced total peripheral resistance
e. Slowed AV nodal conduction velocity

182. Your patient is a 50-year-old man with Type 1 diabetes mellitus, normal renal function, and no microalbuminuria. Although his HbA_{1c} levels are acceptable, because of his lifestyle and eating habits he has experienced more than a few episodes of symptomatic hypoglycemia following insulin injections. He currently has asymptomatic hyperuricemia, but he has had several attacks of acute gout over the last 5 years. Which of the following drugs would be the most rational first choice for starting his antihypertensive therapy?

a. Angiotensin-converting enzyme (ACE) inhibitor or angiotensin receptor blocker
b. β-Adrenergic blocker
c. Nifedipine
d. Thiazide diuretic
e. Verapamil or diltiazem

183. A coronary artery sample was removed from a healthy animal, put in a suitable oxygenated salt and nutrient solution, and connected to a transducer that measured increases (contraction) or decreases (relaxation) of smooth muscle tension (force). Acetylcholine (ACh) was then added to give the cumulative concentrations shown in the figure on the next page.

As expected, in the control setting (left) ACh caused concentration-dependent vasorelaxation (equivalent to vasodilation in the intact animal). The ACh was washed out several times; control conditions returned. The conditions were manipulated, and then the ACh dose-response experiment was repeated (right). Now the data show increased tension developed by the muscle sample (vasoconstriction in vivo) in response to ACh and incremental increases of its concentration.

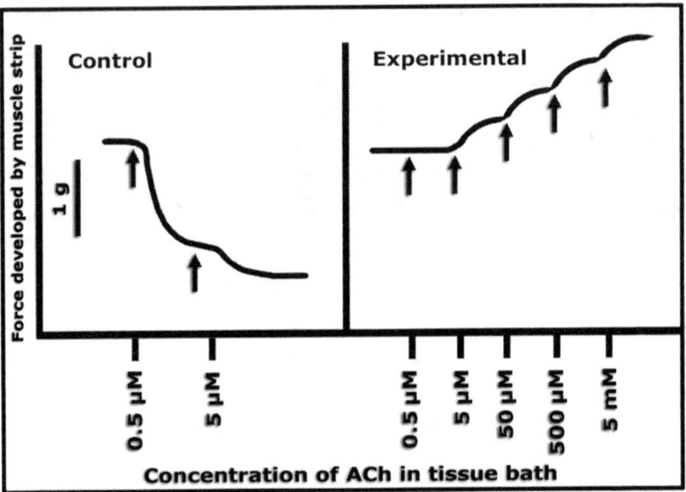

Assume that the vascular responses in this animal model are identical to those that would occur in a human. Which of the following summarizes what was most likely done to the vessel under the experimental conditions, before retesting the responses to added ACh?

a. Endothelium was removed mechanically.
b. Isoproterenol was added right before ACh.
c. Muscarinic receptors were blocked with atropine.
d. Sample was pretreated with prazosin.
e. Tissue was pretreated with botulinum toxin.

184. A 50-year-old man has a long history of asymptomatic hyperuricemia, and you are about to start therapy for newly diagnosed essential hypertension (BP 136/94 mm Hg, based on repeated measurements with the patient supine and at rest). Which antihypertensive drug is most likely to increase his uric acid levels further, and in doing so, be most likely to cause the most common clinical presentation of the hyperuricemia—gout?

a. Hydrochlorothiazide
b. Labetalol
c. Losartan
d. Ramipril
e. Verapamil

185. We conduct an experiment to assess the effects of other drugs on the anti-platelet aggregatory effects of aspirin. In each case we sample venous blood from an otherwise healthy patient, centrifuge the blood to obtain a platelet-rich fraction, and put samples of the platelets into an aggregometer (spectrophotometric device that measures light transmission through the platelets: when the platelets are resting they block light transmission; when they are activated, the aggregated platelets allow more light transmission). We then activate the platelets in the aggregometer by adding ADP (or collagen; makes no difference).

The control (top line) condition reflects results from the patient's platelets while he/she is taking no drugs at all. The bottom trace shows aggregation of platelets isolated from the patient after they have taken aspirin (*ASA*; 81 mg/d) for 14 days in a row. We wait for 2 weeks to ensure that all aspirin has been eliminated (verified by another aggregometer study). Then we restart the patient on 81 mg/d aspirin plus an unknown drug taken with each aspirin tablet, for the final 2 weeks. The platelets tested at the end of the 14 days show only slight inhibition of platelet aggregation—results not significantly from control.

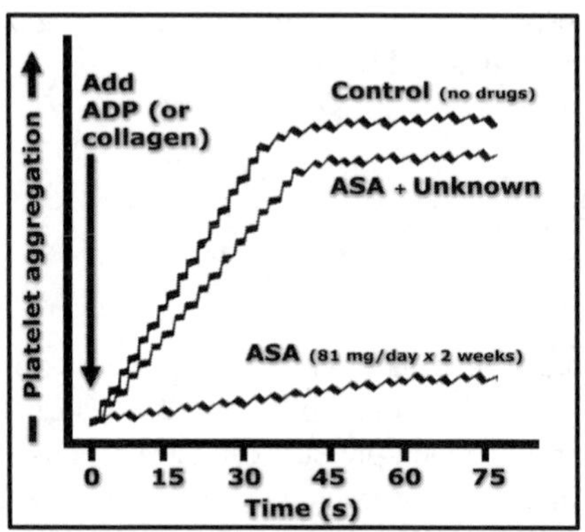

Which of the following drugs was taken with the aspirin and inhibited its antiaggregatory effects in response to ADP or collagen?

a. Acetaminophen
b. Clopidogrel
c. Hydrochlorothiazide
d. Ibuprofen
e. Warfarin

186. Your newly diagnosed hypertensive patient has vasospastic angina. Which drug or drug class would be most rational for starting antihypertensive therapy because it not only exerts antihypertensive effects, but also directly lowers myocardial oxygen demand and consumption and tends to inhibit cellular processes that otherwise favor coronary vasospasm? Assume there are no other specific contraindications to the drug you choose.

a. Angiotensin-converting enzyme (ACE) inhibitor or angiotensin receptor blocker
b. β-Adrenergic blocker
c. Nifedipine
d. Thiazide diuretic
e. Verapamil (or diltiazem)

187. A patient with newly diagnosed essential hypertension starts treatment with a commonly used antihypertensive drug at a dose that is considered to be therapeutic for the vast majority of patients. Soon after starting therapy the patient experiences crushing chest discomfort. ECG changes show myocardial ischemia. Studies in the cardiac cath lab show episodes of coronary vasospasm, and it is likely the antihypertensive drug provoked the vasospasm. Which antihypertensive drug or drug class most likely caused the ischemia and the angina?

a. Atenolol
b. Diltiazem
c. Hydrochlorothiazide
d. Losartan
e. Metolazone

188. A 28-year-old woman is receiving drug therapy for essential hypertension. She subsequently becomes pregnant. You realize that the drug she's been taking for her high blood pressure can have serious, if not fatal, effects on the fetus (it is in pregnancy category X). As a result, you stop the current antihypertensive drug and substitute it with another drug that is deemed to be equiefficacious in terms of her blood pressure, and safer for the fetus. Which of the following drugs was she most likely taking before she became pregnant?

a. α-Methyldopa
b. Captopril
c. Furosemide
d. Labetalol
e. Verapamil

189. A 30-year-old man who has a history of asthma has just been diagnosed with Stage 2 essential hypertension. He regularly uses an inhaled corticosteroid, which seems to work well as a control medication, but also needs to use an albuterol inhaler about once every 3 weeks for suppression of asthma attacks (rescue therapy). Which antihypertensive drug or drug class poses the greatest risk of exacerbating the patient's asthma and counteracting the desired pulmonary effects of the albuterol, even though it might control his blood pressure well?

a. Diltiazem
b. Hydrochlorothiazide
c. Labetalol
d. Ramipril
e. Verapamil

190. We treat a patient with a drug that affects the clotting-thrombolytic systems for a time sufficient to let the drug's effects and blood levels stabilize at a therapeutic level. We then isolate platelets from a blood sample and test their in vitro aggregatory responses to ADP, collagen, PAF, and thromboxane A_2 (TXA_2). Aggregatory responses to ADP are inhibited; responses to the other platelet proaggregatory agonists are unaffected. Which of the following drugs exhibits these properties?

a. Aspirin
b. Bivalirudin
c. Clopidogrel
d. Heparin
e. Warfarin

191. A healthy adult subject is given an intravenous injection of a test drug. Both blood pressure and total peripheral resistance rise promptly. This is followed immediately by a reduction in heart rate. In repeated experiments we find that the vasopressor response is not affected by pretreatment with prazosin. However, pretreatment with atropine prevents the cardiac chronotropic response. The test drug is most likely which of the following?

a. Angiotensin II
b. Dobutamine
c. Isoproterenol
d. Norepinephrine
e. Phenylephrine

192. Nebivolol is a new oral nonselective β_1/β_2-adrenergic blocker that is indicated for managing essential hypertension. The drug allegedly causes fewer side effects than most other β-blockers, and orthostatic hypotension does not occur even with full therapeutic doses. The drug has no effects on changes of total peripheral resistance induced by infusion of phenylephrine or mixed- or indirect-acting sympathomimetics (eg, ephedrine or amphetamine, respectively). Nebivolol's antihypertensive mechanism of action clearly involves those common to all β-blockers, but another mechanism contributes to the overall effect. Given your general knowledge of blood pressure control and of autonomic/cardiovascular pharmacology, which of the following is the other "most likely" mechanism by which nebivolol helps lower pressure?

a. Competitively blocks postsynaptic (α_1) adrenergic receptors
b. Competitively blocks presynaptic (α_2) adrenergic receptors
c. Increases nitric oxide formation
d. Increases synthesis of TXA_2
e. Inhibits catechol-*O*-methyltransferase (COMT)

193. You are reviewing the medication history of a 59-year-old man. He has been taking ramipril and pravastatin for the last 5 years. Other medications include metformin for Type 2 diabetes mellitus, and escitalopram to help manage his depression. At his last clinic visit, a year ago, he was told to continue his current medications but he was also started on slow-release niacin because diet, exercise and other lifestyle modifications, and his current medications, were not adequate. What was the most likely reason for adding the niacin?

a. Counteract deficiencies of B-vitamin absorption caused by the antidepressant
b. Counteract polyphagia, and overeating caused by the metformin.
c. Lower HDL and triglyceride levels that did not respond adequately to the statin
d. Prevent statin-induced neuropathy
e. Slow the progression of diabetic nephropathy caused by the ACE inhibitor

194. Quinidine is ordered for a patient with recurrent atrial fibrillation and who refuses any interventions other than drugs in an attempt to control the arrhythmia. He has some pulmonary fibrosis and a thyroid disorder—both leading you to conclude that amiodarone therapy might not be the best approach. Which of the following statements applies to the quinidine?

a. Decreases SA nodal automaticity due to a strong anticholinergic/vagolytic effect
b. Is likely to increase blood pressure via a direct vasoconstrictor effect
c. Is contraindicated if the patient also requires anticoagulant therapy
d. Tends to increase electrical impulse conduction velocity through the AV node
e. Will increase cardiac contractility (positive inotropic effect) independent of its antiarrhythmic effects

195. A woman has received a cardiovascular drug that is absolutely contraindicated (category X) in pregnancy, but in the absence of pregnancy would have been deemed beneficial because of a particular cardiovascular disorder she has. Unfortunately, neither she nor her physician (whom she rarely visits) knew she was pregnant until she had just started the second trimester. The drug is stopped (and a suitable and safer alternative is started), but it is too late. Her baby is delivered prematurely, and stillborn. It is obvious from examination of the baby that there is a nasal deformity: the nose is flattened into the face, with no apparent bridge. Standard x-rays reveal epiphyseal stippling. These responses are characteristic of which of the following drugs?

a. Clonidine
b. Heparin, low molecular weight (eg, enoxaparin)
c. Hydrochlorothiazide
d. Nitroglycerin
e. Warfarin

196. A patient who has been taking an oral antihypertensive drug for about a year develops a positive Coombs test, and now you are worried about the possibility (although low) that hemolytic anemia may develop if the drug is continued. Which of the following drug is the most likely cause?

a. Captopril
b. Clonidine
c. Labetalol
d. Methyldopa
e. Prazosin

197. A patient presents with severe hypertension and tachycardia. Blood chemistry results, diagnostic radiologic studies, and the overall clinical presentation point to pheochromocytoma. The tumor appears operable, but the patient will have to wait a couple of weeks for an adrenalectomy. We prescribe phenoxybenzamine in the interim, with the goal of suppressing some of the major signs and symptoms caused by the tumor and the massive amounts of epinephrine it is releasing. Which of the following best summarizes what phenoxybenzamine does, or how it acts?

a. Controls blood pressure by blocking α-adrenergic receptors in the peripheral vasculature
b. Controls heart rate by selectively blocking β_1-adrenergic receptors
c. Inhibits catecholamine synthesis in the adrenal (suprarenal) medulla
d. Lowers blood pressure by inhibiting angiotensin-converting enzyme
e. Stimulates catechol-*O*-methyltransferase, thereby facilitating epinephrine's metabolic inactivation

198. We want to compare and contrast the cardiac and hemodynamic profiles of immediate-acting dihydropyridine-type calcium channel blockers (CCBs) and the nondihydropyridine, verapamil (or diltiazem). Which of the following best summarizes how, in general, a nondihydropyridine CCB differs from nifedipine?

a. Causes a much higher incidence of reflex tachycardia
b. Causes significant dose-dependent slowing of AV nodal conduction velocity
c. Causes significant venodilation, leading to profound orthostatic hypotension
d. Has significant and direct positive inotropic effects
e. Is best used in conjunction with a β-blocker or digoxin

199. Digoxin affects a host of cardiac electrophysiologic properties. Some of its effects are caused directly by the drug. Others are indirect: they may involve increasing "vagal tone" to the heart or other compensations, such as withdrawal of sympathetic tone, that arise when cardiac output is improved in a patient with heart failure. For some parameters the direct and indirect effects may be qualitatively (but not quantitatively) opposing, but one will predominate over the other. Which of the following is an expected and usually predominant effect of the drug when plasma levels of digoxin are in the therapeutic range, and electrolyte concentrations are within normal limits?

a. Increased rate of SA nodal depolarization
b. Increased atrial automaticity
c. Increased ventricular automaticity
d. Slowed AV nodal conduction velocity
e. Slowed conduction velocity through the atrial myocardium and His-Purkinje system

200. A patient has Stage 2 essential hypertension. After evaluating the responses to many other antihypertensive drugs, alone and in combination, the physician places the patient on oral hydralazine. Which of the following drug or drug combinations is likely to be needed, adjunctively, to manage the expected and unwanted cardiovascular and renal side effects of the hydralazine?

a. Captopril plus nifedipine
b. Digoxin plus spironolactone
c. Digoxin plus vitamin K
d. Diuretic and a β-blocker
e. Nitroglycerin
f. Triamterene plus amiloride

201. Your class just completed a minireview of the physiology and pathophysiology of blood pressure control and something finally dawned on a classmate: bradykinin, an endogenous vasodilator, contributes to keeping blood pressure low; and its metabolite, formed by an enzyme cleverly called bradykininase (kininase II), lacks vasodilator activity. Another colleague says "wouldn't it be great if we had a drug that could inhibit bradykinin's metabolic inactivation? We could probably use it as an antihypertensive!" You reply that we already have a drug—several, in fact—that does that very thing. Which of the following drugs or drug groups would that be?

a. Atenolol or metoprolol
b. Captopril or other "prils"
c. Hydrochlorothiazide or similar diuretic-antihypertensives
d. Labetalol or carvedilol
e. Losartan or other "sartans"

202. Nitroprusside is being infused intravenously to control blood pressure during surgery. The dose has gotten too high, and the drug has been administered too long. Refractoriness to the antihypertensive effects has occurred. Blood pressure is rising, and other signs and symptoms of potentially severe toxicity develop. What nitroprusside metabolite accounts for or at least contributes to these problems?

a. A highly efficacious α-adrenergic agonist
b. An extraordinarily potent and irreversible Na-K-ATPase inhibitor
c. An irreversible antagonist for angiotensin at the A-II receptors
d. Cyanide
e. Nitric oxide

203. A 66-year-old man who lives in a small rural town, and who has been treated by his family doctor for decades, presents at your medical center. He has coronary artery disease and "mild" heart failure that has been treated for the last 10 years with digoxin and several other drugs. His chief complaints upon arrival at your medical center are nausea, vomiting, and diarrhea. His ECG reveals a bigeminal rhythm and second-degree heart block. A drug-drug interaction is suspected. Which of the following coadministered drugs most likely provoked the problem?

a. Captopril
b. Cholestyramine
c. Furosemide
d. Lovastatin
e. Nitroglycerin

204. At high (but not necessarily toxic) blood levels, a cardiovascular drug causes many signs and symptoms that resemble what you see with "low-grade" aspirin toxicity (salicylism): light-headedness, tinnitus, and visual disturbances such as diplopia. Which of the following drugs most likely caused these responses?

a. Atropine
b. Captopril
c. Dobutamine
d. Propranolol
e. Quinidine

205. A patient is diagnosed with variant (vasospastic or Prinzmetal) angina. Which of the following drugs would be most appropriate, and generally regarded as most effective, for long term therapy aimed at reducing the incidence or severity of the coronary vasospasm?

a. Aspirin
b. Atorvastatin
c. Diltiazem
d. Nitroglycerin
e. Propranolol

206. It is generally acceptable and common to administer unfractionated heparin along with other classes of drugs that affect some aspect of the coagulation or thrombolytic processes. The proviso, of course, is to monitor closely all drug dosages, the appropriate blood tests, and the patient's responses overall, since the main risk is uncontrolled or excessive bleeding, if not frank hemorrhage.

There is one main exception. With which of the following drugs is concomitant administration of heparin contraindicated because of an extremely high risk of excessive bleeding or frank hemorrhage, relative to alternatives that would be preferred instead?

a. Alteplase (tPA)
b. Aspirin
c. Clopidogrel
d. Streptokinase
e. Warfarin

207. A 56-year-old man has a heart failure. His family doctor, who has been treating him since he was a young lad, has been treating him with digoxin, furosemide, and triamterene for several years. The patient now develops atrial fibrillation, and so his doctor starts quinidine and clopidogrel. Which of the following is the most likely outcome of adding the quinidine?

a. Development of signs and symptoms of quinidine toxicity (cinchonism)
b. Hyponatremia due to quinidine's ability to enhance diuretic-induced sodium loss
c. Onset of signs and symptoms of digoxin toxicity
d. Precipitous development of hypokalemia
e. Prompt suppression of cardiac contractility, onset of acute heart failure

208. Flecainide and propafenone are in Vaughan-Williams (antiarrhythmic) Class I-C. What is the clinically relevant "take home" message about this class of drugs?

a. Are only given for arrhythmias during acute myocardial infarction (MI)
b. Are particularly suited for patients with low ejection fractions or cardiac output
c. Are preferred drugs (drugs of choice) for relatively innocuous ventricular arrhythmias
d. Cause pulmonary fibrosis and a hypothyroid-like syndrome when given long term
e. Have a significant pro-arrhythmic effect (induction of lethal arrhythmias)

209. A patient has received excessive doses of nitroprusside, and toxic manifestations are developing in response to a metabolite. Which of the following drugs should be given to help nitroprusside's metabolism proceed further, leading to the formation of a less toxic metabolite?

a. Epinephrine
b. Sodium thiosulfate
c. Thrombin
d. Vitamin C
e. Vitamin E
f. Vitamin K

210. A 52-year-old woman with essential hypertension, hypercholesterolemia, and chronic-stable angina, develops severe constipation. It is attributed to one of her medications. Which one of the following is the most likely cause?

a. Atorvastatin
b. Captopril
c. Labetalol
d. Nitroglycerin
e. Verapamil

211. A patient with Stage 2 essential hypertension is treated with usually effective doses of an ACE inhibitor. After a suitable period of time blood pressure has not been lowered satisfactorily. The patient has been compliant with drug therapy and other recommendations (eg, weight reduction, exercise). A thiazide is added to the ACE inhibitor regimen. Which of the following is the most likely (but usually transient) untoward outcome of this drug add-on, for which you should monitor closely?

a. Excessive fall of blood pressure sufficient to cause syncope
b. Hypokalemia due to synergistic effects of the ACE inhibitor and the thiazide on renal potassium excretion
c. Onset of acute heart failure from depression of ventricular contractility
d. Paradoxical hypertensive crisis
e. Sudden prolongation of the PR interval and increasing degrees of heart block

212. A 45-year-old man post-myocardial infarction is being treated with several drugs, including unfractionated heparin. Stool guaiac on admission was negative, but is now 4+, and he has had several episodes of epistaxis. It turns out that he had received a significant overdose of the anticoagulant. Which of the following would be the best drug to administer to counteract the excessive effects of the heparin?

a. Aminocaproic acid
b. Aprotinin
c. Dipyridamole
d. Protamine sulfate
e. Vitamin K

213. A 45-year-old man asks his physician for a prescription for sildenafil to improve his sexual performance. Because of risks from a serious drug interaction, this drug should not be prescribed, and the patient should be urged not to try to obtain it from other sources, if he is also taking which of the following drugs?

a. Angiotensin-converting enzyme inhibitor
b. β-Adrenergic blocker
c. Nitrovasodilator (eg, nitroglycerin)
d. Statin-type antihypercholesterolemic drug
e. Thiazide or loop diuretic

214. A physician is preparing to administer a drug for which there is a label warning: "Do not administer this drug to patients with second-degree or greater heart block, or give with other drugs that may cause heart block." Which finding would be specifically indicative of heart block, and second-degree heart block in particular?

a. Auscultation of the precordium reveals an irregular rhythm.
b. Blood pressure is low.
c. Heart rate is abnormally low (bradycardia), but there is normal sinus rhythm.
d. ECG reveals ventricular ectopic beats.
e. ECG shows an excessively prolonged PR interval, and some P waves are not followed by a normal QRS complex.
f. ECG shows abnormally widened QRS complexes.

215. A 70-year-old woman is treated with sublingual nitroglycerin for occasional bouts of effort-induced angina. Which of the following best describes the main mechanism by which nitroglycerin causes its desired antianginal effects?

a. Blocks α-adrenergic receptors
b. Forms cyanide, much like the metabolism of nitroprusside does
c. Increases local synthesis and release of adenosine
d. Raises intracellular cGMP levels
e. Selectively dilates/relaxes coronary arteries

216. A 57-year-old patient complains of muscle aches, pain, and tenderness. These affect the legs and trunk. There is no fever, bruising, or any recent history of muscle trauma or strains (as from excessive exercise). He has myoglobinuria, a clinically significant fall of creatinine clearance, and a rise of plasma creatine kinase (CK) to levels nearly 10 times the upper limit of normal. Which drug is the most likely cause of these findings?

a. Aspirin (low dose) for its cardioprotective/antiplatelet effects
b. Captopril for hypertension and heart failure
c. Carvedilol for hypertension, heart failure, and angina prophylaxis
d. Furosemide as adjunctive management of his heart failure
e. Rosuvastatin to control his hypercholesterolemia and the associated risks

217. We use standard invasive hemodynamic techniques to measure or calculate the effects of various drugs on such parameters as arterial pressure, total peripheral resistance, and central venous (right atrial) pressures. The goal is to evaluate whether the drugs primarily cause arteriolar or venular dilation, or affect both sides of the circulation. Which of the following drugs exerts vasodilator effects only in the arterial side of the circulation?

a. Hydralazine
b. Losartan
c. Nifedipine
d. Nitroglycerin
e. Prazosin

218. A 20-year-old collegiate varsity hockey player is referred to you by his coach. The young athlete has excessive bruising after a very physical match 2 days before. His knee had been bothering him earlier, so he took two 325 mg aspirin tablets several hours before the next game. He got checked hard into the boards many times during the game, but denies any excessive or unusual trauma. As you ponder the situation you order several blood tests. Which test or finding do you most likely expect to be altered as a result of the prior aspirin use?

a. Activated partial thromboplastin time (APTT)
b. Bleeding time
c. INR (International Normalized Ratio)
d. Platelet count
e. Prothrombin time

219. A patient in the coronary care unit develops episodes of paroxysmal AV nodal reentrant tachycardia. What drug would generally be considered first-line for promptly stopping the arrhythmia?

a. Adenosine
b. Digoxin
c. Edrophonium
d. Phenylephrine
e. Propranolol

220. A 60-year-old man, hospitalized for an acute myocardial infarction, is treated with warfarin (among other drugs). What is the main mechanism by which warfarin causes the effects for which it is given?

a. Increase in the plasma level of factor IX
b. Inhibition of thrombin and early coagulation steps
c. Inhibition of synthesis/activation of prothrombin and factors VII, IX, and X
d. Inhibition of platelet aggregation
e. Activation of plasminogen

221. A 42-year-old man with an acute MI is treated with alteplase, and electrocardiographic and hemodynamic status improves quickly. By what mechanism did the alteplase cause its beneficial effects?

a. Blocked platelet ADP receptors
b. Inhibited platelet thromboxane production
c. Inhibited synthesis or activation of vitamin K-dependent coagulation factors
d. Prevented aggregation of adjacent platelets by blocking glycoprotein IIb/IIIa receptors
e. Promoted conversion of plasminogen to plasmin

222. A patient with atrial fibrillation is placed on long-term arrhythmia control with amiodarone. In addition to "standard" monitoring, what should be assessed periodically in order to detect adverse effects that are rather unique to this drug among virtually all the antiarrhythmics?

a. Blood glucose, triglyceride, cholesterol, and sodium concentrations
b. Hearing thresholds (audiometry) and plasma albumin concentration
c. Prothrombin time and antinuclear antibody (ANA) titers
d. Pulmonary function and thyroid hormone status
e. White cell counts and blood urate concentration

223. A 64-year-old woman with a history of coronary heart disease has several episodes of transient ischemic attacks (TIAs). Low-dose aspirin would be considered a treatment for prevention of thrombosis, but she has a history of severe "aspirin sensitivity" manifest as intense bronchoconstriction and urticaria. Which of the following would you consider to be the best alternative to the aspirin?

a. Acetaminophen
b. Aminocaproic acid
c. Clopidogrel
d. Dipyridamole
e. Streptokinase

224. A patient who has excessively slow AV nodal conduction rates, that unfortunately haven't been recognized, is started on a drug. As soon as blood levels climb toward the usual therapeutic range the patient goes into complete heart block. Which drug most likely provoked this further prolongation of the PR interval, ultimately leading to the cessation of all AV nodal conduction?

a. Captopril
b. Losartan
c. Nifedipine
d. Nitroglycerin
e. Prazosin
f. Verapamil

225. A patient with heart failure, Stage 1 essential hypertension, and hyperlipidemia (elevated LDL cholesterol and abnormally low HDL-C) is taking furosemide, captopril, atenolol, and simvastatin (an HMG-CoA reductase inhibitor).

During a scheduled physical examination, about a month after starting all the drugs, the patient reports a severe, hacking, and relentless cough. Other vital signs, and the overall physical assessment, are consistent with good control of both the heart failure and blood pressure, and indicate no other underlying disease or abnormalities. Results of blood tests are not yet available. Which of the following is the most likely cause of the cough?

a. An expected side effect of the captopril
b. An allergic reaction to the statin
c. Dyspnea due to captopril's known and powerful bronchoconstrictor action
d. Excessive doses of the furosemide, which led to hypovolemia
e. Hyperkalemia caused by an interaction between furosemide and captopril
f. Pulmonary edema from the loop diuretic

226. A patient with a history of hypertension, heart failure, and peripheral vascular disease has been on oral therapy, with drugs suitable for each, for about 3 months. He runs out of the medications and plans to have the prescriptions refilled in a week or so when he goes into town from the remote farm where he lives.

Within a day or two after stopping his medications he experiences an episode of severe tachycardia accompanied by tachyarrhythmias, and an abrupt rise of blood pressure to 240/140 mm Hg—well above pretreatment levels. He complains of chest pain, anxiety, and a pounding headache. Soon thereafter he suffers a hemorrhagic stroke.

Which of the following drugs or drug groups that the man was taking, and stopped taking suddenly, most likely caused these responses?

a. ACE inhibitor
b. Clonidine
c. Digoxin
d. Furosemide
e. Nifedipine (a long-acting formulation)
f. Warfarin

227. A patient develops atrial fibrillation and rapid onset of significant heart failure and is admitted to the hospital's coronary care unit. As of today he has been receiving otherwise "proper" doses of a drug for 5 days straight. Dosing was done correctly, starting with usual maintenance doses; no loading dose strategy was used. Then, and rather precipitously, the patient develops signs and symptoms of widespread thrombotic events, and platelet counts decline significantly concomitant with the thrombosis. The patient dies within 24 hours of the onset of signs and symptoms of thrombosis. Which drug most likely caused these ultimately fatal responses?

a. Abciximab
b. Clopidogrel
c. Heparin (unfractionated)
d. Nifedipine
e. Warfarin

228. Your patient has bipolar illness, hypercholesterolemia, chronic-stable angina, and Stage 1 essential hypertension. He has been taking lithium and an SSRI for the bipolar illness. Cardiovascular drugs include atorvastatin, diltiazem, sublingual nitroglycerin, captopril, and hydrochlorothiazide. Which outcome, due to interactions involving these drugs, should you most likely expect?

a. Development of acute psychosis from an ACE inhibitor-SSRI interaction
b. Development of a hypomanic state from antagonism of lithium's action by the nitroglycerin
c. Lithium toxicity because of hyponatremia caused by the hydrochlorothiazide
d. Loss of cholesterol control from antagonism of the HMG Co-A reductase inhibitor by the antidepressant
e. Worsening of angina because the SSRI counteracts the effects of the calcium channel blocker
f. Worsening of angina because the lithium antagonizes the effects of the nitroglycerin

229. A patient has a history that includes angina pectoris brought on by "modest" exercise and is accompanied by transient electrocardiographic changes consistent with myocardial ischemia. There is no evidence of coronary vasospasm.

He suddenly develops chest discomfort. Heart rate rises to 170 to 190 beats/min, but rhythm is normal except for infrequent ventricular ectopic beats that quickly stop on their own. His blood pressure varies between 180/110 and 200/120 mm Hg. He has been taking low-dose aspirin (81 mg) daily, sublingual nitroglycerin as needed, and a statin. An ambulance is called. Before he arrives at the hospital he receives one sublingual nitroglycerin tablet and IV morphine, plus oxygen via nasal cannula, from the EMTs on the ambulance.

Although there are several things that need to be done for immediate care once he reaches the hospital, which drug would you administer to reduce heart rate, blood pressure, and the risk of more ventricular ectopy?

a. Aspirin (high dose)
b. Captopril
c. Furosemide
d. Labetalol
e. Lidocaine
f. Nitroglycerin (increased dose as a bolus)
g. Prazosin

230. A first-year house officer notices that a patient is experiencing significant and rapidly rising blood pressure (currently 180/120 mm Hg). One of the medications the patient had been taking is immediate-acting nifedipine oral capsules. There is a dose of this nifedipine formulation at the bedside, so the physician pricks the capsule open and squirts the contents into the patient's mouth. This technique avoids "first-pass" metabolism of the drug and causes rapid absorption and all the effects associated with this calcium channel blocker. What is the most likely outcome of giving nifedipine as described here?

a. AV nodal block
b. Further rise of heart rate, worsening of the ventricular arrhythmia
c. Hypotension and bradycardia
d. Normalization of blood pressure and heart rate
e. Return of blood pressure toward normal, no significant effect on heart rate or the ECG

231. A 55-year-old patient with multiple cardiovascular diseases is being treated with low-dose (81 mg/d) aspirin, digoxin, furosemide, triamterene, atorvastatin, and nitroglycerin—all prescribed by the family physician he's had for decades. The patient now experiences nausea, vomiting, and anorexia, and describes a "yellowish-greenish tint" (chromatopsia) to white objects and bright lights. These signs and symptoms are most characteristic of toxicity due to which drug?

a. Atorvastatin
b. Digoxin
c. Furosemide
d. Nitroglycerin
e. Triamterene

232. A 28-year-old female patient has Stage 1 essential hypertension (resting BP 144/98), tachycardia, and occasional palpitations (ventricular ectopic beats). Normally we might consider prescribing a β-blocker to control the blood pressure and cardiac responses, but our patient also has asthma, and she is trying to get pregnant. Which drug would be the best alternative to the β-blocker in terms of likely efficacy on pressure and heart rate, and in terms of relative safety?

a. Diltiazem
b. Enalapril
c. Furosemide
d. Phentolamine
e. Prazosin

233. A patient presents with hypertension. The underlying cause—a pheochromocytoma—is not looked-for or detected in the initial work-up. An oral antihypertensive drug is prescribed. We soon find that the patient's blood pressure has risen to levels above pretreatment levels—so much so that we are worried about imminently dangerous effects from the drug-induced worsening of hypertension. Concomitant with the drug-induced rise of blood pressure the patient develops signs and symptoms of heart failure. Which drug was most likely administered?

a. Captopril
b. Hydrochlorothiazide
c. Labetalol
d. Losartan
e. Propranolol
f. Verapamil

234. A patient on long-term warfarin therapy has an INR that is excessive (6.5; normal, not anticoagulated, is 1.0; the target for this patient was 2.5). She reports episodes of epistaxis over the last 2 days and now there is a great risk of serious bleeding episodes. In addition to stopping warfarin administration for a day or more, which drug would you want to administer to counteract warfarin's excessive effects that led to spontaneous bleeding?

a. Aminocaproic acid
b. Epoetin alfa
c. Ferrous sulfate
d. Phytonadione (vitamin K)
e. Protamine sulfate

235. A patient with hypertension and heart failure has been treated for 2 years with carvedilol and lisinopril. He has just had hip replacement surgery, but because he is not ambulating he is started on unfractionated heparin, postoperatively, for prophylaxis of deep venous thrombosis. Oral antacids and esomeprazole (gastric parietal cell proton pump inhibitor) have been added for prophylaxis of acute stress ulcers. Five days post-op, he experiences sudden onset dyspnea and electrocardiographic and other indications of an acute MI. The patient's platelet counts are dangerously low and there are signs and symptoms of reduced blood flow to the distal extremities. Which of the following is the most likely underlying problem?

a. Accidental substitution of low-molecular-weight heparin (LMWH) for unfractionated heparin
b. Accidental/inadvertent aspirin administration
c. Hemolytic anemia from a carvedilol-ACE inhibitor interaction
d. Heparin-induced thrombocytopenia
e. Reduced heparin effects by increased metabolic clearance (caused by esomeprazole)

236. A patient with angina pectoris is started on a nitroglycerin transdermal delivery system (skin patch) for prophylaxis of his angina. He wears the patch 24 hours a day, 7 days a week, except for the few minutes when he showers each day. What is the main concern with "around-the-clock" administration of this or other long-acting formulations of nitrovasodilators?

a. Cyanide poisoning
b. Development of tolerance to their vasodilator actions
c. Gradual development of reflex bradycardia in response to successive doses
d. Onset of delayed, characteristic adverse responses including thrombosis and thrombocytopenia
e. Paradoxical vasoconstriction leading to hypertension

237. For many hypertensive patients we can prescribe either lisinopril (or an alternative in the same class) or losartan. What statement correctly summarizes how losartan differs from lisinopril or other lisinopril-like drugs?

a. Lisinopril competitively blocks catecholamine-mediated vasoconstriction, losartan does not
b. Lisinopril effectively inhibits synthesis of Angiotensin II, losartan does not
c. Losartan causes a higher incidence of bronchospasm and hyperuricemia
d. Losartan is preferred for managing hypertension during pregnancy, whereas captopril is contraindicated
e. Losartan is suitable for administration to patients with heart failure, whereas captopril and related drugs should be avoided

238. A 46-year-old man has Stage 1 essential hypertension (resting BP 150/98), primary hypercholesterolemia, and modestly elevated fasting glucose levels (130 mg/dL) measured on several occasions. His cholesterol levels (total, HDL, LDL) have not been acceptably modified by dietary changes and daily use of a statin. The physician adds ezetimibe to the regimen. Which of the following statements summarizes ezetimibe's actions, or what would be expected in response to its use?

a. Exerts profound cardiac negative inotropic effects that poses a risk of heart block
b. Frequently causes orthostatic hypotension that in turn triggers reflex cardiac stimulation
c. More likely than other drugs to increase the risk of severe statin-induced myopathy
d. Reduces intestinal cholesterol uptake, has no direct hepatic effect to inhibit cholesterol synthesis
e. Significantly increases risk of atherosclerotic plaque rupture

239. A 58-year-old man presents in the emergency department with his first episode of acute coronary syndrome (ACS) and all evidence points to a myocardial infarction. Angioplasty and stenting are not possible because the cardiac cath lab is busy with other higher-priority patients, so administration of a thrombolytic drug is the only option. Which of the following is the most important determinant, overall, of the success of thrombolytic therapy in terms of salvaging viable cardiac muscle (or other ischemic tissues)?

a. Choosing a "human" (cloned) plasminogen activator (eg, tPA), rather than one that is bacterial-derived
b. Infarct location (ie, anterior wall of left ventricular vs another site/wall)
c. Presence of collateral blood vessels to the infarct-related coronary artery
d. Systolic blood pressure at the time the MI is diagnosed
e. Time from onset of infarction to administration of the thrombolytic agent

240. A patient with an acute coronary syndrome is given a variety of cardiovascular drugs as he is being readied for transport to the cath lab for possible placement of a stent. One of the meds is abciximab. Which of the following best describes the mechanism of action of this drug?

a. Blocks thrombin receptors selectively
b. Blocks ADP receptors
c. Blocks glycoprotein IIb/IIIa receptors
d. Inhibits cyclooxygenase
e. Inhibits prostacyclin production

241. A patient presents in the emergency department with acute hypotension that requires treatment. Hypovolemia is ruled-out as a cause or contributor, and information gathered from the patient and family indicates the cause is overdose of an antihypertensive drug.

One approach to treatment is to administer a pharmacologic (ordinarily effective) dose of phenylephrine, an α-adrenergic agonist. You do just that, because blood pressure fails to rise at all—and a second dose doesn't work either. On which antihypertensive drug did the patient most likely overdose?

a. Captopril or another ACE inhibitor
b. Hydralazine
c. Prazosin
d. Thiazide diuretic (eg, hydrochlorothiazide)
e. Verapamil

242. An elderly man who has just been referred to your practice has been taking an oral drug for symptomatic relief of benign prostatic hypertrophy (BPH). In addition to its effects on smooth muscles of the prostate and urethra, this drug can lower blood pressure in such a way that it reflexly triggers tachycardia, positive inotropy, and increased AV nodal conduction, at least for a short time after treatment is started. Initial oral dosages of this drug also have been associated with a high incidence of syncope. The drug neither dilates nor constricts the bronchi. It causes the pupils of the eyes to constrict and interferes with mydriasis in dim light.

Which prototype is most similar to this unnamed drug in terms of the pharmacologic profile?

a. Captopril
b. Hydrochlorothiazide (prototype thiazide diuretic)
c. Labetalol
d. Nifedipine
e. Prazosin
f. Propranolol
g. Verapamil

243. You are contemplating starting ACE inhibitor therapy for a patient with essential hypertension. Which of the following patient-related condition(s) contraindicates use of any ACE inhibitor and so should be ruled out before you prescribe this drug?

a. Asthma
b. Heart failure
c. Hyperlipidemia, coronary artery disease
d. Hypokalemia
e. A woman who is pregnant or may become pregnant

244. A patient develops sinus bradycardia. Heart rate is dangerously low, and an effective and safe drug needs to be given right away. Which drug would be the best choice for normalizing heart rate without initiating any other arrhythmias?

a. Atropine
b. Amiodarone
c. Edrophonium
d. Lidocaine
e. Phentolamine

245. A patient presents in the emergency department with severe angina pectoris, and acute myocardial ischemia is confirmed by electrocardiographic and other clinical indicators. Unknown to the ED team is the fact that the ischemia is due to coronary vasospasm, not to coronary occlusion with thrombi. Given this etiology, which drug, administered in usually effective doses, may actually make the vasospasm and the resulting ischemia worse?

a. Alteplase (tPA)
b. Aspirin
c. Captopril
d. Nitroglycerin
e. Propranolol
f. Verapamil

246. Many clinical studies have investigated the benefits of daily aspirin use in the primary prevention of coronary heart disease and sudden death in adults. The results have been somewhat inconsistent, in part because different dosages were studied, and there were important differences in the populations that were studied. Nonetheless, many (if not most) of the studies have revealed that for some patients aspirin increased the incidence of a particularly unwanted adverse response, even when dosages were kept within the range typically recommended for cardioprotection (eg, 81-162 mg/d). What is the most likely adverse response associated with aspirin prophylaxis, particularly in patients who have a low risk of an acute coronary syndrome or cardiovascular disease in general?

a. Centrolobular hepatic necrosis
b. Hemorrhagic stroke
c. Nephropathy
d. Tachycardia and hypotension leading to acute myocardial ischemia
e. Vasospastic angina

247. A patient with essential hypertension has been treated with a fixed-dose combination product that contains hydrochlorothiazide and triamterene. Blood pressure and electrolyte profiles have been kept within acceptable limits for the last 18 months. Now, however, blood pressure has risen to the point where the physician wants to add another antihypertensive drug. The drug is started; after several weeks blood pressure falls into an acceptable range, but the patient has become hyperkalemic. What drug was added and was most likely responsible for the desired blood pressure fall and the unwanted rise of potassium levels?

a. Diltiazem
b. Prazosin
c. Propranolol
d. Ramipril
e. Verapamil

248. A patient has a supraventricular tachycardia. We inject a drug and heart rate falls to a normal (or at least more acceptable) level. Although this drug caused the desired response, it did so without any direct effect in or on the heart. Which drug was most likely used?

a. Edrophonium
b. Esmolol
c. Phenylephrine
d. Propranolol
e. Verapamil

249. A 69-year-old man presents with NYHA Stage II (mild) heart failure. His symptoms failed to improve adequately in response to captopril and carvedilol so the physician stops the carvedilol and adds usual therapeutic doses of digoxin and furosemide. At a follow-up examination 3 months later, we find good symptomatic relief of the heart failure. Blood electrolytes and all other lab tests are within normal limits. At this time, which electrocardiographic change would you expect to see in response to the digoxin, compared with a baseline (pretreatment) ECG?

a. P waves widened, amplitude increased
b. PR intervals prolonged
c. QRS complexes widened
d. RR intervals shortened
e. ST segments elevated

250. A 23-year-old nonpregnant woman has been using a preparation of oral ergotamine to manage her frequent migraine headaches. She consumes an excessive dose of the drug while trying to abort a particularly severe and refractory attack. Which adverse cardiac or cardiovascular consequences are most likely to occur as a result of the ergot overdose?

a. Myocardial and peripheral (eg, limb) ischemia due to intense vasoconstriction
b. Renal failure secondary to rhabdomyolysis
c. Spontaneous bleeding due to direct inhibition of platelet activation/aggregation
d. Syncope secondary to acute hypotension
e. Tachycardia, tachyarrhythmias from β_1-adrenergic receptor activation

251. A patient presents with a blood pressure of 220/120 and a heart rate of 90 beats/min despite usually effective antihypertensive drug therapy. Further work-up indicates the patient has a rare cause of these and other signs and symptoms: pheochromocytoma. You realize that β-adrenergic blockers are useful as antihypertensive drugs, and for helping to normalize heart rate in patients with supraventricular tachycardia. As a result of the diagnosis, and your knowledge, you administer a usually effective dose of propranolol. What is the most likely outcome of doing this?

a. Blood pressure falls promptly, followed by reflex tachycardia.
b. Epinephrine release from the tumor is suppressed, hemodynamics normalize.
c. Heart rate and cardiac function rise quickly because the β-blocker has triggered additional epinephrine release from the tumor.
d. Left ventricular afterload is decreased, cardiac output rises via increases of both left ventricular stroke volume and heart rate.
e. Total peripheral resistance rises, cardiac output falls, and the patient goes into cardiogenic shock

252. A 59-year-old man presents in the emergency department with crushing chest discomfort. An ECG indicates a small transmural left ventricular free wall infarction, and prompt cardiac catheterization and assessment of prior lab results indicate significant hypercholesterolemia. The patient is given all the drugs listed below, for both immediate management of the ischemia and its symptoms and for long-term prevention of a subsequent, and potentially fatal, MI. Which of the following drugs would provide immediate relief of the consequences of myocardial ischemia, but has no long-term effects to reduce the risk of sudden death or ventricular dysfunction from another MI?

a. Aspirin
b. Atorvastatin
c. Captopril
d. Nitroglycerin
e. Propranolol

253. A 65-year-old woman is transferred to the thoracic surgery ICU after cardiac surgery. She has diffuse rales bilaterally, a pulse of 90 beats/min, an elevated central venous pressure, and a blood pressure of 160/98 mm Hg. The surgery resident wants to inject an otherwise-correct dose of an IV drug to control heart rate and blood pressure, but grabs a syringe that contains another drug. The patient's heart rate increases to 150 beats/min and her blood pressure rises to 180/106. Which of the following drugs did this patient most likely receive in error?

a. Dobutamine
b. Esmolol
c. Neostigmine
d. Propranolol
e. Verapamil

254. A 50-year-old man is aware of the benefits of aspirin in terms of reducing the risk of death from an acute myocardial infarction, mainly because he has seen many of the ads and internet posts about this. He notices that the usual recommended dose of aspirin for cardioprotection is 81 mg/d, but reasons that the bigger the dose, the bigger and better the protective effect. He has taken "at least" 1000 mg of aspirin (three "regular strength" aspirin tablets) twice a day for the last 6 months. While he is fortunate in terms of having no apparent gastrointestinal (GI) adverse effects that are associated with long-term, high-dose aspirin use, he suffers an MI. Autopsy results show considerable platelet occlusion of several coronary vessels. Which of the following summarizes the most likely mechanism by which high-dose aspirin caused these adverse events?

a. Inhibited TXA_2 synthesis in platelets
b. Favored adhesion of platelets to the coronary vascular endothelium
c. Ruptured atherosclerotic plaque in the coronaries, exposing platelets to collagen
d. Suppressed hepatic synthesis of vitamin K-dependent clotting factors
e. Triggered excessive activation of platelets by ADP

255. You and a colleague are discussing which α-blocker to use, adjunctively, to control blood pressure in a pheochromocytoma patient. Your colleague correctly states that phenoxybenzamine is the "preferred" drug. You state that prazosin would be a better choice. Which of the following statements about prazosin is correct in comparison with phenoxybenzamine, and might actually support your proposal that it would be a better choice?

a. Causes not only peripheral α-blockade but also suppresses adrenal epinephrine release
b. Has a longer duration of action, which enables less frequent dosing
c. Has good intrinsic β-blocking activity, phenoxybenzamine does not
d. Overdoses, and the hypotension it may cause, are easier to manage pharmacologically
e. Will not cause orthostatic hypotension, which is a common consequence of phenoxybenzamine

256. In clinic you meet a 55-year-old man who is described by the attending as having metabolic syndrome, including high LDL and low HDL cholesterol levels, essential hypertension, Type 2 diabetes mellitus, and anginal attacks upon stress about once every 2 months. He currently has asymptomatic hyperuricemia, but has a gout attack about once a year. The patient is obese (92 kg), 6 ft tall, and has a body mass index (kilogram per square meter of body surface area) of 40 (normal or desirable no more than 24.9 kg/m^2). He has a 20-year history of smoking a half pack of cigarettes a day, and both parents died in their late 50s—the father from an acute MI, the mother from hemorrhagic stroke. The gentleman is taking medications deemed appropriate for each of the conditions noted above. One is colesevelam. What is the probable reason why the colesevelam was given?

a. Counteracts hypokalemia caused by a thiazide diuretic
b. Lowers LDL-cholesterol levels
c. Lowers plasma urate levels, lowers of gout
d. Prevents myocardial ischemia, angina, by reducing myocardial oxygen demand
e. Provides antihypertensive and natriuretic effects

257. A man has an aneurysm in the aortic root, a consequence of Marfan syndrome. He experiences a hypertensive crisis that requires prompt blood pressure control. Nitroprusside will be infused for its immediate antihypertensive effects. Which of the following drugs would we administer along with the nitroprusside to minimize the risk of aneurysm rupture due to increases of left ventricular dP/dt as blood pressure falls?

a. Atropine
b. Diazoxide
c. Furosemide
d. Phentolamine
e. Propranolol

258. In 2001, Zoccali and colleagues published (Lancet 358:2113) an article entitled Plasma Concentration of Asymmetrical Dimethylarginine (ADMA) and Mortality in Patients with End-stage Renal Disease: A Prospective Study. They concluded that increased plasma levels of ADMA are a strong predictor of all-cause mortality, and especially negative cardiovascular outcomes, in their study population. Several other studies (eg, Krempl, Elevation of Asymmetric Dimethyl Arginine in Patients with Unstable Angina and Recurrent Cardiovascular Events, Eur Heart J., 26:1846, 2005) had similar outcomes, and now there is considerable interest in therapeutic agents that might beneficially affect ADMA's cellular actions or metabolic roles. Which of the following properties applies to ADMA?

a. Inhibits angiotensin-converting enzyme, blocks A-II receptors
b. Inhibits nitric oxide synthase (NOS)
c. Inhibits TXA_2 synthesis
d. Mimics tumor necrosis factor
e. Stimulates leukotriene synthesis via lipoxygenases

259. Nicotinic acid (niacin), in the relatively large doses that are used to treat certain hyperlipoproteinemias, causes an often-disturbing cutaneous flush and pruritus. What mechanism or action contributes to the vasodilatory response and the flushing?

a. Activation of α-adrenergic receptors on vascular smooth muscle
b. Calcium channel blockade in vascular smooth muscle
c. Local production of prostaglandins
d. Release of angiotensin II
e. Release of histamine

260. The figure below shows typical cardiovascular responses to the slow intravenous injection of four adrenergic drugs into a normal, resting subject. Assume the doses of each are sufficient to cause the effects we see here, but not so high that toxic effects occur. No other drugs are present, and sufficient time has been allowed to enable complete dissipation of the effects of any prior drugs. The dashed line between the systolic and diastolic pressure traces approximates mean arterial pressure.

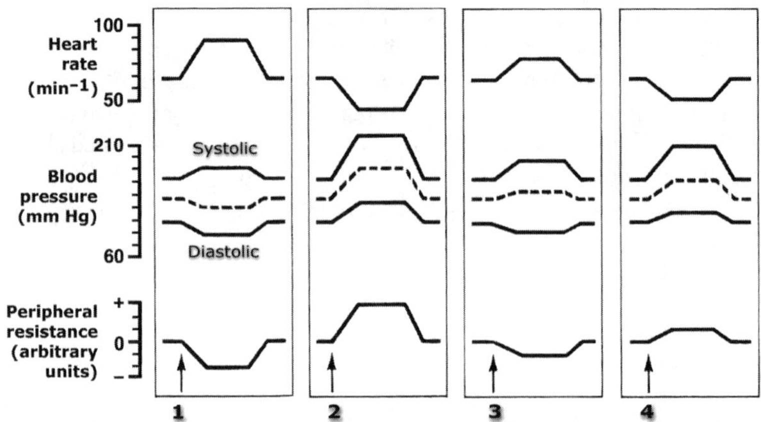

Abbreviations used, and answer choices, are

EPI, epinephrine
ISO, isoproterenol
NE, norepinephrine
PHE, phenylephrine
PHN, phentolamine
PRO, propranolol

Select the letter that indicates the drugs that are ordered in the sequence shown (1, 2, 3, 4).

a. EPI, NE, PHE, ISO
b. ISO, EPI, NE, PHE
c. ISO, PHE, EPI, NE
d. NE, ISO, PHE, EPI
e. PHE, EPI, NE, PRO
f. PHE, ISO, NE, EPI
g. PRO, PHN, PHE, ISO

261. You've diagnosed essential hypertension in a 55-year-old man. He has adhered well to your instructions with respect to diet, losing weight, and exercising, but now, at a follow-up visit, you believe some drug therapy would be beneficial. When you initially took his history you learned that he is a pipe smoker and an avid motorcyclist. Lab tests indicate his uric acid levels are elevated; he has had five acute gout attacks over the prior 10 years. He also reported a Raynaud-like problem: even when ambient temperatures are in the 50°F range, while riding his motorcycle the wind and the "cold" cause his fingers to blanch and become numb because of cold-induced vasoconstriction. Which drug or drug group would be the most logical to try to manage his blood pressure and reduce the incidence or severity of the hyperuricemia and peripheral vasospasm? Assume there are no contraindications or precautions, other than those mentioned above, for the drug you choose.

a. Angiotensin-converting enzyme inhibitor
b. Angiotensin receptor blocker
c. Atenolol (or metoprolol)
d. Calcium channel blocker
e. Propranolol
f. Thiazide diuretic

Questions 262 to 264

Look at the ECG below and answer the following three (3) questions, 262-264. It shows an uninterrupted tracing of lead V1, before and after carotid sinus massage (at arrow).

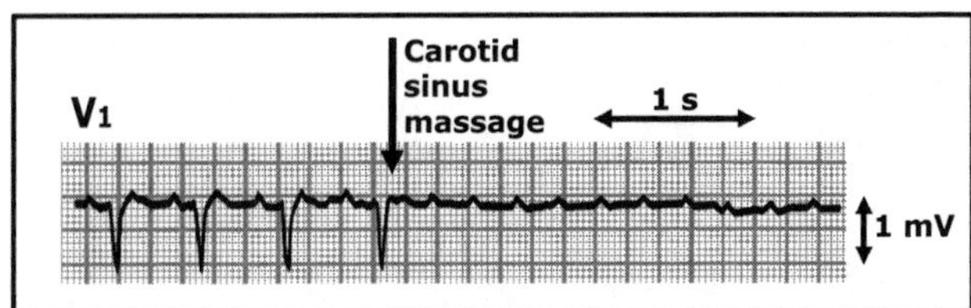

262. What is the mechanism by which carotid massage exerted its effect?

a. Activated what is tantamount to the baroreceptor reflex, increasing vagal tone and acetylcholine release considerably
b. Caused catecholamine release
c. Directly stimulated the parasympathetic ganglion that ultimately innervates the SA node
d. Induced atrial fibrillation (atrial rate > 300/min)
e. Occluded venous return to the heart, thereby interfering with filling and contraction of all heart chambers "downstream" of the right atrium

263. Based on the outcome of carotid sinus massage, what can you say about the origin of the aberrant electrical activity that leads to the tachycardia you see before the massage?

a. Bundle of Kent (ie, anomalous or accessory pathway for AV conduction) yielding retrograde and antegrade conduction
b. His-Purkinje system
c. Left bundle branch
d. Multiple ectopic ventricular foci
e. Supraventricular

264. What drug, given as an intravenous bolus, might be used as an alternative to carotid massage, causing essentially the same outcome and, therefore, the same interpretation of the origin of the arrhythmia?

a. Adenosine
b. Atropine
c. Epinephrine
d. Isoproterenol
e. Lidocaine

Cardiovascular Pharmacology

Answers

178. The answer is c. *(Brunton, pp 823-832. Katzung, pp 191, 195-196, 199t.)* At usual therapeutic doses, nitroglycerin (NTG) acts primarily as a peripheral venodilator. At higher doses arterial dilation also occurs. The net effect is that, particularly with excessive doses, peripheral vasodilation occurs and blood pressure (BP) falls. Critical among these pressure changes is a fall of diastolic BP. I say critical because DBP is the main driving force for blood flow through the coronary vasculature. Up to a point autoregulation of coronary flow may help maintain cardiac perfusion, but once DBP reaches a certain level coronary blood flow is inadequate to meet the oxygen demands of the myocardium (ie, ischemia has developed). Add to the underperfusion of the heart by reduced DBP the fact that if BP falls by a sufficient amount, and sufficiently fast, the baroreceptor reflex is activated. That, in turn, increases heart rate and contractility—an increase of myocardial oxygen demand simultaneous with reduced oxygen supply due to the decreased coronary perfusion.

NTG does not, and cannot, induce coronary vasoconstriction directly (a). Deteriorated (old and/or improperly stored) nitroglycerin (b)—particularly sublingual tablet forms—will not provoke ischemia or angina, as described here. It simply will exert less (or no) peripheral vasodilation. NTG is often used, with success and usually with other antianginal drugs (usually a CCB, but not β-blockers) for patients with coronary vasospasm (c). Finally, for patients with angina that is not vasospastic in etiology, NTG is frequently prescribed with a β-adrenergic blocker (e), the sublingual NTG for acute symptom control and the β-blocker for prophylaxis.

Note: There is an interesting and somewhat controversial phenomenon ascribed to NTG and some other vasodilator drugs: coronary steal. In essence, vasodilation shunts or diverts (steals) blood flow from areas of low perfusion (eg, a stenotic coronary vessel) to areas of high perfusion. The postulated outcome is that poorly perfused vessels (and the tissues served by them) become even less well perfused, thereby causing or worsening distal tissue ischemia.

179. The answer is d. (*Brunton, pp 886-887. Katzung, pp 214-215, 219, 1023.*) Digoxin inhibits the sarcolemmal Na^+,K^+-ATPase (sodium pump). This reduces the active (ATP-dependent) extrusion of intracellular Na^+. The relative excess of intracellular Na^+ competes with intracellular Ca^{2+} for sites on a sarcolemmal 2Na-Ca exchange diffusion carrier, such that less Ca^{2+} is extruded from the cells. The net results include a rise of free $[Ca^{2+}]_i$ and greater actin-myosin interactions (ie, a positive inotropic effect that increases cardiac output through an increase of stroke volume).

Digoxin has no direct agonist or antagonist effects on β-adrenergic receptors (a), nor does it directly facilitate G protein-related processes (b). Very high concentrations of digoxin can increase mitochondrial Ca^{2+} release, but this has been demonstrated only in in vitro models of isolated mitochondria. Whether it occurs in vivo as an element of digoxin toxicity isn't known. Regardless, it is not the main mechanism by which digoxin-induced positive inotropy, or the symptomatic relief it affords, occur. Stimulation of cAMP synthesis in the heart applies to β-adrenergic agonists, but not to digoxin.

180. The answer is e. (*Brunton, pp 832-838, 914. Katzung, pp 199-201, 236-237, 243, 283.*) Verapamil, a nondihydropyridine calcium channel blocker (CCB), depresses both the SA node and the AV node and would be effective for prophylaxis of paroxysmal atrial or supraventricular tachycardia. Nifedipine (c), the prototypic dihydropyridine CCB, has little effect on PSVT because it and the other dihydropyridines lack cardiac depressant effects. Moreover, if we chose a fast-/immediate-acting dosage form of nifedipine, it might trigger substantial reflex cardiac stimulation. The increased sympathetic tone to the heart could worsen the PSVT. Nitroglycerin (d) is mainly a venodilator, but it can cause falls of arterial blood pressure sufficient to trigger reflex cardiac activation that would exacerbate the tachycardia. Adenosine (a) may be useful in diagnosing whether ventricular tachycardia is of supraventricular or ventricular origin, because it effectively slows AV nodal conduction. It is also used as acute therapy for PSVT. However, it is a fast- and short-acting parenteral drug, which renders it unsuitable for the condition I stated: outpatient prophylaxis. Lidocaine (b) is mainly used for ventricular tachyarrhythmias, not those of supraventricular origin. Both adenosine and lidocaine are parenteral drugs with short half-lives; neither property makes them suitable for outpatient prophylactic use.

181. The answer is a. *(Brunton, pp 271-276, 838. Katzung, pp 175-177, 203-205, 216-218, 235, 240, 1021-1022.)* Metoprolol is primarily a β_1-adrenergic blocker at low doses, but at high doses can block β_2 receptors also. Thus, it is sometimes called a "cardioselective" β-blocker, much like atenolol. Most of the β-blockers have no vasodilating activity (noteworthy exceptions are labetalol and carvedilol, which have α-blocking activity; and nebivolol, which vasodilates via a nitric oxide-dependent process).

β-Adrenergic receptor blockers slow resting heart rate and reduce contractility, both of which reduce myocardial oxygen demand. They also blunt cardiac stimulatory responses that increase oxygen demand, whenever the sympathetic nervous system is activated (eg, in response to exercise or drugs that tend to cause reflex sympathetic activation). These all involve blockade of β_1 receptors.

Metoprolol does not cause coronary vasodilation (and may favor constriction, which can become clinically significant in patients with variant angina, by "unmasking" α-mediated coronary vasoconstriction; see Question 187; thus answer b is incorrect); and it may increase (not decrease, d) total peripheral resistance by blocking β_2-mediated dilation in some vascular beds. This effect is usually slight. All the β-blockers slow AV nodal conduction velocity, but that effect per se contributes little to the reduced oxygen demand that is mainly derived from the drugs' effects on overall rate and contractility. Thus, answer e is incorrect.

All the β-blockers reduce angiotensin II synthesis (c), but it is an indirect effect, involving β_1 blockade, due to reduced renin release from the juxtaglomerular apparatus of the kidneys. Although that effect clearly occurs, it is not a major mechanism by which β-blockers exert their antianginal effects, nor is the magnitude of the inhibition of angiotensin II synthesis on par with that caused by ACE inhibitors.

182. The answer is a. *(Brunton, pp 858-860. Katzung, pp 181-183, 217, 219.)* ACE inhibitors are often selected first for hypertensive patients who also have diabetes mellitus (Type 1 or 2)—provided their renal function is satisfactory (specifically, no severe bilateral renal arterial stenosis, or no inadequate blood flow to one kidney if the other was removed; no albuminuria). Recall that angiotensin II constricts the efferent arterioles in the kidneys, which increases glomerular filtration. So, by reducing angiotensin II synthesis, an ACE inhibitor will block this effect and reduce filtration even further. Angiotensin receptor blockers (ARBs, eg, losartan) will do the same but by blocking angiotensin receptors rather than by inhibiting angiotensin synthesis.

ACE inhibitors (and ARBs) do not cause any problems with glycemic control or the responses to antidiabetic drugs, and they seem to exert some protective effect that slows or delays diabetes-related nephropathy.

β-Adrenergic blockers (b) would not be a good choice if hypertension is accompanied by diabetes mellitus, particularly when insulin is used for glycemic control. Should the diabetic patient experience an episode of hypoglycemia, a β-blocker may delay recovery of blood glucose levels, mask tachycardia that is one symptom of hypoglycemia development, and interact with some antidiabetic drugs (even those used for Type 2; excessive blood glucose-lowering). (If the diabetes is well controlled, and if the patient has other disorders for which benefits of β-blockade may outweigh potential problems, such as mild-moderate heart failure or recent myocardial infarction, then a β-blocker may be considered.)

Thiazides (d) can elevate blood glucose levels, or at least antagonize the desired effects of antidiabetic drugs (probably by reducing parenchymal cell responsiveness to insulin). Nonetheless, they might not be a first-choice in the setting of diabetes—at least not for the patient described in the scenario. (Some clinicians disagree, of course, and consider a thiazide or thiazide-like diuretic [eg, metolazone] a first choice drug for essential hypertension in most patients.)

Nifedipine (c) or verapamil or diltiazem (e) seem not to complicate glycemic control or interact with antidiabetic drug therapy. Nonetheless, they lack other benefits offered by ACE inhibitors (especially the renal-protective effects) in the setting of diabetes and so would not be a first choice or of special value.

183. The answer is a. (*Brunton, pp 183-185. Katzung, pp 98, 101, 331, 334f.*) ACh causes vasodilation only when the vascular endothelium is intact functionally and anatomically. The normal response, initiated by ACh acting as an agonist on muscarinic receptors, involves endothelium-derived relaxing factor/nitric oxide (EDRF/NO) that is generated in and released from the endothelium (that is why it's called "endothelium-derived"). The NO diffuses into the adjacent vascular smooth muscle cells and increases cGMP formation. That, in turn, causes extrusion of Ca^{2+} and relaxation of the muscle (vasodilation in the intact animal). When the endothelium is removed (actually quite easy to do experimentally) or damaged, ACh causes concentration-dependent increases of smooth muscle tension.

Isoproterenol (b) is a β_1/β_2 agonist. Added to an in vitro preparation such as the one used here, it would only cause smooth muscle relaxation (β_2 effect) unless the β-receptors were blocked; and has no way to alter the contractile responses to added ACh. Blockade of muscarinic receptors (c) cannot be correct. If that were the case, particularly under control conditions, contractile response to ACh would be diminished or abolished, and contraction shown under the experimental conditions would not be changed from what is shown in the figure. Prazosin (d) cannot be correct. It is an α_1-receptor blocker, and there is no way pretreating with it would cause vasoconstriction with or without added ACh. Botulinum toxin (e) blocks ACh from cholinergic nerves. Although there may be some postganglionic parasympathetic (and sympathetic) nerve "endings" in the tissue sample, the responses shown in the figure were caused by adding ACh directly to the tissue bath and so they are independent of any residual autonomic neural influences.

184. The answer is b. (*Brunton, pp 753-757, 847-850. Katzung, pp 171, 184, 260-261.*) Thiazide diuretics tend to raise uric acid concentration in the blood, probably by reducing urate's tubular secretion. This may be of little concern for patients with no history of hyperuricemia or gout, but for those with such a history it can be a problem that is not associated with any of the other answer choices given. Thiazides can be administered to hyperuricemic/gouty patients, but that may require another drug (allopurinol or febuxostat; both xanthine oxidase inhibitors) to counteract diuretic-induced rises of urate levels. If we can avoid the problems by avoiding the thiazide, and the possible need for adding a second drug to counteract the hyperuricemia, why not do just that?

None of the other answer choices (β-adrenergic blockers of any sort, b; angiotensin receptor blockers or ACE inhibitors, c and d; or traditional calcium channel blockers such as verapamil, e) have any appreciable, desired, or untoward effects on urate levels, renal handling of urate, or the incidence or severity of gout.

185. The answer is d. (*Brunton, pp 674, 688, 699, 1482. Katzung, pp 598, 624, 627.*) These in vitro responses, showing that ibuprofen (or another

NSAID, naproxen) can significantly antagonize the antiplatelet effects of aspirin, is clinically relevant. Both ibuprofen and aspirin compete for the same binding sites on both COX-1 and COX-2. Aspirin's interaction is covalent, and irreversible. Ibuprofen, however, binds to the same COX sites as aspirin. Its antiplatelet effects are comparatively weak and reversible. More importantly, the bound ibuprofen prevents the ability of aspirin to bind to same critical enzyme site. If aspirin therapy is stopped, overall platelet COX-1 activity will increase by about 10% per day, and just 20% of baseline COX activity—that is, skipping aspirin for more than 2 to 3 days—may be enough to enable sufficient COX activity to be restored such that the protective antiplatelet effects are lost. Using ibuprofen for more than a few days in a row is likely to do the same. In short, the interaction should be avoided. And remember: Ibuprofen (and naproxen) is available OTC, and unless you explicitly tell your patients to avoid it, your pharmacologic efforts to afford cardioprotection may be for naught.

186. The answer is e. (*Brunton, pp 837-840. Katzung, pp 181, 191, 199-203, 219, 1022.*) The vascular calcium channel-blocking actions of verapamil or diltiazem (nondihydropyridine class) will not only lower systemic blood pressure, but also tend to counter coronary arterial calcium influx that favors vasospasm. Thus, in this setting we can expect both antihypertensive and antianginal effects from one drug.

One might argue that nifedipine (answer c) would be a reasonable alternative. However, recall that the dihydropyridines (the class to which nifedipine belongs) lack cardiac depressant actions. Rapidly acting formulations of a dihydropyridine, even if given orally, are likely to lower blood pressure (the desired antihypertensive effect), but lacking cardiac-depressant actions are liable to trigger reflex (sympathetic/baroreceptor) cardiac stimulation. The resulting increases of either or both cardiac rate and contractility (mediated, reflexly, by sympathetic activation) necessarily may raise myocardial oxygen demand sufficient to cause myocardial ischemia, and/or may trigger coronary vasospasm. (The degree to which a dihydropyridine will cause unwanted reflex cardiac stimulation depends on the drug, the dose, and even the dosage form [eg, immediate-acting vs extended-acting]) Nonetheless, a nondihydropyridine would have a much better overall profile of cardiac/vascular actions.

ACE inhibitors or an ARB (a), or a thiazide (d), might cause no particular problems for a patient with vasospastic angina, but they also have no direct actions that would help that comorbidity. Why select one of them when a nondihydropyridine calcium channel blocker might be beneficial for both problems?

β-Blockers (b) would be a poor choice. Recall that the coronary vasculature constricts in response to α-adrenergic influences, while vascular β_2-receptor activation tends to cause coronary vasodilation. Patients with vasospastic angina depend on β-mediated vasodilatory influences, and are at greater risk of ischemic events if the β-receptors are blocked.

187. The answer is a. *(Brunton, pp 143t, 272-275, 824-826, 837-840. Katzung, pp 156-158, 160-161, 204-205.)* β-Blockers (represented in this question by atenolol) should not be administered (especially by a systemic route) to patients with vasospastic angina unless for a medical emergency that requires β-blockade as a life-saving measure. Recall the dual roles of adrenergic receptors in the coronary vasculature. Activation of β_2-adrenergic receptors causes vasodilation. Activation of α-adrenergic receptors in the coronary (and other) vasculature favors vasoconstriction or—in the setting of variant angina—vasospasm. Normally these receptors are exposed to circulating epinephrine, which causes the opposing vasodilator (β_2) and vasoconstrictor (α) effects. Norepinephrine is also activating α-adrenergic receptors. Block only the β_2 (vasodilator) effects in the coronaries and the constrictor (and spasm-favoring) effects of the α-receptors are left unopposed.

Diltiazem (b), a nondihydropyridine calcium channel blocker, would not only lower blood pressure but also suppress the tendency for coronary vasoconstriction or spasm by blocking vascular smooth muscle calcium influx. Hydrochlorothiazide (c) is the prototype thiazide diuretic, and metolazone (e) is thiazide-like in terms of most of its pharmacologic profiles. Neither is at all likely to cause or favor vasoconstriction in the coronary vessels or elsewhere. Losartan (d) is an angiotensin receptor blocker. It not only has good antihypertensive activity, but also is apt to suppress any coronary vasoconstrictor influences of circulating angiotensin.

188. The answer is b. *(Brunton, p 809. Katzung, pp 181-183, 217-219, 297, 1028t.)* ACE inhibitors (and angiotensin receptor blockers [ARBs], eg, losartan) are contraindicated in pregnancy (category X), and should not be administered to "women of childbearing potential"—not just women who are pregnant—in the first place. Normal in utero development of the kidneys and other urogenital structures seems to be angiotensin-dependent.

ACE inhibitors, or ARBs, given during the second or third trimesters have been associated with severe and sometimes fatal developmental anomalies of these structures. Cranial hypoplasia, and neonatal hyperkalemia and hypotension, have also been reported.

α-Methyldopa (a) is considered one of the preferred antihypertensive drugs for pregnant women. It not only controls maternal blood pressure well, but also is remarkably free of adverse effects on the fetus. (Indeed, it is the most likely drug that we would prescribe for this hypertensive and now pregnant woman.)

β-Blockers such as labetalol (d) are sometimes used during pregnancy, posing no specific or significant risks to the mother or the fetus, provided adequate perinatal care is given and blood pressure doesn't fall excessively. None of the calcium channel blockers (including verapamil, e) seem to have any significant cardiovascular benefits or risks during pregnancy, compared with other drugs. (Verapamil, for example, is in pregnancy category C.) One theoretical concern with verapamil and diltiazem is a prolongation of labor as parturition draws near, due to suppression of uterine contractility.

There are concerns with using diuretics during pregnancy. Furosemide (c) or other loop diuretics pose relatively significant fetal risks. However, that is related to potential maternal hypovolemia and hypotension that may lead to placental underperfusion. There is no teratogenic or embryopathic risk on par with that associated with the angiotensin modifiers (ACE inhibitors or ARBs). Moreover, when the goal is treating essential hypertension in the absence of pregnancy, hypervolemia, edema, ascites, and so on, loop diuretics are seldom used. Instead, thiazide or thiazide-like diuretics are the ones usually chosen. Nevertheless, the thiazides also pose a risk of placental underperfusion, and so they are not the preferred or ideal antihypertensives for the pregnant woman.

Note: It is not necessary (now) for you to memorize the pregnancy classifications of the non-teratogenic drugs listed above. What you need to know is that ACE inhibitors and ARBs are absolutely contraindicated. So is warfarin, at least during the first 12 weeks of gestation, which is addressed in Question 195.

189. The answer is c. *(Brunton, pp 287-288. Katzung, pp 158, 339-356.)* No β-blocker ordinarily should be administered to patients with asthma, because of a great risk of severe and potentially fatal bronchoconstriction or bronchospasm (unless the β-blocker is being given for a medical emergency that requires β-blockade, and likely benefits outweigh likely risks). This applies to all classes of β-blockers: nonselective, like propranolol; β_1 "selective," that is, atenolol or metoprolol; those with intrinsic sympathomimetic/partial agonist activity, such as pindolol; and those that also have α-blocking activity, that is, labetalol and carvedilol. The contraindication applies to all administration routes, including topical (ophthalmic); there are clinical reports of fatal bronchospasm induced by topical ophthalmic administration of "just one drop" of β-blockers.

The reason? Airways of persons with asthma are exquisitely sensitive to a host of bronchoconstrictor stimuli and exquisitely dependent on the bronchodilator effects of circulating epinephrine (β_2 receptors). Block those β-receptors, and that sets the stage for bronchoconstriction or bronchospasm. Another important factor is that this patient needs albuterol for occasional relief of bronchospasm. The drug works, of course, by activating β_2-adrenergic receptors in the airways. Any of the β-blockers will antagonize albuterol's desired effects, the so-called cardioselective agents included, because their selectivity for β_1 receptors is only relative, not absolute; and it is highly dose-dependent.

Diltiazem (a) and particularly verapamil (e), both nondihydropyridine calcium channel blockers, might be a good choice for this patient. They not only lower blood pressure by blocking calcium influx into vascular smooth muscle, but also (theoretically, at least) do the same in airway smooth muscle, thereby preventing or at least reducing bronchoconstriction. Hydrochlorothiazide possibly could exacerbate the problems by causing excessive fluid loss (which could favor bronchoconstriction), but the chances of this are low. (Loop diuretics such as furosemide would be of more concern, owing to their greater efficacy in terms of causing loss of circulating fluid volume.) There are no specific concerns with using ramipril, an angiotensin-converting enzyme inhibitor. (Remember: drugs with generic names ending in "-pril" are ACE inhibitors, so even if you learned about only captopril as an ACE inhibitor, you should have realized that ramipril is in the same class.)

Note: It's fair to say that the "Big 4" classes of antihypertensive drugs can be summarized as A, B, C, D: **A**CE inhibitors or angiotensin receptor blockers; β-blockers; **C**alcium channel blockers; and **D**iuretics (thiazides or thiazide-like agents such as metolazone). Which is "best" for a particular patient depends on a host of patient-related factors that may weigh in favor of selecting a drug from a particular class (A, B, C, D) or weigh against a particular class. There has been resurgence in the use and recommendation of thiazides or thiazide-like drugs for initiating antihypertensive therapy. Likewise, much more recently, and for a variety of reasons, some experts are stating that β-blockers should be dropped from the Big 4 list for many patients.

190. The answer is c. *(Brunton, pp 1468f, 1482f-1483. Katzung, pp 598-599.)* Clopidogrel (and the much lesser-used drug ticlopidine), is a noncompetitive antagonist of ADP. This prodrug (it must be metabolically activated) causes largely irreversible (ie, for the lifetime of the platelet) inhibition of platelet aggregation by blocking ADP binding to the G_i-coupled P2Y (AC) receptor. It has no effect on platelet activation and amplification caused by such other proaggregatory agonists as collagen, TXA_2, thrombin, PAF, serotonin, or epinephrine.

Aspirin (a) inhibits platelet aggregation caused by TXA_2 only, and does so only by inhibiting TXA_2 synthesis via cyclooxygenase, not by blocking TXA_2 receptors.

Bivalirudin (b) is a synthetic hirudin derivative (you may recall that hirudin is produced by the medicinal leach, *Hirudo medicinalis*). It is classified as an anticoagulant, not as an antiplatelet drug. It is a direct-acting inhibitor of free and clot-bound thrombin, which leads to two main effects: (1) decreased conversion of fibrinogen to fibrin; and (2) reduced activation of factor XIIIa, which in turn decreases conversion of soluble fibrin monomers to insoluble (polymerized) fibrin.

Bivalirudin is given IV as an alternative to heparin (both drugs bind to free thrombin, but bivalirudin also interacts with clot-bound thrombin), mainly along with aspirin for patients with unstable angina who are undergoing angioplasty. It is also used to help treat heparin-induced thrombocytopenia; and seems to be more effective than heparin when given post-myocardial infarction. A related drug is argatroban.

Heparin and warfarin (d, e) have no direct effects on platelets. (You should also recall that since warfarin's site of action is the liver, it has no anticoagulant effects when tested in vitro [ie, added to a tube of whole blood].)

Note: I mentioned that ticlopidine is much lesser-used than clopidogrel. Actually, it's seldom used. The reason? A greater risk of thrombotic thrombocytopenic purpura (TTP) and/or neutropenia.

191. The answer is a. *(Brunton, pp 795-800. Katzung, pp 294-297.)* The bradycardia caused by the unknown drug is reflex-mediated by baroreceptor activation in response to the rise of blood pressure. Angiotensin II, by activating vascular A-II receptors, raises blood pressure and peripheral resistance, and that response would not be inhibited by pretreatment with prazosin (selective α_1-adrenergic antagonist), nor any other adrenergic blocker for that matter.

The bradycardia, of course, involves reflex parasympathetic activation (and simultaneous withdrawal of sympathetic tone to the heart), release of ACh from the vagus, and activation of muscarinic receptors on the SA node. Atropine pretreatment indeed prevents that response, as described in the question—and regardless of whether the original pressor response was caused by A-II, or any other vasopressor drug for that matter.

Dobutamine (b) doesn't fit the bill; it is largely a selective β_1 agonist. For all practical purposes it causes no vasoconstriction (an α_1 response if we limit things to adrenergic drugs), and via the β_1 activation will directly increase heart rate, contractility, automaticity, and electrical impulse conduction (eg, through the AV node). No α activation occurs (rises of blood pressure, if they occur in response to dobutamine, are due to the positive inotropic effect), and so prazosin would have no direct effect on responses to dobutamine. Isoproterenol (c) can be ruled out for largely similar reasons; it activates both β_1 and β_2 receptors and lacks vasoconstrictor activity, whether due to activation of α-adrenergic receptors or by other mechanisms.

Could norepinephrine (d) be a reasonable answer? It certainly causes a vasopressor response and reflex bradycardia (at usual doses). However, the question stated that the unknown drug's pressor response is not inhibited by α blockade. Since a major element of NE's pressor effect depends on α activation, it's not a reasonable choice. The same applies to phenylephrine (e): this nonselective α agonist also causes a pressor response that would be reduced or blocked altogether by prazosin pretreatment.

192. The answer is c. *(Brunton, pp 276t, 286-289. Katzung, pp 156t, 157t, 159-177.)* Even if you know nothing specifically about nebivolol you should be able to conclude that increased formation or activity of nitric oxide (a vasodilator, among other things) is the only reasonable answer. A drug that competitively blocks α_1 receptors (a; for example phentolamine or prazosin) would, indeed, lower blood pressure (BP). However, the question stated that nebivolol had no effect on the vasoconstrictor effects of either phenylephrine (direct α agonist) or amphetamines (indirect-acting sympathomimetics; release neuronal norepinephrine). (Recall that labetalol and carvedilol are the β-blockers that also block α_1-adrenergic receptors.) Competitive blockade of α_2 receptors (b) cannot be correct. Blocking the presynaptic α-receptors would inhibit released norepinephrine's usual ability to "feedback inhibit" further NE release upon an action potential. Had nebivolol blocked the α_2 receptors, then, the most likely response would be a rise, not a fall, of peripheral resistance and BP. TXA_2 (d) is a vasoconstrictor (among other things). Increasing its synthesis would tend to raise BP/peripheral resistance also. COMT (e) inhibits the metabolic inactivation of catecholamines in the GI tract, liver, and elsewhere (outside of neurons). In theory, COMT inhibitors also would raise BP caused by its substrates. β-Blockers are not catecholamines, and so are not substrates for COMT.

193. The answer is c. *(Brunton, pp 955-956. Katzung, pp 613-614.)* Answering this question correctly indeed depends on your knowledge of several drugs, and their prototype or representative agents, that goes beyond "cardiovascular" (since I included a diabetes drug [metformin] and an antidepressant [escitalopram] as possible answer choices).

Nonetheless, niacin (nicotinic acid; vitamin B_3) is often added-on—in dosages higher than those recommended for vitamin supplementation—mainly to lower HDL and triglyceride levels, particularly in patients with the classic mixed hyperlipidemia characterized by elevated cholesterol and triglyceride levels (Type IIb) and who aren't adequately managed with a statin. The primary effect of niacin is to decrease production of VLDLs (mainly by inhibiting lipolysis in adipocytes). Since LDLs are by-products of VLDL degradation, the fall in VLDL levels causes LDL levels to fall as well. Lastly, recall that VLDLs deliver triglycerides to and increase their storage in adipose tissue. By decreasing VLDL production, then, niacin indirectly counters triglyceride accumulation and favors triglyceride clearance (elimination). See the answer for Question 259 for more information about niacin's more common side effects.

Pravastatin and other statins (HMG CoA reductase inhibitors), while mainly used for hypercholesterolemia (to lower LDL-cholesterol levels), often concomitantly raise HDL and lower triglyceride levels adequately. When statins and lifestyle modifications fail to control triglyceride levels adequately, adding niacin is usually a reasonable next step.

Citalopram (a), escitalopram, and other SSRI-antidepressants, have no known effects on altered vitamin absorption or on the cardiovascular system. Metformin (b), the prototype biguanide often used for managing Type 2 diabetes mellitus (Chapter 9), typically suppresses (not increases) appetite. Statins do not cause peripheral neuropathy (d); and ACE inhibitors (ramipril and others; e) do not cause diabetic nephropathy, although they are clearly contraindicated for patients with severe bilateral renal arterial stenosis, such as that associated with severe and poorly controlled diabetes mellitus.

194. The answer is d. *(Brunton, pp 928-929. Katzung, pp 236-238, 901t, 905-906.)* Quinidine is becoming an outmoded drug, but it is, of course, still being used. It may be described as a broad-spectrum antiarrhythmic (but that does not mean it is indicated or safe for all arrhythmias and all etiologies). It is mainly used for long-term management of supraventricular and ventricular arrhythmias: atrial flutter and fibrillation and sustained ventricular tachycardia. The drug's effects reflect direct ion channel-blocking actions plus a variety of receptor-blocking effects that may counteract the direct effects.

Direct blockade of sodium channels (a "major" action of Class I antiarrhythmics) slows impulse conduction in the atria, ventricles, and His-Purkinje system. Repolarization at those sites tends to be delayed, presumably by blockade of potassium channels. Among other changes, the ECG shows widened QRS complexes and prolonged QT intervals (which may predispose patients, particularly those with long QT syndrome, to some serious arrhythmias, including torsades).

Quinidine has strong anticholinergic (vagolytic) effects that are particularly apparent at the SA node (increased automaticity, tends to predominate over direct depressant effects from sodium channel blockade) and the AV node (increased conduction velocity; correct answer d). (Recall that vagal tone on the SA node slows spontaneous depolarization and heart rate; the vagolytic effects of quinidine will therefore do the opposite.) The effects on AV conduction are a main reason why, when quinidine therapy is to be started and atrial rates are still high, we pretreat the patient with a dose of a drug that "blocks down" the AV node: digoxin, sometimes verapamil, and occasionally a β-blocker. The main reason why ventricular rates aren't identical to (or close to) atrial rates during atrial fibrillation is because the AV node cannot transmit impulses at such high rates. This protective effect depends on AV nodal refractoriness and a relative inability to transmit too many impulses per time. If we did not suppress the AV node before giving quinidine, the AV nodal "conduction-stimulating" effects of the quinidine might increase AV nodal transmission; ventricular rates might rise to dangerous levels as atrial rate slows in response to the quinidine.

Quinidine is not likely to increase blood pressure (b), or worsen preexisting hypertension. Quite the contrary: the predominant vascular effect of the drug is dilation, and blood pressure falls, due to peripheral vascular α-adrenergic blocking activity. Likewise, quinidine exerts a negative inotropic effect—not a positive one (e)—on ventricular muscle. That, too, can contribute to a fall of blood pressure. For long-term management of a patient with atrial fibrillation, anticoagulants are important (not contraindicated; c) for prophylaxis of venous thrombosis; the use of quinidine does not contraindicate that.

195. The answer is e. *(Brunton, pp 1475-1480. Katzung, pp 594-597, 600, 1029t.)* The scenario describes the classic findings with "warfarin embryopathy:" nasal deformities and epiphyseal stippling. The drug is, as noted, absolutely contraindicated during pregnancy. The fetal risks are greatest if warfarin is taken at any time during the first 12 or so weeks of gestation, but adverse fetal effects can occur later. They are irreversible, sometimes fatal; there is no drug or vitamin (eg, vitamin K, folate) therapy that will be of benefit. All the other drugs listed pose some pregnancy-related risks (but lower and with less supporting data than with warfarin), and they do not share the characteristics of warfarin embryopathy. Clonidine (a) is in pregnancy category C. Its antihypertensive mechanism is largely identical to that of methyldopa, which is in category B, and usually is a preferred drug for hypertension during pregnancy. Low-molecular-weight heparin (b) is also pregnancy category B. If anticoagulation is required during pregnancy, it is the drug that most likely will be used. Hydrochlorothiazide (or thiazide diuretics in general) has no known human teratogenic effects (category B). Nitroglycerin is not contraindicated because of teratogenesis (category C).

Note: I'll kindly ask you to review the answers and explanations for Question 188, and recall that even though a cardiovascular drug may not be teratogenic nor absolutely contraindicated in pregnancy, it can cause adverse (potentially fatal) fetal effects if, for example, it causes hypotension and/or hypovolemia, which can significantly reduce placental blood flow.

196. The answer is d. *(Brunton, pp 852-854. Katzung, p 173.)* Among all the common oral antihypertensives, a Coombs-positive test is associated only with methyldopa. It occurs in up to about 20% of patients taking this drug long term. It may progress to hemolytic anemia, but that rarely occurs. The probable cause is an immune reaction (IgG antibodies) directed against and potentially lysing the red cell membrane. Other drugs with the potential to cause an immunohemolytic anemia are penicillins, quinidine, procainamide, and sulfonamides, but not captopril or other ACE inhibitors (a), clonidine (b), labetalol or other β-blockers (c), or prazosin or other α-receptor blockers (e).

197. The answer is a. *(Brunton, pp 267-268. Katzung pp 150, 152, 177, 285.)* Phenoxybenzamine is a long-acting and noncompetitive α-adrenergic blocker. It works by alkylating (rather than merely occupying and "blocking") α-adrenergic receptors, thereby rendering them incapable of interacting with α-adrenergic agonists such as epinephrine (which is being released in abundance by the pheochromocytoma). The drug has no ability to block β-adrenergic receptors (b), inhibit catecholamine synthesis (c), inhibit angiotensin-converting enzyme (d), or affect any of the major enzymes involved in catecholamine degradation (COMT, answer e; or MAO).

198. The answer is b. *(Brunton, pp 832-836. Katzung, pp 181, 199-203, 219, 243-244.)* Let's deal with the nondihydropyridines first. Verapamil (especially) and diltiazem cause not only arteriolar dilation (via calcium channel blockade in vascular smooth muscle; dilation on the venous side does not occur; answer c), but also direct cardiac depressant effects (due to calcium channel blockade in cardiac tissues, and so answer d is incorrect). These cardiac effects oppose, or blunt (not cause; answer a) reflex sympathetic cardiac activation that otherwise would occur in response to only peripheral vasodilation. Such problems as reflex tachycardia and positive inotropy are much less—usually nonexistent—with the nondihydropyridines. In fact, when reflex cardiac stimulation caused by other drugs (eg, nitroglycerin) is problematic and must be controlled, either verapamil (probably preferred) or diltiazem may be a reasonable alternative to the traditional agents for blocking the unwanted cardiac responses: the β-adrenergic blockers. Moreover, a nondihydropyridine CCB is usually the drug of choice for controlling cardiac stimulatory responses when a β-blocker is contraindicated (eg, in asthma).

In contrast, the dihydropyridines (consider nifedipine as the group prototype) are "selective" for their vascular effects and cause no direct cardiac effects. They cause significant arteriolar (but not venular) dilation, which can activate the baroreceptor reflex that increases sympathetic influences on the heart: positive inotropy, positive chronotropy (reflex tachycardia can be severe), and increased automaticity and conduction velocity (dromotropic effects). Of course, how strongly the reflex response will be, if it occurs at all, depends on how quickly and by how much blood pressure falls. That, in turn, depends on the dose of the dihydropyridine, how it is administered (orally? intravenously?) and, for oral dosage forms, whether the product is formulated as an immediate-acting one or a slow- or long-acting one.

Be aware that combined use of diltiazem or verapamil with a β-blocker is risky (and so answer e is incorrect) due to the possibility of additive or stronger inhibitory effects on cardiac rate, contractility, and especially AV nodal function. And, whether used alone or in combination, β-blockers and the nondihydropyridine CCBs (verapamil, diltiazem) should not be administered to patients with severe heart failure due to the added risks from further suppression of cardiac output.

Notes: Diltiazem is classified, chemically, as a benzothiazepine (similar to but not to be confused with benzodiazepines—diazepam, midazolam, and many other drugs used for their CNS effects). Verapamil is, chemically, a phenylalkylamine. However, memorizing the names of these chemical groups is probably a waste of your time: these drugs are almost always referred to simply as nondihydropyridines.

199. The answer is d. *(Brunton, pp 886-889, 921-923. Katzung, pp 211f, 214-216, 219-220.)* Before explaining the answers, it's important to reiterate several elements in the question: the digoxin is being used in the presence of heart failure; blood levels of the drug are in the therapeutic range; and plasma electrolytes are normal. This is important because what happens depends on these and other conditions, and responses that can be characterized as part of digoxin toxicity will differ.

Of the effects listed here, you would expect to find slowed AV nodal conduction velocity in response to digoxin. This is a common and, in many situations useful, effect. For example, when the drug is used as part of the pharmacologic management of atrial fibrillation or flutter, the main desired response is not suppression of the arrhythmia per se, but rather to "block down" the AV node so that as atrial rates fall (but are still high), the AV node will be unable to transmit the same frequency of impulses to the ventricles. That is, dig "protects" the ventricles from excessive acceleration by inducing a degree of AV block. In terms of more specific effects on the AV node, digoxin slows conduction velocity and increases AV nodal refractory periods.

Other predominant electrophysiologic effects on the heart—all concentration-dependent and often secondary to improved cardiac output—include decreases (not increases; answers b, c, and e) of both SA nodal, atrial and ventricular automaticity. Conduction rates through those structures and the His-Purkinje system tend to increase (not decrease; e). Through direct and indirect effects, digoxin can increase or decrease Phase 4 (spontaneous) depolarization of the SA node. However, the prominent effect is a reduction of SA depolarization as an indirect consequence of reduced sympathetic and increased parasympathetic tone in response to improved cardiac output.

Note: Various texts, and people, often use the terms digitalis, cardiac glycoside, or simply dig (not pronounced as you would when talking about making a hole with a shovel). *Digitalis purpura* (purple foxglove) entered the medical limelight around 1776, when William Withering (both a physician and botanist) published *A Botanical Arrangement of All the Vegetables Naturally Growing in Great Britain*. Thus, the term digitalis, which actually contained a variety of digoxin-like chemicals that included a sugar moiety (thus, the glycoside) and that affected the heart (thus, cardiac). As time passed several of these chemicals were isolated and later synthesized, and for a time used clinically. Two that you may find in a text, mentioned in lecture, or included in an exam (I sure hope not!) are digitoxin and ouabain (pronounced WAA-bane). They are no longer used clinically (they haven't been for a long time), so ignore them. When anyone uses the term digitalis, cardiac glycoside, or dig in modern clinical context, they are referring to digoxin: it's the only game in town. And if someone should test you on digitoxin or ouabain on a cardiac pharmacology exam...well, I won't tell you what I'd do.

200. The answer is d. *(Brunton, pp 860-862. Katzung, pp 177-181, 191-208, 213, 219.)* Hydralazine predominately dilates arterioles, with negligible effects on the venous side of the circulation. It typically lowers blood pressure "so well" and quickly that it can trigger the following two unwanted cardiovascular responses that need to be dealt with:

1. Reflex cardiac stimulation (involving the baroreceptor reflex) is common, and it is typically managed with a β-adrenergic blocker (unless it is contraindicated). An alternative approach would be to use either

verapamil or diltiazem (but not a dihydropyridine-type calcium channel blocker such as nifedipine, which would not suppress—and, in fact might aggravate—the reflex cardiac stimulation).

2. The renin-angiotensin-aldosterone system is activated. One consequence of this unwanted compensatory response would be increased renal sodium retention that would expand circulating fluid volume and counteract hydralazine's blood pressure-lowering effects. This is typically managed with a diuretic. A thiazide may be sufficient to combat the renal sodium retention, but a more efficacious diuretic (loop diuretic) may be necessary.

Captopril (or another ACE inhibitor, or an angiotensin receptor blocker such as losartan) might be a suitable add-on (it would cause synergistic antihypertensive effects and prevent aldosterone-mediated renal effects). However, combining it with nifedipine (dihydropyridine) is irrational (a). As noted above, given the "pure" vasodilator actions of nifedipine and no cardiac-depressing activity whatsoever (as we get with verapamil or diltiazem), the net effect on heart rate would be either no suppression of the tachycardia or a worsening of it. Also, it is irrational in most cases to use two vasodilators together, that is, hydralazine and nifedipine.

Digoxin, alone or with virtually any other drug (b, c), is not rational. There is no indication that there is need for inotropic support in this patient.

Spironolactone (b), alone or with digoxin, would be of little benefit. One could argue that by virtue of the spironolactone's ability to induce diuresis by blocking aldosterone's renal tubular effects, it would counteract hydralazine's ability to lead to renal sodium retention. That may be true, but spironolactone (with or without digoxin) will do nothing desirable to the unwanted tachycardia.

Nitroglycerin (e) would add to hydralazine's antihypertensive effects (like hydralazine and calcium channel blockers, it is a vasodilator), but it would probably aggravate the reflex cardiac stimulation and also increase the unwanted renal response (via a hemodynamic mechanism).

Both triamterene and amiloride (f) are potassium-sparing diuretics. The combination of these two diuretics, which are in the same class and work by identical aldosterone-independent mechanisms, is irrational whether or not they are added to a hydralazine regimen. Either might beneficially combat a propensity for renal sodium retention in response to hydralazine. But, as with any diuretic alone, either or both would do nothing to control the cardiac responses to hydralazine.

If you are associating hydralazine with some vitamin-related problem, you should be thinking not of Vitamin K but of vitamin B_6 (pyridoxine): hydralazine can interfere with B_6 metabolism, causing such symptoms as peripheral neuritis, and so prophylactic B_6 supplementation is often used along with long-term hydralazine therapy.

Note: Nowadays many physicians consider hydralazine to be (at best) a 5th or 6th line agent for chronic hypertension. Regardless, the drug certainly is not a "go to" drug unless, essentially, hypertension is severe and other reasonable antihypertensive drug options have been tried and shown to be ineffective.

201. The answer is b. *(Brunton, pp 643, 648-649, 800-810. Katzung, pp 181-183, 217, 295-296.)* Angiotensin-converting enzyme (ACE) and bradykininase (also known as kininase II) are exactly the same enzymes. We use the former name when the substrate is angiotensin I (the product, of course, is angiotensin II); we call it bradykininase when the substrate is bradykinin. None of the other drugs listed inhibit the enzymatic conversion of either A-I to A-II, or of bradykinin to its inactive products: β-blockers such as atenolol, metoprolol (a), labetalol, carvedilol (d); or thiazide or thiazide like diuretics (c; or any other diuretics for that matter). Losartan (e) and other "sartans" (valsartan, for example) block angiotensin II receptors, but have no catalytic activity with respect to angiotensin or bradykinin metabolism.

202. The answer is d. *(Brunton, pp 863-865. Katzung, pp 179-180, 335, 1023.)* Cyanide is the ultimate toxic metabolite of nitroprusside sodium. The drug is initially metabolically reduced to nitric oxide (e), which is responsible for the arteriolar and venular dilation. However, it is another metabolite, CN^- (and to a lesser extent the next metabolite, thiocyanate) that is the main cause of or contributor to toxicity.

When CN^- accumulates to sufficiently high levels (as from excessive or excessively prolonged administration of the drug), the vasculature develops what amounts to a tolerance to the drug's vasodilator effects, and so blood pressure usually starts to rise despite the presence of high drug levels. Toxic cyanide accumulation can also lead to severe lactic acidosis: the CN^- reacts with Fe^{3+} in mitochondrial cytochrome oxidase, inhibiting oxidative phosphorylation. Other characteristic signs and symptoms of the toxic syndrome include a cherry red skin (because mitochondrial oxygen consumption is blocked, venous blood remains oxygenated and as "bright red" as normal arterial blood), hypoxia, and, ultimately, seizures and ventilatory arrest.

Neither nitroprusside nor any of its metabolites have any adrenergic agonist (a) or antagonist activity; stimulatory or inhibitory effects on the sodium pump (b); or actions on angiotensin synthesis or angiotensin receptors (c).

Note: Nitroglycerin and other similar nitrovasodilators are not metabolized to CN^- and so manifestations of CN^- poisoning are not elements of their toxicity profile.

203. The answer is c. *(Brunton, pp 886-889, 921-923. Katzung, pp 258-260.)* The patient's signs and symptoms are consistent with digoxin toxicity. Hypokalemia due to the effects of potassium-wasting diuretics such as furosemide increase susceptibility to digoxin toxicity, and they are probably the most common cause of it. How does this occur? Digoxin binds to a K^+ binding site on the sodium pump (ATPase). That is, there is competition between digoxin molecules and K^+ for the same binding sites. When potassium levels are low (as can occur with any potassium-wasting diuretic, that is, a loop, thiazide, or thiazide-like diuretic, or even a carbonic anhydrase inhibitor such as acetazolamide), more digoxin molecules are able to bind to the ATPase—even though the actual digoxin concentration in the bloodstream hasn't changed. More binding leads to greater ATPase inhibition: an intensified digoxin effect that, quite often, can lead to adverse responses rather than better therapeutic effects.

Captopril (a) has no direct effects on digoxin's actions. (We might add that an ACE inhibitor such as captopril, along with a β-blocker and a diuretic—not digoxin—are now considered the preferred therapy for most patients with recent onset and mild heart failure.) Cholestyramine (b), a cholesterol-binding resin, interacts with concomitantly administered (oral) digoxin to reduce digoxin absorption. It would not increase the risk of digoxin toxicity; quite the opposite, it would reduce digoxin's plasma concentrations and therapeutic effectiveness. Lovastatin (d; an HMG-Co-A reductase inhibitor/"statin") and nitroglycerin (e) are not likely to cause the observed toxicity either.

204. The answer is e. *(Brunton, pp 690, 928. Katzung, pp 237-238, 624, 1021.)* Many of the signs and symptoms of salicylism (low-grade aspirin toxicity) are similar to those caused by high blood levels of quinidine (antiarrhythmic, no longer a first line agent) or quinine (mainly used as an antimalarial). Quinidine, quinine, and related drugs are called cinchona alkaloids, and the relatively mild toxicity syndrome caused by these drugs is called cinchonism. (These drugs were originally obtained from a plant known, generically, as *Cinchona*.) Aspirin and the cinchona alkaloids are chemically similar in some important chemical and pharmacologic ways. The common signs and symptoms include light-headedness, tinnitus, and visual disturbances such as diplopia.

The signs and symptoms described here are not at all like those caused by atropine (a) or other antimuscarinic drugs; captopril (b) or other ACE inhibitors; dobutamine (c); or propranolol (d) or any other β-adrenergic blockers. Indeed, of all the cardiovascular drugs you could possibly think of, the syndrome is unique to quinidine.

205. The answer is c. *(Brunton, p 837. Katzung, pp 191-204.)* The etiology involves coronary vasospasm, and that can be blocked well with a calcium channel blocker (CCB): diltiazem, verapamil, or dihydropyridines (eg, nifedipine, for which slow-/extended-acting oral formulations are used). The CCBs block coronary vascular smooth muscle influx of calcium, which is a critical process in triggering vasospasm.

Nitroglycerin (d) seems to be marginally effective in terms of long-term symptom relief, although it may be the only rapidly acting drug that will be efficacious for acute angina and self-medication.

Aspirin (a), through its antiplatelet aggregatory effects, would be beneficial, prophylactically, if coronary thrombosis were part of the etiology of variant angina, but thrombosis isn't the main problem with coronary vasospasm. Aspirin has no intrinsic vasodilator or antispasmodic activity.

Atorvastatin (b, or other statins) are useful for primary prevention of coronary heart disease, but coronaries that undergo spasm may be remarkably free of atherosclerotic plaque, and the statins have no antispasmodic effects per se.

The β-blockers (e), which are important drugs for many patients with ischemic heart disease and chronic-stable angina, can do more harm than good in vasospastic angina. In essence, β-receptor activation in the coronaries tends to cause vasodilation, an effect that to a degree counteracts simultaneous and opposing α-mediated constriction. Block only the β-receptors, and the α-mediated constrictor effects—vasospasm-favoring effects—are left unopposed. Variant angina, then, is likely to be made worse, not better, with β-blockers. (You might ask whether a combined α-/β-blocker like labetalol or carvedilol might be better than a nonselective or cardioselective β-blocker. Perhaps in theory, but not in practice. Remember that the α-blocking effects of these drugs are comparatively weak; their β-blocking, spasm-favoring effects will predominate.)

206. The answer is d. *(Brunton, pp 1472, 1480-1481. Katzung, pp 597-598.)* Heparin is commonly (but not without risk) administered with thrombolytic drugs, but should not be used if the thrombolytic drug is streptokinase (SK). Streptokinase has been aptly described as "non-clot-specific" in terms of its sites of action. It forms an SK-plasminogen complex that converts plasminogen into plasmin, which degrades the fibrin network that holds clots intact. That is the basis of its thrombolytic effects. However, the site of action of this prototype thrombolytic drug is not "confined" to clots, as is the case with such drugs as alteplase (a) or tenecteplase (and several others synthesized using recombinant DNA techniques). The systemic formation of plasmin caused by SK leads to degradation or otherwise decreased levels of fibrinogen and other essential clotting factors throughout the circulatory system. This leads to a markedly increased risk of hemorrhage. There is an increased risk of bleeding when heparin is used with any thrombolytic, but proper dosing and monitoring can reduce the risks dramatically. The risks are too great, however, to use heparin concomitant with SK.

Clearly, aspirin (b), clopidogrel (c) and warfarin (e) exert antiplatelet or anticoagulant effects, and concomitant use of aspirin may increase the bleeding risk. However, with proper (and necessary) monitoring of coagulation parameters and proper adjustments of doses, these drugs can be safely used with aspirin, as they often are.

207. The answer is c. *(Brunton, 921-923, 929. Katzung, pp 214-216, 220.)* Digoxin toxicity is likely to occur within 24 to 48 hours unless the digoxin dose is adjusted down. The reason is that quinidine will reduce the renal excretion of digoxin, the drug's main elimination route. This is probably due to some mechanism by which quinidine inhibits P-glycoprotein transport of digoxin in the kidneys. (See the answer for Question 7, for a short table listing some drugs that are substrates, inducers, and inhibitors of P-glycoprotein.)

There is no "reverse interaction"—that is, an ability of digoxin to cause signs and symptoms of quinidine toxicity (a). Quinidine has no significant impact on the renal actions of any diuretics, whether these actions are expressed in terms of urine output (volume or concentration) or renal handling of sodium or potassium or other electrolytes or solutes (b, d).

Quinidine-induced digoxin toxicity may suppress cardiac contractility, but that would not necessarily be a direct effect of an interaction on the inotropic state of the myocardium. Rather, it would be secondary to potential digoxin-induced arrhythmias, and it would not occur "promptly."

Quinidine does cause some drug-drug interactions by pharmacokinetic mechanisms. It is a potent inhibitor of CYP2D6, and can, for example, inhibit the analgesic effects of codeine by inhibiting its metabolism to morphine. However, this mechanism does not apply to the quinidine-digoxin interaction; digoxin is eliminated completely by the kidneys, with no prior metabolism.

208. The answer is e. *(Brunton, pp 911-915. Katzung, pp 239-240, 247.)* The class I-C antiarrhythmics are associated with a higher incidence of severe proarrhythmic events than virtually any other antiarrhythmics in other classes. This risk partially explains why, when these drugs were first approved, they were indicated only for life-threatening ventricular arrhythmias that failed to respond to all other reasonable (and safer) alternatives. (This risk also contributed to why another I-C agent, encainide, was withdrawn from the market.)

Nowadays, these I-C agents are still used for serious (life-threatening) and refractory ventricular arrhythmias (not for innocuous ones; a), not necessarily those caused by an acute coronary syndrome (a), and clearly not for patients with low ejection fractions or cardiac output (b). Their efficacy arises mainly from significant sodium channel blockade. However, they also block some potassium channels, which accounts for modestly growing interest in and use of these drugs for some atrial or other supraventricular arrhythmias. Regardless of whether the use is for an atrial or ventricular arrhythmia, the proarrhythmic effects should not be overlooked or forgotten.

Pulmonary fibrosis and alterations of thyroid hormone status (typically, a hypothyroid-like state; answer d) are uniquely associated with amiodarone (among all the antiarrhythmics), and amiodarone was not one of the answer choices.

Note: I'll opine that memorizing which antiarrhythmic agents are in which Vaughn-Williams class may not be profitable (except for answering nit-picky and clinically irrelevant exam questions). Among the reasons why (1) this classification is based largely on electrophysiologic effects of the drugs in largely normal, isolated cardiac cells, not in diseased intact human hearts; (2) some antiarrhythmic drugs have electrophysiologic/ionic mechanisms of action that would reasonably place them in more than one Vaughn-Williams class (eg, amiodarone); (3) placement in a particular Vaughn-Williams class does not necessarily predict clinical use of the antiarrhythmic; and (4) side effects profiles and toxicities of drugs in the same Vaughn-Williams class—both cardiac and extracardiac—can differ substantially.

209. The answer is b. *(Brunton, pp 864-865. Katzung, pp 196, 1022-1023.)* Cyanide, whether from nitroprusside metabolism or from other sources (see Question 486 in the toxicology chapter), normally reacts with endogenous sulfur-containing compounds, mainly thiosulfate. Under the influence of mitochondrial rhodanese (a transsulfurase), relatively nontoxic (less toxic than CN^-) thiocyanate is formed and is readily excreted in the urine. With excessive exposure to nitroprusside (or CN^- from other sources), endogenous sulfur-containing substrate stores are depleted. We manage this, then, by IV infusion of an aqueous sodium thiosulfate solution.

Epinephrine (e) or other catecholamines, thrombin (c), vitamin C (d) or E (e; or any other vitamins for that matter), have no roles nor beneficial effects in the context of cyanide poisoning.

Note: To avoid or at least reduce the risks of nitroprusside-induced cyanide toxicity, some agencies add sodium thiosulfate to the nitroprusside before the drug is administered, thereby providing ample exogenous substrate for the detoxification reaction.

210. The answer is e. *(Brunton, p 836. Katzung, pp 201-202, 243-244.)* Constipation is a fairly common and sometimes very bothersome response to some verapamil. The incidence and severity of this GI problem are less with diltiazem, and very uncommon with dihydropyridines. If severe and not managed properly, verapamil-induced effects on the GI musculature can lead to fecal impaction or other significant intestinal problems can occur. The best initial approach—if continued use of the offending drug is needed—is to modify the diet by increasing water and dietary fiber intake.

Constipation (or diarrhea) may occur with statins (a), ACE inhibitors (b, or angiotensin receptor blockers), β-blockers (c), or nitrovasodilators (d) but the incidence for a given patient is extremely low and usually temporary and relatively innocuous.

211. The answer is a. *(Brunton, pp 847-849, 858-859. Katzung, pp 171-172, 181-184.)* Although combined use of an ACE inhibitor (or angiotensin receptor blocker [ARB], eg, losartan) and a diuretic is quite common, great care must be taken when adding one of the drugs to therapy that has been started with the other. The reason is that some patients develop a sudden fall of blood pressure that may be sufficient to cause syncope or other complications. Volume and sodium depletion seem to be among several probable causative factors.

Answer b is incorrect. The effects of ACE inhibitors (or ARBs) and thiazides on renal handling of potassium are the opposite of one another, not synergistic. ACE inhibitors tend to elevate potassium levels (mainly by lowering aldosterone levels); the thiazides (and loop diuretics, eg, furosemide) are potassium-wasting.

There is no evidence that adding one of these drugs to therapy with the other can cause acute (or chronic) heart failure (c); indeed, such a combination is often an essential component in managing chronic heart failure. Blood pressure will fall, not rise, and certainly not cause hypertensive crisis (d); and slowed AV nodal conduction rates (e) due to this drug combination do not occur.

212. The answer is d. *(Brunton, p 1474. Katzung, pp 591-593.)* Administration of protamine sulfate will quickly reverse the bleeding caused by excessive effects of heparin. It binds to heparin, forming a stable complex that abolishes heparin's anticoagulant activity.

Aminocaproic acid (a) binds avidly to plasmin and plasminogen, and so is an effective inhibitor of fibrinolysis and an antagonist of fibrinolytic/thrombolytic drugs. Aprotinin (b) is a bovine pancreatic trypsin inhibitor. It is used to prevent perioperative blood loss (and the need for blood transfusions) because it slows fibrinolysis. The main use is in the setting of coronary bypass or other cardiac surgeries when patients are subjected to cardiopulmonary bypass. Aprotinin can cause anaphylactic reactions and so it should never be given unless the patient is on cardiopulmonary bypass at the time of administration (or can be placed on it quickly) so that circulation can be maintained until the anaphylaxis can be managed. Dipyridamole (c) weakly blocks platelet ADP receptors, and has a long but uninspiring history as an antiplatelet drug. Vitamin K (e) is used as an antidote for excessive effects of such drugs as warfarin, and does nothing for heparin overdoses.

213. The answer is c. *(Brunton, pp 823-892. Katzung, pp 191, 195-196, 199t.)* Nitroglycerin causes its vasodilator effects via a nitric oxide (NO)- and cyclic GMP-dependent mechanism. The NO activates guanylyl cyclase which forms cGMP from GMP. The cGMP, in turn, dephosphorylates myosin light chains, leading to reduced actin-myosin interactions and relaxation of the smooth muscle cells. Normally, this vascular effect is modulated by cGMP degradation (to GMP) by cGMP-specific phosphodiesterases (PDEs). Sildenafil (and the related drugs tadalafil and vardenafil), inhibit the activity of those PDEs, thereby maintaining cGMP levels and potentiating the vasodilator effects. This interaction may lead to severe excessive effects, including life-threatening hypotension and myocardial and cerebral ischemia. Sildenafil and related drugs also increase the risk of symptomatic hypotension if taken by people who are also being treated with α-adrenergic blockers, including those that selectively block α_1 receptors (eg, prazosin and doxazosin) and are used for managing hypertension. The same applies to α-blockers such as tamsulosin, which is used to provide symptomatic relief in some men with benign prostatic hypertrophy.

There are no similar interactions between sildenafil and related drugs with ACE inhibitors (a), β-blockers (b; unless, perhaps, they also have α-blocking activity), statins (d), or diuretics (e).

Note the important mechanistic links between vasodilation/hypotension, sexual intercourse, and potentially fatal cardiac responses. Sexual arousal—and, especially orgasm—causes a massive activation of the sympathetic nervous system. One consequence of that, α-mediated vasoconstriction that tends to keep blood pressure up, is too feeble to overcome the hypotensive effects of the sildenafil-nitroglycerin combination. Along with a fall of blood pressure is a fall of coronary perfusion pressure (diastolic blood pressure), that is, reduced myocardial blood flow/oxygen supply. Yet the sympathetic activation concomitantly causes significant increases of cardiac rate and contractility, that is, increased myocardial oxygen demand. Oxygen demand rises, supply falls, and the stage is set for acute myocardial ischemia.

A final point to consider. It is reasonable to assume that if the patient is taking any or even several of the drugs listed in the question, he has underlying cardiac disease. However, and in contrast with what some students have suggested, underlying cardiac disease per se does not automatically contraindicate or even excessively increase the risks from sexual intercourse and orgasm. (How severe is the patient's cardiovascular disease? It is well controlled? What are the specific diseases and risks he has?) Similarly, none of the drugs listed other than the nitrovasodilators (and some α-blockers mentioned in the previous paragraph) contraindicate the use of any of the ED drugs.

214. The answer is e. *(Brunton, pp 902-904. Katzung, pp 225-233.)* Although you may not consider this question a pharmacology question, being able to answer it correctly is important to the rational and safe use of many drugs.

In general, heart block refers to excessively slowed AV nodal conduction, which you assess by measuring the PR interval on the ECG. Recall that this interval gives information on how long it takes for electrical impulses that originate with SA nodal depolarization to pass through the atrial myocardia and the AV node, ultimately leading to ventricular activation (manifest as the QRS complex). Impulse conduction through the atria is normally quick; it is the AV node that has the slowest intrinsic impulse conduction rate anywhere in the heart, and it is arguably the structure that is most susceptible to drug- (or disease-) induced changes of supraventricular conduction that lead to the diagnosis of AV block.

In first-degree heart block, the main manifestation is a prolonged PR interval, but each P wave is followed by a normally generated QRS complex. In second-degree heart block, the PR interval is prolonged and some P waves are not conducted through the AV node, and so are not followed by a QRS triggered by the prior atrial activation (eg, 2:1 block). In third-degree (complete) heart block, no P waves are conducted normally through the AV node, and ventricular activation is solely dependent on intrinsic automaticity of the ventricles (or conducting tissue therein).

Finding irregularities upon auscultation of the heart (a), the presence of blood pressures that are above or below (b) what is generally regarded as normal, or the presence of sinus bradycardia (c), are not reliable indicators of heart block. Ventricular ectopic beats (d) and/or wide QRS complexes (f) may accompany heart block (especially complete heart block), but are not necessarily indicative of it.

215. The answer is d. *(Brunton, pp 824-826. Katzung, pp 192-194, 331-337.)* Nitric oxide is thought to be enzymatically released from nitroglycerin (and other nitroglycerin-like vasodilators). It then reacts with and activates guanylyl cyclase to increase GMP, which in turn dephosphorylates myosin light chain kinase, causes calcium extrusion, and suppresses smooth muscle tone. Tolerance may develop in part from a decrease in available sulfhydryl groups. The vasodilator effects occur primarily on the venous side of the systemic circulation, and it is not at all "selective" in terms of actions on the coronary vessels (e), which was a popular—but incorrect—explanation of the drug's actions long ago.

Autonomic receptors are not involved in the primary (direct) responses to nitroglycerin. The drug does not block α-adrenergic (or β) receptors (a) or influence the synthesis or actions of adenosine (c). Finally, and importantly, whereas nitroprusside is metabolized to cyanide, nitroglycerin and related drugs are not (b).

216. The answer is e. *(Brunton, p 951. Katzung, pp 612-613, 618t.)* Never been taught specifically about rosuvastatin? Well, the drug name ends in "-statin" so you should automatically know quite a bit about it. The findings described in the question are consistent with statin-induced myositis and myopathy, which seem to have progressed to rhabdomyolysis and renal failure—both potentially fatal. This syndrome (and hepatotoxicity) is the most serious adverse response to the statins. It is more prevalent in older patients, those with multiple illnesses, and especially those with renal or liver disease. Coadministration of most other lipid-lowering drugs (none of which are in the list in Question 216) increases the risk of rhabdomyolysis, hepatotoxicity, or both. As an aside, the risk of rhabdomyolysis (or lesser skeletal muscle changes) is not too much different between the currently available statins. However, it was (allegedly) such a problem with one relatively recent drug, cerivastatin, that the drug was pulled from the market.

The signs and symptoms described in the question, and the underlying mechanisms, do not apply to: aspirin (a) at any dose, or to other traditional nonsteroidal anti-inflammatory drugs; ACE inhibitors (b) or angiotensin receptor blockers; β-adrenergic blockers (c) of any sort; or furosemide (d) or other loop diuretics.

217. The answer is a. *(Brunton, pp 857-858, 860-862, 864-865. Katzung, pp 177-181, 219.)* Hydralazine's primary vasodilator actions occur on arterioles, not on venules. The others have both arteriolar and venular dilator activity, thereby lowering both afterload and central venous pressure (venous capacitance; right atrial pressure). Hydralazine's probable mechanism of action involves a nitric oxide (NO)-mediated process. (There is also some evidence that the drug opens voltage-gated potassium channels on vascular smooth muscle cells, causing muscle cell hyperpolarization and ultimate vasodilation.)

The other drugs listed cause vascular smooth muscle relaxation on both arterioles and venules: losartan (b), by blocking angiotensin II receptors; nifedipine (c) via calcium channel blockade; nitroglycerin (d) by NO as an intermediate; and prazosin (e) by selective α_1-adrenergic blockade. Here is a short table listing the main sites where various drugs or drug classes exert their main or sole vasodilator actions.

	Main Site(s) of Peripheral Vasodilation	
Drug or Drug Class	**Arterioles**	**Veins**
Nitroglycerin[a]		√
Selective α_1 blockers (prazosin, etc.) or phentolamine	√	√
ACE inhibitors, ARBs[b] (captopril, losartan, etc)	√	√
Nitroprusside[a]	√	√
CCBs (dihydropyridine or nondihydropyridine; nifedipine, verapamil, etc)	√	√
Hydralazine, diazoxide[a]	√	

Abbreviations: ACE, angiotensin-converting enzyme; ARB, angiotensin II receptor antagonists; CCB, calcium channel blocker.

[a]Nitric-oxide mediated; [b]vasodilation secondary to inhibited angiotensin II synthesis (ACE inhibitors) or blockade of vascular A-II receptors (ARBs).

218. The answer is b. *(Brunton, pp 688, 1482. Katzung, pp 313-315, 624.)* Aspirin inhibits cyclooxygenases I and II. In terms of clotting, the main effect will be inhibition of platelet aggregation by reduced formation of TXA_2. Bleeding time will be prolonged and will remain that way until sufficient numbers of new platelets have been synthesized and released into the bloodstream, because aggregation of those platelets already exposed to the drug will be inhibited for their lifetime. The APTT (a), which should not be affected by aspirin, is used to monitor effects and adjust the dose of unfractionated heparin (such monitoring is not required with low molecular weight heparin, eg, enoxaparin). Measuring prothrombin time (and its normalized value, the INR; answers c and e) is used to monitor warfarin therapy and adjust dosages as needed. Platelet counts (d), also not affected by aspirin, are used to assess for the development of thrombocytopenic purpura, which may rarely occur during therapy with (for example) the clopidogrel-like drug ticlopidine, or with heparin when thrombocytopenia is anticipated or suspected.

219. The answer is a. *(Brunton, pp 917, 920. Katzung, pp 236-237, 244.)* Nowadays, IV injection of adenosine is generally regarded as first choice for terminating PSVT in which reentry phenomena play an important pathophysiologic role. (If the ECG shows a wide QRS complex, adenosine would be contraindicated.) Among other reasons, it is preferred over another reasonable alternative, verapamil, because of a faster onset of action. Adenosine is also a primary drug for managing episodes of ventricular tachycardia, provided there are no cardiac structural defects (aneurysms, damage to papillary muscles or the chordae tendinae, etc).

Digoxin (b), edrophonium (c; rapidly acting ACh esterase inhibitor), phenylephrine (d; nonselective α-adrenergic agonist), and propranolol or other β-blockers (e), are older therapies falling into relative disuse. In one way or another their effects revolve around causing or unmasking increased parasympathetic influences on the SA and/or AV nodes: digoxin via its predominant effects to slow AV nodal conduction; phenylephrine by increasing blood pressure, which triggers a baroreceptor reflex that reduces sympathetic drive and essentially increases or unmasks parasympathetic tone; propranolol, by blocking β_1-mediated sympathetic influences; and edrophonium, which quickly but briefly raises parasympathetic influences on nodal tissues.

220. The answer is c. *(Brunton, pp 1746-1747. Katzung, pp 594-597, 600.)* Warfarin is a coumarin derivative that is generally used for long-term anticoagulation, and is wholly unsuitable for immediate anticoagulation because it takes at least 5 days of administration for meaningful inhibition of prothrombin time (reported as the International Normalized Ratio [INR]) to develop and stabilize. It antagonizes the gamma carboxylation of several glutamate residues in prothrombin and the coagulation Factors II,

VII, IX, and X. This process is coupled to the oxidative deactivation of vitamin K. The reduced form of vitamin K is essential for sustained carboxylation and synthesis of the coagulation proteins. It appears that warfarin inhibits the action of the reductase(s) that regenerate the reduced form of vitamin K. The prevention of the inactive vitamin K epoxide from being reduced to the active form of vitamin K results in decreased carboxylation of the proteins involved in the coagulation cascade.

Warfarin does not increase factor IX levels (a), inhibit thrombin (b), inhibit or otherwise directly affect platelet function (d), or alter plasminogen levels or activity (e).

221. The answer is e. *(Brunton, pp 1469f, 1480-1481. Katzung, p 597.)* Alteplase, a thrombolytic drug, is an unmodified tissue plasminogen activator (tPA). It activates plasminogen that is bound to fibrin (ie, it is "clot-specific," unlike streptokinase which acts throughout the circulatory system). The plasmin that is formed in response to the drug acts directly on fibrin. This results in dissolving the fibrin into fibrin-split products, followed by lysis of the clot.

Clopidogrel exerts antiplatelet effects by blocking platelet ADP receptors (a); aspirin exerts antiplatelet effects by inhibiting thromboxane production (b) via cyclooxygenase; warfarin, neither a thrombolytic nor an antiplatelet agent, inhibits hepatic synthesis (activation) of vitamin K-dependent clotting factors (c); abciximab is an example of an antiplatelet drug that blocks the platelet Gp IIb/IIIa receptors (d)—the "final common step" in platelet aggregation, regardless of which ligand initiated platelet activation (eg, collagen, ADP, TXA_2).

222. The answer is d. *(Brunton, pp 920-921, 1526t, 1527, 1532t. Katzung, pp 240-241, 678.)* Pulmonary fibrosis has been reported with long-term amiodarone therapy, but not in response to other antiarrhythmics. Pulmonary function tests may remain normal for months and then decline quickly and to significant degrees as irreversible fibrosis develops. Changes of thyroid hormone status—occasionally reflecting hypothyroidism and, for more patients (about 3% of all who take amiodarone long-term), hyperthyroidism—are also uniquely associated with amiodarone: this drug is structurally related to the thyroid hormones and contains iodine. Changes of thyroid hormone status may be subclinical and detectable only with suitable blood tests or may lead to typical signs and symptoms of hyper- or hypothyroidism.

Keep in mind that some adverse responses that are unique to other antiarrhythmic drugs were listed as possible answers. For example, low-grade quinidine toxicity (cinchonism) often includes tinnitus (but that manifestation of ototoxicity cannot be detected with audiometry), and procainamide commonly causes a lupus-like syndrome, for which monitoring of ANA titers is important.

Amiodarone has no significant or direct effects on blood glucose, lipid, or sodium concentrations (a); is not ototoxic (b); has no effects on the various elements of the coagulation cascade or the production of antinuclear antibodies (c; remember that the antihypertensive drug, methyldopa, may increase ANA titers); and does not affect white cell (or red cell) counts or serum urate levels (e). Of course, it's likely that a patient with atrial fibrillation will be placed on warfarin (at least for a while), and so monitoring the prothrombin time (reported as the INR) would be essential in that case. And, since this patient may have multiple cardiovascular "risk factors," periodic monitoring of lipid profiles would be essential too. Nonetheless, these do not apply specifically or uniquely to amiodarone.

223. The answer is c. *(Brunton, pp 1481-1483. Katzung, pp 598-599.)* Clopidogrel (ticlopidine is a related but seldom used drug, and prasugrel is the newest member of the class) decreases platelet aggregation by blocking platelet ADP receptors (which dipyridamole, d, also seems to do, but very weakly, and it is not a "preferred" alternative to aspirin or other antiplatelet drugs), thereby inhibiting ADP-induced platelet activation. It has no direct platelet effects involving activation by TXA_2, collagen, or other mediators, nor does it inhibit platelet aggregation by any actions on the platelet glycoprotein IIb/IIIa receptors.

Acetaminophen (a) has no antiplatelet effects. Aminocaproic acid (b) prevents activation of plasminogen and inhibits plasmin directly. It may be used to counteract the effects of thrombolytic drugs given in relative or absolute overdoses. Streptokinase (e) is a bacterial derived, "non-clot-specific" thrombolytic drug.

224. The answer is f. *(Brunton, pp 834-835, 914, 916t. Katzung, pp 181, 200-202, 236-237, 243-244.)* In essence, we are asking "which drug can suppress AV nodal conduction velocity?" Verapamil and the similar nondihydropyridine calcium channel blocker, diltiazem, do that. Recall the profile of verapamil and diltiazem: a vasodilator effect plus a direct cardiac "depressant" effect that includes slowing of AV conduction (and potential depression of other cardiac contractile and electrophysiologic phenomena).

Be sure you can contrast this dual vasodilator/cardiac depressant profile for verapamil and diltiazem with that of the dihydropyridines (eg, nifedipine; answer c). The dihydropyridines cause vasodilation, but lack any cardiac depressant actions. Indeed, with dihydropyridine dosages sufficient to lower blood pressure enough, and quick enough, there will be baroreceptor reflex activation of the sympathetic nervous system. One consequence of increased norepinephrine release at the heart would be increased AV nodal conduction velocity, which could be construed as an "unblocking" of the AV node—precisely the opposite of what may happen with verapamil or diltiazem.

Captopril (a; ACE inhibitor) and losartan (b; angiotensin receptor blocker) have no significant effects on AV nodal conduction.

Nitroglycerin (d; nitrovasodilator) and prazosin (e; vasodilator that acts by competitive α_1 blockade) also have no direct effect on the AV node, but are likely to lead to an indirect acceleration of AV conduction via baroreceptor activation if blood pressure falls enough and quickly enough.

On a final and important note, be sure you understand that all β-adrenergic blockers (including those with some α-blocking activity, eg, labetalol and carvedilol) can slow AV nodal conduction and can cause or worsen heart block.

225. The answer is a. *(Brunton, pp 808-809, 879. Katzung, pp 181-183.)* Captopril and some of the other ACE inhibitors, may cause severe, hacking, and relentless cough in some patients. One theory is that it is due to increased levels of bradykinin in smooth muscles in the throat. (Recall that angiotensin-converting enzyme, which forms angiotensin II, is the same enzyme as bradykininase, which metabolically inactivates bradykinin.) Many patients receiving captopril (or other ACE inhibitors) experience no problems of this sort. Still other patients, mainly taking other ACE inhibitors, may develop swelling of the oropharyngeal mucosae, and some may develop life-threatening angioedema.

There are no likely allergic reactions (b) triggered by any of the drugs, statins included. Captopril is not a bronchoconstrictor and is not at all likely to cause dyspnea (c) by that mechanism or others. Hyperkalemia (e) is not a likely explanation. Note that by indirectly lowering aldosterone levels (angiotensin II is the main stimulus for aldosterone release, and we have inhibited angiotensin II synthesis), the main renal effects would be increased sodium excretion and increased potassium retention. However, we are administering furosemide (a loop diuretic), which causes renal potassium-wasting. Thus, we would not expect hyperkalemia (e) from this combination of drugs (as we would if the diuretic was a potassium-sparing one such as amiloride, triamterene, or spironolactone). Moreover, loop diuretics are usually part of the treatment regimen for acute pulmonary edema, not a cause of it (f).

226. The answer is b. *(Brunton, pp 255-256, 854-885. Katzung, pp 145, 173-174.)* Abrupt discontinuation of clonidine has been associated with a rapidly developing and severe "rebound" phenomenon that includes excessive cardiac stimulation and a spike of blood pressure that may be sufficient to cause stroke or other similar complications. Recall that clonidine is a "centrally acting α_2-adrenergic agonist." Through its central effects it reduces sympathetic nervous system tone. This, in turn, appears to cause supersensitivity of peripheral adrenergic receptors to direct-acting adrenergic agonists, including endogenous norepinephrine and epinephrine. Once, and soon after, the drug is stopped, endogenous catecholamines trigger hyperresponsiveness of all structures under sympathetic control.

When ACE inhibitors (a; or angiotensin receptor blockers), furosemide (d), or nifedipine (e; long-acting or otherwise) are abruptly stopped, blood pressure (and blood volume, depending on the drug) will begin to rise from treatment levels, but there will be no sudden "spike" of pressure nor an "overshoot" of it. Digoxin (c) discontinuation is not associated with the symptoms noted in the question. Besides, the half-life of digoxin (about 36-40 h if renal function is normal) is such that stopping the drug abruptly would not likely lead to any significant "withdrawal" events occurring within a day or two of discontinuation.

There is no reason to predict that suddenly stopping warfarin (f) would cause tachyarrhythmias, hypertension, or hemorrhagic stroke—and certainly not within 24 to 48 hours.

Important note: A similar, and dangerous, rebound phenomenon occurs when β-blockers are stopped after continuous use for more than a couple of weeks. If the drug blocks only β-receptors, then excessive cardiac stimulation will be the main excessive response. (Remember: BP = CO × TPR, cardiac output and therefore BP will rise from increases of both heart rate and stroke volume.) If α-receptors are also blocked, for example by carvedilol or labetalol, rebound vasoconstriction (a rise of TPR) may occur too. The take-home messages: (1) don't stop β-blockers abruptly unless you have a readily available means to control the potentially life-threatening responses; (2) make sure your patients understand that they must not abruptly stop β-blockers or clonidine or related antihypertensives.

227. The answer is c. *(Brunton, p 1474. Katzung, pp 591-593.)* The scenario describes heparin-induced thrombocytopenia (HIT). It is an immune-mediated thrombocytopenia that is accompanied by a paradoxical increase in thrombotic events (eg, in limbs, brain, lungs, heart). It affects about 1% to 3% of patients receiving heparin for more than about 4 days in a row. The cause appears to involve formation of antibodies that develop into heparin-platelet complexes. This leads to substantial increases of platelet activation that, in turn, leads to, thrombosis, vascular damage, and eventually significant declines in the number of functional circulating platelets (since platelets have been consumed in widespread thrombotic events). This phenomenon is not associated with any of the other drugs listed in the question: abciximab (a; glycoprotein IIb/IIIa blocker); clopidogrel (b; platelet ADP receptor blocker); heparin (c); or nifedipine (d; or other calcium channel blockers.)

Important note: Warfarin can also cause a paradoxical prothrombotic state, probably due to suppressed protein C activity. It is most likely to occur if loading doses are used, rather than starting with the anticipated maintenance dose, but the onset with warfarin doesn't fit the description in the question. If you do some checking on the web or in medicine texts, you will probably find several algorithms for calculating warfarin loading doses. The safest advice is not to use any loading doses: always get the initial anticoagulation with a heparin, start warfarin maintenance doses simultaneously, then continue the heparin for at least 5 days and until the INR reaches the desired range. Using warfarin loading dose strategies does not hasten warfarin's antithrombotic effect.

228. The answer is c. *(Brunton, pp 487-488, 753. Katzung, pp 502-503.)* There is a clinically important relationship between plasma sodium concentrations and the concentration-dependent effects of lithium. In essence, Li^+ and Na^+ compete with one another, such that in the presence of hyponatremia the effects of the lithium may be increased, potentially to the point of causing toxicity. (Conversely, hypernatremia can counteract lithium's therapeutic effects.) Of the drugs listed, hydrochlorothiazide (and all other thiazides or thiazide-like diuretics) poses the greatest risk of causing hyponatremia. (And you should consider the ultimate renal effects of ACE inhibition to lower Na^+ levels further when used with a diuretic. ACE inhibitors used without a diuretic are not likely to cause hyponatremia.)

Angiotensin-converting enzyme inhibitors (a) do not interact with SSRIs to increase the risk of acute psychosis (a). Nitroglycerin or other nitrovasodilators do not counteract the effects of lithium (b), nor does lithium counteract the effects of the vasodilators (f). SSRIs do not antagonize the effects of statins (d) or of calcium channel blockers (e).

229. The answer is d. *(Brunton, pp 838, 850-851, 884, 914-915. Katzung, pp 153, 159, 177.)* Labetalol is the best choice, assuming no contraindications (eg, to β-blockade, such as asthma or 2nd degree or complete heart block). Given its combination of both α- and β-adrenergic (β_1 and β_2) blocking effect, it offers the best approach for managing the hypertension, the tachycardia, the resulting oxygen supply-demand imbalance that leads to both chest discomfort and the ischemic ST-changes, and the ventricular ectopy (which is probably a reflection of excessive catecholamine stimulation of β_1 receptors). If the patient is having an acute myocardial infarction, starting β-blocker therapy early is also decidedly beneficial short term and for the long run. (Almost any other β-blocker might be a suitable alternative, but labetalol has the combined α-/β-blocking actions that are likely to be of greatest benefit. Carvedilol has the same profile, but it is given orally and in this setting that would not be ideal because of slow onset of action.)

Aspirin in high doses (a), or an ACE inhibitor (b) will do no harm in this situation, but they will also do no good for the short term. Nonetheless, neither aspirin nor an ACE inhibitor will do much, if anything, to control heart rate, blood pressure, or the ECG changes.

Nothing in the scenario suggests this patient is volume-overloaded or suffering acute pulmonary edema. Therefore, administering furosemide (c) in such a situation seems not to be indicated. Moreover, giving it is likely to cause prompt reductions of blood volume and, along with it, of blood pressure. The latter effect is likely to lead to further—and unwanted—reflex sympathetic activation that would make matters worse.

Lidocaine (e) might be suitable for ischemia-induced arrhythmias, but the question identified several other important signs and symptoms that would not be relieved by this antiarrhythmic drug. As noted above, the profile of labetalol offers the greatest likelihood of managing multiple problems with one drug.

Increasing the dose of nitroglycerin (f; and especially giving it as a bolus) is likely to drop blood pressure acutely, but it would trigger reflex (baroreceptor) stimulation of the heart. The usual "anti-ischemic" effects of the drug, at low doses, would be counteracted by such "pro-ischemic" changes as further rises of heart rate and stroke volume, and a probable increase in the frequency of premature ventricular beats. Prazosin (g) would lower blood pressure nicely. However, once again we have to worry about excessive pressure lowering, triggering the baroreceptor reflex from a very quick pressure fall, and worsening many of the already worrisome findings.

230. The answer is b. *(Brunton, pp 835-838. Katzung, pp 181, 191, 199-203.)* A good way to arrive at the answer is to remember the rather narrow cardiovascular profile of nifedipine, the prototype dihydropyridine calcium channel blocker, and perhaps to compare it with the two main nondihydropyridines, diltiazem and verapamil.

The nondihydropyridines block vascular smooth-muscle calcium channels, and so cause vasodilation. Any of these drugs, therefore, would help lower this patient's blood pressure.

However, nifedipine (and other dihydropyridines) lack any cardiac-depressant effects. The implication is that as the nifedipine drives blood pressure down (and it will, quite promptly and in an uncontrolled fashion with this sometimes-used but wholly inappropriate and unsafe administration method), there will be intense baroreceptor activation and resulting cardiac stimulation. There are no drug-induced negative inotropic, chronotropic, or dromotropic (conduction velocity) effects to counteract the excessive cardiac stimulation as there would be if we had used either diltiazem or verapamil.

So, in the presence of reflex-mediated increases of catecholamines affecting the heart, AV conduction would increase (not be slowed or blocked); there would be further increases of heart rate (at least; certainly, no fall) to accompany lowering of blood pressure (possibly to hypotensive levels); and the current episodes of ventricular ectopy might convert to longer runs, or to ventricular tachycardia or fibrillation.

231. The answer is b. *(Brunton, p 889. Katzung, p 220.)* This collection of signs and symptoms is characteristic of digoxin toxicity, regardless of the cause (eg, frank overdose or the development of hypokalemia, which increases the risk of digoxin toxicity). Although a possible cause of the hypokalemia is the furosemide (but the patient was receiving triamterene, which counteracts furosemide's potassium-wasting effect), it is not correct to say that furosemide per se is the cause, because signs and symptoms of furosemide toxicity, whether acute or chronic, are not similar at all to those described here.

Although some of the other drugs the patient was taking may have contributed to the digoxin toxicity syndrome, none of them cause those signs and symptoms in their own right: statins (a); furosemide or other diuretics (c), including triamterene (e); or nitroglycerin (d) or other nitrovasodilators.

232. The answer is a. *(Brunton, pp 832-837, 857-858. Katzung, pp 175-177, 181, 183-185.)* The main goals are to safely lower blood pressure and help normalize heart rate. If we cannot use a β-blocker for that, a nondihydropyridine calcium channel blocker, either diltiazem or especially verapamil, would be an excellent choice. In addition to controlling the cardiovascular problems they are unlikely to exacerbate the asthma.

Enalapril (b), one of many ACE inhibitors, might nicely and gradually lower blood pressure, and should have no adverse effects on airway function. Nonetheless it is unlikely that it or any other ACE inhibitor would have much of a beneficial impact on the tachycardia. More important is the fact that ACE inhibitors, and angiotensin receptor blockers such as losartan, should not be administered to women who are pregnant or likely to become pregnant. Furosemide (c) would transiently lower blood pressure, but our patient has essential hypertension: she is not volume-overloaded, and so this diuretic would not be a good choice. Moreover, if circulating fluid volume fell sufficiently, and sufficiently fast, the baroreceptor reflex might be activated, causing even further rises of heart rate.

Phentolamine (d) and prazosin (e) are both α-adrenergic blockers. Phentolamine is rapidly acting, given parenterally, and nonselectively blocks both α_1 and α_2 (presynaptic) receptors. Even with small doses, the blood pressure fall is usually sufficient, and sufficiently fast, to reflexly increase heart rate (and contractility) even more. A parenteral drug such as this simply is not appropriate therapy in this situation. Prazosin is given orally, works relatively slowly, and blocks only α_1 receptors. While its effects are more gradual, perhaps slow enough that the baroreceptors are not activated, this drug will do nothing to control the patient's tachycardia.

233. The answer is e. *(Brunton, pp 143t, 164, 256, 1643. Katzung, pp 153-154.)* Pheochromocytomas—rare cause of hypertension—generally involve excessive levels of circulating catecholamines from tumors of the adrenal (suprarenal) medulla. (In adults, only about 10% of all cases of pheochromocytoma are due to catecholamines released from non-adrenal sites.) Regardless of the site(s) of the tumor(s), the main factor in leading to an increase of blood pressure and heart rate in this condition is α-mediated vasoconstriction arising from excessive levels of epinephrine, norepinephrine, or both. Epinephrine (but not norepinephrine) will cause β_2-mediated dilation of some vascular beds. However, that vasodilator effect, which might be construed as a mechanism to keep blood pressure from rising too much, is slight in comparison with the opposing vasoconstrictor (α mediated) influences of the catecholamines elsewhere in the peripheral vasculature. Even if you consider the vasodilator influences to be slight, they will be blocked by propranolol or any other β-adrenergic blocker that lacks vasodilator activity (ie, all but carvedilol, labetalol, nebivolol), such that diastolic and mean blood pressures will rise further, at least initially. The so-called cardioselective β_1 blockers such as atenolol and metoprolol will block β_2 receptors in the vasculature, and elsewhere, at blood levels that are not too far above the usual "therapeutic" range. In essence, blockade of β_2 receptors in the vasculature will leave α-mediated constrictor effects unopposed, and blood pressure will rise (concomitant with suppression of cardiac contractility and rate). The problem is not likely to happen, or the outcome be as severe, with labetalol (c). It is, indeed, a β-blocker, but it also has intrinsic α-blocking activity that should blunt the vasoconstrictor influences of circulating epinephrine and neuronally-released norepinephrine at the same time it is blocking all the β-adrenergic receptors.

None of the other drugs would raise blood pressure further, and while none of them is indicated as primary therapy for pheochromocytomas, ultimately any of them are more likely to lower, not raise, blood pressure, although not by much in the face of catecholamine excess: angiotensin "modifiers" such as captopril (a) or losartan (d); hydrochlorothiazide (b) or any other common diuretic; and verapamil (f) or other calcium channel blockers, dihydropyridine or not.

234. The answer is d. *(Brunton, pp 1484-1486. Katzung, pp 595-597.)* Phytonadione (vitamin K_1) is the antidote. It overcomes (reverses, antagonizes) warfarin's hepatic anticoagulant effects, which involve inhibited vitamin K-dependent synthesis/activation of clotting factors (II, VII, IX, X, and prothrombin).

Aminocaproic acid (a) is an adjunct (to whole blood, packed red cells, or fresh-frozen plasma) for managing bleeding in response to excessive effects of thrombolytic drugs (eg, alteplase [tPA]). It is not indicated for warfarin-related bleeding. Epoetin alfa (b) is a hematopoietic growth factor that stimulates erythrocyte production in peritubular cells in the proximal tubules of the kidney. Its uses include management of anemias associated with chronic renal failure, chemotherapy (of nonmyeloid malignancies), or zidovudine therapy in patients with acquired immunodeficiency syndrome. It is inappropriate for this patient. Ferrous sulfate (b; or fumarate or gluconate) is indicated for prevention or treatment of iron-deficiency anemias. It will do nothing to lower the patient's INR or alleviate related symptoms. Protamine sulfate (e) is the antidote for heparin overdoses. It interacts with and neutralizes heparin in the blood to form a complex that lacks anticoagulant activity. It does nothing to the hepatic vitamin K-related problems that are at the root of excessive warfarin effects.

235. The answer is d. *(Brunton, p 1474. Katzung, p 592.)* This patient's presentation is fairly typical of heparin-induced thrombocytopenia (HIT) in terms of both physical findings and time-course of onset. If heparin administration lasts for more than about a week, platelet counts should be checked several times a week for the first month or so and then monthly thereafter, because this is a potentially fatal response. It is immune-mediated: antibodies form against a heparin-platelet complex; platelets are activated (thus, the thrombosis and such complications as pulmonary and/or coronary occlusion, as I described); the vascular endothelia are damaged; and ultimately the number of platelets that can be detected in a venous blood sample declines markedly (and so, the thrombocytopenia). The overall incidence of HIT is about 10 times higher with unfractionated heparin than with LMW heparin, and so answer a is not the best or most likely choice. Should HIT occur or be suspected, the approach includes stopping the heparin and substituting other anticoagulants. A good choice would be a direct thrombin inhibitor (eg, bivalirudin).

Aspirin (b), by virtue of its antiplatelet effects, should not induce thrombosis. ACE inhibitors and β-blockers do not interact to cause hemolytic anemia (c) or other blood dyscrasias. There is no known and clinically relevant interaction between heparin and proton pump inhibitors, esomeprazole (e) or others.

236. The answer is b. *(Brunton, pp 828-829. Katzung, pp 194-198.)* Using long-acting nitrovasodilators "24-7" is not a good idea, because it ultimately leads to tolerance to the desired vasodilator effects. This is of concern in part because, by definition, when a system or function develops tolerance to a drug, we must increase the dose in order to achieve effects of the same intensity as occurred before. With nitroglycerin patches, or other long-acting oral nitrovasodilators, increasing the dose to restore the response ultimately accelerates or otherwise intensifies the tolerance, such that further dosage increases seem warranted. More importantly, with the development of tolerance, the vasodilator/antianginal efficacy of sublingual (or transmucosal) nitrate is diminished too. So, should the patient develop angina, usual dosages of immediate-acting nitrates may not provide relief of either the symptoms or the underlying myocardial ischemia.

If you thought cyanide poisoning (a) you were probably thinking of nitroprusside toxicity. Cyanide is not a metabolite of nitroglycerin or other drugs traditionally used for angina. Doses of nitrates that are too high, or that otherwise lower peripheral resistance too quickly, may trigger reflex tachycardia. This is, for some patients, a problem early-on in therapy with rapidly acting nitrates. It usually becomes less problematic as therapy continues, of if the dosage is titrated down a bit. It is rarely a problem with long-acting nitrates. We do not see bradycardia (c), reflex or otherwise, in response to these drugs. Nitrovasodilators, short- or long-acting, and regardless of the administration route, do not cause thrombosis or affect any other aspects of the coagulation-thrombolysis processes (d). Paradoxical vasoconstriction leading to hypertension (e) does not occur.

237. The answer is b. *(Brunton, pp 800-805, 813-814. Katzung, pp 182, 217-219, 297.)* Losartan, an angiotensin receptor blocker (ARB) has no effect on angiotensin II synthesis (as do the ACE inhibitors such as lisinopril, captopril, and others). Its main antihypertensive actions, therefore, include only blockade of angiotensin II-mediated aldosterone release from the adrenal cortex, and of angiotensin II's vasoconstrictor effects.

Lisinopril and the other ACE inhibitors inhibit angiotensin II synthesis, and that effect accounts (indirectly) for reduced aldosterone release and AII-mediated vasoconstriction. They also inhibit metabolic inactivation of bradykinin, an endogenous vasodilator (bradykininase, angiotensin-converting enzyme, and kininase II are synonyms for essentially the same enzyme). However, the ACE inhibitors and the angiotensin receptor blockers do not antagonize catecholamine-mediated vasoconstriction (a). Nonetheless, there is growing evidence that angiotensin II enhances (not inhibits) sympathetic-mediated vasoconstriction (by increasing neuronal norepinephrine release and/or blocking neuronal norepinephrine reuptake). Either an ACE inhibitor or an ARB should be equivalent in attenuating that blood pressure-elevating effect.

Neither an ACE inhibitor nor an ARB is associated with an increased incidence of bronchospasm (c; although some ACE inhibitors may cause cough, presumably from locally increased bradykinin levels, and angioedema, perhaps by the same mechanism). Both ACE inhibitors and ARBs are contraindicated during pregnancy (e).

ACE inhibitors are considered to be an "essential" part of therapy (along with β-blockers and a diuretic) for most patients with heart failure. Angiotensin receptor blockers such as losartan may prove to be equally effective alternatives. Thus, answer e is incorrect.

By the way: You didn't learn explicitly about lisinopril and so didn't recognize its classification? Remember: drugs with generic names that end in "-pril" are ACE inhibitors.

238. The answer is d. *(Brunton, pp 959-960. Katzung, p 616.)* Ezetimibe inhibits absorption of dietary cholesterol through the gut. It has no hepatic or other direct effects that contribute to its clinically desired effect. The drug lacks cardiac effects (a) or vascular effects (b). There is no good evidence that ezetimibe increases the risks of plaque rupture and the often devastating consequences of that. Other lipid-lowering drugs, such as niacin, the fibrates, and perhaps some of the cholesterol-binding resins, seem to increase the risks of statin-induced myopathy, rhabdomyolysis, or liver dysfunction. Such increased risks are the major problems to be faced when statins are used in combination with other lipid-lowering agents. However, this seems not to be a problem with ezetimibe. It is said to be a reasonable drug to combine with a statin, and one proprietary fixed-dose combination that contains ezetimibe and a statin is available and quite widely used. There are, however, questions about whether ezetimibe alone or in combination with other lipid-lowering drugs, is actually as efficacious as it was thought to be.

239. The answer is e. *(Brunton, pp 831-841, 1480-1481. Katzung, p 597.)* "Time is muscle," some say when addressing the issue of thrombolysis for coronary occlusion. Ideally, the "door to needle" time should be 90 minutes or (preferably) much less. It is true that choosing alteplase (a) or some other tPA variant may be associated with a lower risk of bleeding, owing to their clot-specific site of action; and that it is relatively safer to use them with heparin. In contrast, streptokinase administration once may lead to antibodies that, if the patient is retreated with the same drug (within about 5 days to 2 years), may either neutralize the drug (rendering it ineffective) or trigger an allergic reaction, or do both. However, I stated this was our patient's first MI. (You could argue that the patient may already have anti-SK antibodies from a prior streptococcal infection, but did you think of that?)

The key point, then, is starting thrombolysis as quickly as possible, not which drug is chosen (a), where the infarct is (b), the presence of absence of collaterals (c), or within reason what blood pressure (d) is. There seems to be maximum benefit (salvaging tissue, reducing ultimate infarct size, maintaining reasonable cardiac function, and reducing mortality) if a thrombolytic—any thrombolytic—is administered within 1 hour of symptom onset. According to many studies, benefits of thrombolysis become comparable to placebo if the drug isn't started until around 6 hours after symptom onset, and in terms of mortality thrombolytics may actually increase the risk of morbidity or death if given after about 12 hours or so.

240. The answer is c. *(Brunton, pp 1468f, 1483. Katzung, pp 588f, 599.)* Abciximab, and such related drugs as tirofiban and eptifibatide, block the glycoprotein IIb/IIIa receptor on platelets. Abciximab is an antibody raised against the IIb/IIIa receptor. It binds to the receptor, and in doing so blocks the formation of fibrinogen bridges between the IIb/IIIa receptors on adjacent platelets. That is, otherwise, the final critical and common step in causing platelets to aggregate with their neighbors.

Recall that platelet activation can be triggered by TXA_2, thrombin, collagen, ADP, and platelet-activating factor (PAF) (among other agonists). Block the activating effects of just one of those factors and the proaggregatory effects of the other activators are left unchecked. Platelet activation ensues; some platelet-derived activators are released, thereby recruiting the activation of more platelets—the amplification process. For example, clopidogrel blocks ADP receptors (b); aspirin inhibits cyclooxygenases (d) that leads to reduced TXA_2 formation and, at higher than the usual antiplatelet doses can also inhibit prostacyclin synthesis (e). Finally, bivalirudin is a drug that inhibits thrombin's activity by binding directly to thrombin (not thrombin receptors; a), and that mechanism of action does not apply to abciximab.

241. The answer is c. *(Brunton, pp 254, 269-270. Katzung, pp 135-140, 142-143, 150-153.)* Phenylephrine, as noted, causes vasoconstriction through its agonist activity on α-adrenergic receptors. Prazosin competitively blocks those receptors, and since we have a patient who has taken an excessive dose of the antagonist it should be no surprise that usually effective (or even higher) doses of phenylephrine will not be able to overcome that blockade. None of the other drugs listed (ACE inhibitors, a; hydralazine, b; thiazides, d; or verapamil or any other calcium channel blocker for that matter) have any direct effects on α-adrenergic receptors, nor the ability of phenylephrine to activate them. (Thiazides probably exert their antihypertensive effects by causing some net sodium depletion, which reduces vascular responsiveness to adrenergic agonists, angiotensin II, and any other vasoconstrictors you may conjure. However, it is highly unlikely that a thiazide would completely eliminate any vasopressor effects of one usual dose of phenylephrine, let alone repeated doses.)

242. The answer is e. *(Brunton, pp 269-271. Katzung, pp 150-155, 186t.)* This is an apt description of an α-adrenergic blocker, and not at all descriptive of the actions or effects of any other drug listed. Prazosin can be considered the prototype of the α-adrenergic blockers, at least those that selectively block α_1 receptors (in comparison with phentolamine and several other drugs, which block both α_1 and α_2 receptors) and are given orally. It's not likely your patient with BPH was taking prazosin itself (or a related drug like doxazosin or terazosin). That is because those drugs not only exert significant inhibitory effects on smooth muscle of the prostate capsule and urethra, but also on the peripheral vasculature. Thus, they could cause a fall of BP, which we don't want if our only goal is managing BPH. However, if the patient is also hypertensive, one drug may help both conditions. If blood pressure is normal, or controlled well with other antihypertensives, then prazosin or other α-blockers used for hypertension may lower pressure too much (unless we lower the dosage). More likely your benign prostatic hypertrophy patient is taking tamsulosin. It's in the same general class as prazosin, but seems to have more selectivity for smooth muscles in the urinary tract, and fewer or milder peripheral vascular (α-blocking) actions that would tend to lower blood pressure and trigger the other responses I noted.

Let's take a quick look at why the other answers don't fit the description completely. Captopril (a) or other ACE inhibitors aren't used for BPH, and they do not change pupil size or interfere with mydriasis in dim light. And, like the description of the unknown drug, they have no effects on airway smooth muscle, either excitatory or inhibitory. ACE inhibitors do lower blood pressure, but when given orally the fall of pressure is so slow that the baroreceptors don't sense such a gradual fall. These same statements would apply to a thiazide diuretic (b) too.

What about labetalol (c)? Its α-blocking activity probably would cause mydriasis and peripheral vasodilation. However, given orally the vasodilator response is relatively weak and the fall of blood pressure it would cause (in conjunction with reductions of heart rate and stroke volume from β-blockade) isn't likely to occur quickly enough for the baroreceptors to sense and respond to it. Even if pressure fell enough, and fast enough, and the baroreceptors were activated, the stronger β-blocking effects of labetalol would blunt, if not prevent altogether, reflex cardiac stimulation. And effects of labetalol on the airways? None, just like the unknown drug, but if the patient had asthma (we did not say he did) then bronchoconstriction due to β-blockade is liable to occur.

Finally, what about nifedipine (d; or other dihydropyridine calcium channel blockers)? Oral nifedipine can cause such prompt and significant changes of blood pressure that the baroreceptor reflex is activated. That's not desirable, but it can happen. The drug also lacks significant bronchodilator or (especially) constrictor effects. However, its effects on smooth muscles in the urinary tract are slight, and the drug is not indicated for managing BPH; and lacking direct autonomic agonist or antagonist effects it does not change pupil size or prevent changes of pupil size in response to increases or decreases of ambient light.

243. The answer is e. *(Brunton, p 809. Katzung, pp 181-183, 1028t.)* ACE inhibitors (and angiotensin receptor blockers [ARBs] eg, losartan) are contraindicated in women who are pregnant or of child-bearing potential. ACE inhibitors and ARBs do not exacerbate asthma (a), they are considered first-line adjunctive drugs for managing most patients with heart failure (b), which may or may not be an accompaniment of hyperlipidemias or coronary artery disease (c). We would want to normalize potassium levels if the patient were hypokalemic (d; but it depends on what the absolute potassium levels are, and whether the hypokalemia is symptomatic), before we gave an ACE inhibitor, but one would want to be very careful in terms of how to go about doing that. ACE inhibitors and ARBs ultimately lower circulating aldosterone levels, which in turn favors more renal potassium retention. One of these drugs, alone, might correct potassium levels. Giving an ACE inhibitor or ARB along with a potassium-sparing diuretic may not merely correct the hypokalemia but, eventually and more likely, cause hyperkalemia.

244. The answer is a. *(Brunton, pp 192, 197. Katzung, pp 116, 119-122.)* Sinus bradycardia can be conceptually viewed as an imbalance of two opposing factors on the SA node: (1) too great an influence of the parasympathetic nervous system, specifically, of ACh acting on muscarinic receptors; or (2) too little activation of β_1-adrenergic receptors. We can address either, or both, imbalances pharmacologically. According to current ACLS guidelines, using atropine to block excessive parasympathetic influences, allowing heart rate to go up, is the recommended first approach.

An alternative approach would be to activate β_1-adrenergic receptors, for example, with isoproterenol. Amiodarone (b) is neither effective nor indicated for sinus bradycardia. It is used as a first-line drug for cardiac arrest; is indicated for managing some serious and life-threatening ventricular arrhythmias; and has gotten growing attention for its apparent efficacy to manage atrial fibrillation—a rather unusual use given the seriousness of the other arrhythmias for which the drug is given. Edrophonium (c) would be among the worse drugs you could give to this bradycardic patient. This rapidly acting ACh esterase inhibitor will cause accumulation of even more ACh at the SA node (and elsewhere in the autonomic nervous system where ACh is the neurotransmitter activating smooth muscles and various exocrine glands). If the patient's heart doesn't stop in response to edrophonium, assuming we give a usual dose, it is mere luck. Lidocaine (d) is effective for a host of ventricular arrhythmias, including those associated with an MI. It will do nothing good for the bradycardia. You might argue that phentolamine (e), the prototype α-adrenergic blocker, would work. It might, but probably at great cost to this patient's hemodynamic status. When we inject "usual" doses of phentolamine heart rate indeed goes up. That is mediated by the baroreceptor reflex: and to elicit that response we have to give enough drug to rapidly and markedly drop blood pressure via the drug's vasodilator actions. That, in turn, "withdraws" central parasympathetic tone and causes a relative increase in sympathetic outflow. Both effects would increase heart rate. Unfortunately, our bradycardic patient probably already has a blood pressure and cardiac output that are on the low side of conducive to a long and happy life. Even if he didn't, causing blood pressure to promptly and markedly fall often doesn't lead to a favorable outcome.

245. The answer is e. *(Brunton, pp 143t, 272-275, 824-826, 837-884. Katzung, pp 192-196, 203-205.)* In terms of autonomic control of coronary vascular tone, envisage a "balance" between the vasoconstrictor influences of α-adrenergic activation and the opposing vasodilator influences of β_2-receptor activation. Spasm-prone coronaries appear to be very dependent on the β-mediated vasodilator influences to reduce the incidence and severity of spasm. Any β-blocker will remove those favorable influences, and tend to provoke (or intensify or prolong) spasm and the resulting ischemia in distal tissues. This vascular effect is likely to overshadow any beneficial effects attributed to reductions of myocardial oxygen demand via suppression of heart rate and contractility.

You could correctly argue that in the absence of demonstrated coronary occlusion the administration of tPA (a) would be inappropriate. However, that drug is not likely to make matters worse. Captopril (c), the prototype ACE inhibitor, should have no negative or positive effects on vasospasm. Nitroglycerin (d) might reduce the incidence or severity of spasm through nitric-oxide-mediated vasodilation. Verapamil (f) would probably be one of the most rational drugs to give, since its vascular calcium channel-blocking activity would help suppress spasm. Its negative inotropic and chronotropic effects would, additionally, reduce myocardial oxygen demand and be beneficial.

246. The answer is b. *(Brunton, pp 177-178, 395-397. Katzung, pp 246, 598, 622-624.)* That aspirin might increase the risk of stroke should not be surprising. The same mechanism by which the drug exerts protective effects against MI, by inhibiting platelet aggregation, explains why some patients who otherwise might develop a cerebral bleed are at increased risk of doing so. There is no good evidence that aspirin ingestion causes hepatotoxicity of any sort (a); tachycardia and/or hypotension (d; other than via blood loss and hypovolemia due to excessive bleeding); nor causes or provokes coronary vasospasm (e). Long-term use of many nonsteroidal anti-inflammatory drugs may cause nephropathy, but that is typically associated with high-dose use, and rarely with aspirin itself.

247. The answer is d. *(Brunton, pp 797-798, 780. Katzung, pp 170-171, 181-183, 217-219, 221t, 260-266.)* The patient has been taking two diuretics, one potassium-wasting (the thiazide), the other potassium-sparing. Ramipril is an ACE inhibitor (recall: drugs with generic names ending in "-pril" are members of that class) that ultimately will lower aldosterone levels. This will, in essence, counteract the sodium-retaining effects of aldosterone, and also its potassium-wasting effects. So by adding the ACE inhibitor to the regimen we will now be treating the patient with two drugs that tend to elevate potassium levels to a degree that cannot be compensated for by the thiazide.

Adding an ACE inhibitor to our patient's regimen would be a good idea (provided there are no contraindications to doing so) in terms of getting additional blood pressure control, but it would probably require eliminating the triamterene at some point (if not from the start) to avoid the hyperkalemia.

Prazosin (b), a selective α_1-adrenergic blocker, is not at all likely to have elicited the hyperkalemia. Diltiazem (a) and verapamil (e), both nondihydropyridine calcium channel blockers, are not likely to affect potassium levels in a measurable way. Adrenergic blockers (eg, propranolol; c) may lower serum potassium levels, presumably by enhancing K^+ uptake into skeletal muscle. But, overall these drugs are not, however, the most likely cause of the hypokalemia, even when used in combination with the diuretics.

248. The answer is c. *(Brunton, pp 242, 254, 263-264. Katzung, pp 169, 225-227.)* Phenylephrine is the prototypic α-adrenergic agonist. It terminated the arrhythmia reflexly, via the baroreceptors, in response to a vasopressor effect. (Raising blood pressure quickly and markedly is a risky way of terminating this tachycardia, of course, due to such risks as causing a hemorrhagic stroke.) All the other drugs would also terminate the arrhythmia, but by actions on the heart. Edrophonium (a) is an ACh esterase inhibitor with a fast onset of action and a brief duration. It would slow heart rate by increasing the effects of ACh on the SA node, slowing the spontaneous rate of phase 4 depolarization. Esmolol is a β-blocker (nonselective) that also has a fast onset and short duration of action. It and propranolol (d) would slow heart rate via direct β-blocking effects on the

SA node. Verapamil (e) will do the same by blocking AV nodal calcium channels.

249. The answer is b. *(Brunton, pp 912, 921-922. Katzung, pp 214-216, 219-220, 225-233.)* Answering this question, of course, requires that you not only know the expected effects of digoxin, but also that you can "translate" those effects into interpretations of findings from a most useful diagnostic tool, the electrocardiogram.

An expected and important effect of digoxin is slowed atrioventricular nodal conduction velocity, manifest as prolongation of the PR interval. The effect, which can lead to increasing degrees of heart block, depends on the plasma concentration of digoxin and on the concentrations of several ions, potassium arguably the most important.

Digoxin tends to speed electrical impulse velocity through the atrial myocardium, and so widening of P waves (a) would be the opposite of the expected response. There is no good reason to expect increased P-wave amplitude due to the digoxin. (Atrial enlargement, a result of the heart failure and not the drug, is likely.)

Digoxin also speeds electrical impulse conduction velocity through the ventricles (eg, the His-Purkinje system), and so widened QRS complexes, compared with baseline, would be the opposite of the expected effect.

RR intervals essentially reflect ventricular rate. Before treatment of heart failure there are varying degrees of compensatory "sympathetic drive" over the heart, leading to tachycardia and shortened RR intervals (d). Once digoxin starts increasing cardiac output, there is a lessening of sympathetic drive (and the physiologic need for it). Thus, compared with baseline heart rate, posttreatment heart rate is slower; this is manifest as a longer RR interval compared with baseline.

ST segment changes are among the manifestations of acute coronary syndrome and regional myocardial ischemia. Based on the description of the patient, who appears to have normal blood profiles and no evidence of acute ischemia, ST elevation (e) is not a reasonable answer.

250. The answer is a. *(Brunton, pp 308-311. Katzung, pp 285-289.)* Although ergotamine, and the ergot alkaloids in general, may not be considered typical cardiovascular drugs, they clearly can cause significant, cumulative, and sometimes dangerous cardiovascular effects. Ergotamine can cause intense and prolonged vasoconstriction in both the peripheral and coronary vasculatures. Thus, of the answer choices given, myocardial ischemia and ischemia of, for example, one or more extremities are the most likely outcomes. These vascular responses pose particular problems for patients with ischemic heart disease, especially those who have vasospastic, or variant, angina; or patients with peripheral vascular disease. (One ergot alkaloid, ergonovine, is such a powerful coronary vasoconstrictor that it is sometimes used in angiographic studies of the heart to diagnose vasospastic angina.) The coronary effects may be rapidly fatal; limb ischemia may be sufficiently intense and prolonged to induce gangrene and require amputation of the affected limb(s).

Rhabdomyolysis, with or without renal failure (b), is unlikely, at least as a direct consequence of ergotamine, as the ergot compounds in general have no appreciable effects on skeletal muscle structure or function. There are no direct effects on platelet activation or aggregation that would lead to spontaneous bleeding (c). However, platelet activation and thrombotic events certainly may occur secondary to stasis in vascular beds that have been intensely constricted by the drug. Hypertension, not hypotension with or without syncope (d), is a likely consequence of peripheral vasoconstriction. Sudden rises in blood pressure are likely to cause bradycardia (not tachycardia; e) *via* baroreceptor reflex activation. Members of the ergot alkaloid class (eg, ergotamine, ergonovine) have variable agonist or antagonist effects (direct or indirect) on α-adrenergic, dopaminergic, and serotoninergic receptors, but not on β-adrenergic receptors.

(For study purposes in other areas of pharmacology you may want to recall the following: (1) Triptans [eg, sumatriptan] or methysergide tend to be used more than ergotamine or similar drugs for migraine. (2) Ergonovine is sometimes used as an alternative or backup to oxytocin for controlling postpartum uterine bleeding or hemorrhage: it causes intense and prolonged uterine smooth muscle contraction, and relatively slight cardiovascular effects. (3) Another ergot drug, bromocriptine, is used to manage hyperprolactinemia [due to its strong dopaminergic effects] such as that which may occur with pituitary tumors, and is also sometimes used for managing Parkinson disease.)

251. The answer is e. *(Brunton, pp 143t, 164, 269-270. Katzung, pp 153-154.)* Pheochromocytomas are epinephrine-secreting tumors, and so the worrisome and dangerous consequences are due to excessive vasoconstriction (α-mediated) and cardiac chronotropic and inotropic responses (β_1).

A β-adrenergic blocker is an essential component of pharmacotherapy. It must be administered along with another drug that blocks α-adrenergic receptors, but should not be given before the α-adrenergic blocker is given. Activation of β_2-adrenergic receptors in the peripheral vasculature plays a small but important role in blood pressure control (since β_2 activation in some vascular beds causes vasodilation). Block that effect in a patient with epinephrine excess—a pheochromocytoma—and any potentially blood pressure-lowering effects are lost. Blood pressure will, therefore, either rise or stay the same in terms of peripheral vascular effects.

In the face of this still-high blood pressure and total peripheral resistance the β-blocker will reduce both heart rate and contractility, and so cardiac output will fall (recall that CO = HR × SV). The outcome may be not merely a fall of cardiac output, but a considerable fall in a very short time that might well put the patient into acute heart failure.

Blood pressure is not at all likely to fall promptly due to any peripheral vasodilator effects; if it did (and it won't), the β-blocker would prevent reflex tachycardia (a) via direct actions on cardiac β_1 receptors. The β-blockers do not inhibit catecholamine release (b), whether from a catecholamine-secreting tumor or from a normal sympathetic nervous system. A β-blocker will not trigger catecholamine release from a pheochromocytoma (c), nor will it normalize cardiovascular status in any other way if given without an α-blocker. A β-blocker alone, in this situation, will raise left ventricular afterload, and reduce cardiac output by effects on both heart rate and stroke volume. Thus, answer e is wrong.

252. The answer is d. *(Brunton, pp 830-832. Katzung, pp 194-198.)* Nitroglycerin and other nitrovasodilators provide immediate symptom relief in most patients with an acute coronary syndrome or MI. However, there is no evidence that these drugs provide long-term preventative effects against sudden death from an acute MI. In contrast, aspirin (a; antiplatelet drug), a lipid-lowering drug such as atorvastatin (b), ACE inhibitors such as captopril (c), and β-blockers such as propranolol (e), have documented protective effects to reduce the risk of death from a subsequent MI.

253. The answer is a. *(Brunton, pp 250-251, 889-894. Katzung, pp 140, 216-217.)* Intravenous infusion of dobutamine, a β_1 agonist, was the most likely cause of the increased heart rate. Blood pressure probably rose secondary to positive chronotropic and inotropic effects of the drug; it cannot be by any direct effect on total peripheral resistance, since even at high doses dobutamine has no vasoconstrictor activity. Esmolol (b) is a nonselective β-blocker with a rapid onset of action, and a brief duration of action (due to rapid hydrolysis by plasma esterases. Being a β-blocker, neither it nor propranolol (d) would raise heart rate or blood pressure. Neostigmine (c) is an ACh esterase inhibitor. It and verapamil (e), a nondihydropyridine calcium channel blocker, would be expected to reduce heart rate. Verapamil would also tend to lower, not raise, blood pressure by virtue of its peripheral vasodilator action.

254. The answer is b. *(Brunton, pp 655, 657-658, 660, 1470, 1482. Katzung, pp 313-320, 326.)* At the usual low cardioprotective doses of aspirin, the main and therapeutically useful effect of the drug is inhibition of TXA_2 synthesis via the COX-1 pathway. Recall that TXA_2 is one important—but certainly not the only—trigger of platelet activation, amplification, and aggregation. However, at high(er) doses, aspirin also inhibits synthesis of other eicosanoids, of which PGI2 (prostacyclin), synthesized in the vascular endothelium, is of most importance here. Endothelial prostacyclin synthesis helps prevent platelets from adhering to the vascular wall. Suppress PGI2 in the endothelium, and platelet adherence is increased, despite the fact that platelet TXA_2 synthesis has already been blocked. It's important to remember here that aspirin does nothing to inhibit platelet activation by such other agonists as collagen or ADP. By lowering endothelial PGI2 levels we've increased the likelihood that platelets activated by eicosanoid-independent agonists will adhere to the lining of blood vessels, and potentially occlude them.

Aspirin has no effect on Gp IIb/IIIa receptors (a); it does not rupture or otherwise damage vascular plaques (c) to expose collagen; inhibit synthesis of any liver-based clotting factors (d); or amplify or otherwise enhance the effects of ADP (e) or of other platelet activators.

255. The answer is d. *(Brunton, pp 264-269, 851-852. Katzung, pp 150-152, 177, 285.)* Prazosin causes competitive α blockade. This is in stark contrast to phenoxybenzamine, which causes insurmountable (noncompetitive) and long-lasting blockade of α-receptors by alkylating them. This covalent interaction, in comparison with typical weak ionic interactions between most drugs and their receptors, accounts for phenoxybenzamine's long-lasting (not shorter-acting; a) and noncompetitive blockade. As a result of altering receptor conformation, not merely occupying them as prazosin and most other α-blockers do, phenoxybenzamine renders largely ineffective the α agonists that ordinarily would be used to counteract effects of excessive receptor blockade. Thus, if the patient became hypotensive in response to phenoxybenzamine, raising pressure with typical and usually effective drugs may not succeed. Neither drug has intrinsic β-blocking activity (b), and so regardless of which of these drugs we use for the pheochromocytoma patient, a β-blocker will need to be used adjunctively to control (primarily) heart rate and contractility. Neither drug suppresses epinephrine release from the adrenal/suprarenal medulla (c); both tend to cause orthostatic hypotension by blocking peripheral α-mediated vasoconstriction that occurs upon standing up suddenly.

256. The answer is b. *(Brunton, pp 953-955. Katzung, pp 615, 1081.)* Colesevelam is the newest bile-acid sequestrant, and is the drug of choice when a bile acid-sequestrant is indicated. The older agents are cholestyramine and colestipol. These drugs, which are given orally, are nonabsorbable resins that bind (sequester, adsorb) many substances that are present in the GI tract (eg, bile salts) at the same time as the drug, prevents them from being (re)absorbed, and facilitates their elimination in the feces. None of these drugs have any effects on renal handling of electrolytes, nonelectrolytes, or free water (a, e); no effects on urate levels (c); no direct antianginal effects, and certainly no negative inotropic or chronotropic effects; and are not antihypertensive (e).

Colesevelam may be used alone, but usually it is in combination with a statin. On average, colesevelam alone can lower LDL cholesterol by about 20% (the typical range is between 15% and 30%). In contrast, combined therapy with a statin can reduce LDL cholesterol by up to 50%. Similar results can be obtained by combining a sequestrant with niacin. LDL-lowering effects begin soon after dosing starts, but it may take a month or so for effects to peak.

All the bile-acid sequestrants lower LDL cholesterol through a mechanism that ultimately depends on increasing LDL receptors on hepatocytes, and that occurs via a sequence of related steps. Bile salts and the cholesterol from which they are made are excreted into the intestines. Normally, thereafter, a good portion of the excreted bile salts and cholesterol is reabsorbed and recycled in a process usually called enterohepatic recirculation. The bile acid sequestrants interrupt the recycling. They adsorb the cholesterol-rich bile acids in the intestine and form an insoluble complex that prevents the bile salts and cholesterol from being returned to the circulation. As a result, the excretion of cholesterol-laden bile salts increases. This increased fecal excretion creates a demand for increased bile acid formation in the liver; and that, in turn, requires increased cholesterol supply to the liver. That cholesterol comes from LDL. In order to use more LDL cholesterol the liver cells increase their number of LDL receptors. That increases their capacity for LDL uptake. The result is an increase in LDL uptake from plasma, and a decrease of circulating LDL levels. With continued administration of the sequestrant, the cycle repeats itself as bile salt excretion continues to increase, and over time the eventual result is a fall of LDL levels.

Bile-acid sequestrants may increase VLDL levels in some patients. In most cases, the elevation is temporary and mild. However, if VLDL levels are elevated before treatment, the bile-acid sequestrants may cause further sustained and substantial VLDL increases. Therefore, bile-acid sequestrants are not drugs of choice for lowering LDL cholesterol in patients with high VLDL levels.

Colesevelam is now the preferred bile acid sequestrant because it differs from cholestyramine and colestipol in at least four main ways: (1) colesevelam is better tolerated (less constipation, flatulence, bloating, and cramping); (2) It does not reduce the absorption of fat-soluble vitamins (A, D, E, and K), whether from foods, beverages, or from vitamin supplements; (3) It does not significantly reduce oral absorption of statins, digoxin, warfarin, and most other drugs studied that are present in the GI tract at the same time as the sequestrant. (4) Finally, it is of course very common for patients with CHD risk to have hypercholesterolemia and diabetes. Colesevelam also causes desirable glucose-controlling effects for many patients with Type 2 diabetes (ie, about 90% of all cases of diabetes) when used in combination with such other antidiabetic medications as metformin, sulfonylureas, or insulin. It is the only bile acid sequestrant approved for use as an antidiabetic adjunct.

257. The answer is e. *(Brunton, pp 272-275, 864. Katzung, pp 177-181.)* Nitroprusside (or any other IV vasodilator, eg, nitroglycerin) is likely to elicit baroreceptor reflex-mediated rises of heart rate and contractility. It may be significant and dangerous for any patient, more so for patients with ischemic heart disease, and potentially deadly for patients with aneurysms, such as our patient. For aortic aneurysm patients, the problem is not the rise of heart rate, but rather of left ventricular contractility (left ventricular dP/dt). The bounding aortic pressure pulse with each systole favors expansion or rupture of the aneurysm, and use of a β-blocker such as propranolol is an effective and common way to minimize the risk (and, of course, reflex cardiac stimulation overall). Atropine (a) is an illogical choice. It will increase heart rate (and, indirectly, contractility) further by removing parasympathetic tone on the SA node. Diazoxide (b) is a rapidly-acting antihypertensive/vasodilator, given as an IV bolus in situations where safe nitroprusside use (and the invasive monitoring it normally requires) is not practical. Diazoxide, like nitroprusside, triggers reflex cardiac stimulation as blood pressure falls. The drug also has some direct cardiac-stimulating effects (not involving antimuscarinic or adrenergic-agonist effects). Diazoxide also tends to cause hyperglycemia (an oral dosage form of the drug is sometimes prescribed to manage blood glucose levels in patients prone to developing hypoglycemia). Furosemide (c) is a loop diuretic that is an important adjunct in such conditions as hypertensive crisis, but only if due to or accompanied by volume overload, heart failure, and acute pulmonary edema. However, the volume depletion and hypotension it would cause would exacerbate the clinical situation I have described. The prompt diuresis and fall of blood pressure may also trigger unwanted baroreceptor-mediated cardiac stimulation. Phentolamine (d), an α-adrenergic blocker, would be irrational. It is a powerful vasodilator (indeed, it is often used for vasoconstrictor drug-induced hypertensive emergencies) that would add to—unfavorably—nitroprusside's prompt antihypertensive effect and the reflex cardiac stimulation that is so dangerous for our patient.

258. The answer is b. Our knowledge about asymmetrical dimethyl arginine (ADMA) is quite new, particularly in terms of clinical consequences, and so you're not likely to read anything about it in current pharmacology texts. (It will be in newer editions, not only because of its clinicopathologic roles but also because ADMA inhibitors are being studied intensively).

ADMA inhibits the ability of nitric oxide synthase (NOS) to incorporate L-arginine moieties, which is required for NO synthesis by the synthase. Some of the main actions of NO include causing vasodilation, inhibiting platelet aggregation and adhesion, inhibiting vascular smooth muscle cell proliferation, and inhibiting LDL oxidation. In the presence of ADMA, less NO is formed and the usually beneficial or protective effects of

NO are diminished or lost. Elevated plasma ADMA levels have been documented in patients with hypertension, hypercholesterolemia, peripheral arterial occlusive disease, women who are preeclamptic, and tobacco smokers. There's also a strong link (not necessarily causal) between ADMA, diabetes, and adverse cardiovascular outcomes: diabetics who remain hyperglycemic despite drug therapy and lifestyle modifications—and especially those who have insulin resistance (ie, most patients with Type 2 diabetes)—tend to have elevated ADMA levels.

ADMA does not inhibit ACE or block angiotensin receptors (a); it does not inhibit TXA_2 synthesis (c) or any other aspect of the cyclooxygenase or lipoxygenase (e) pathways; and it does not mimic tumor necrosis factor (d).

259. The answer is c. *(Brunton, p 956. Katzung, pp 613-614.)* The cutaneous flushing and the underlying vasodilation (and pruritus) caused by niacin almost certainly involves prostaglandins. We can reach this conclusion rather empirically, based on the fact that these responses may be prevented by the prior administration of aspirin, which of course blocks prostaglandin synthesis. (Using sustained-release niacin preparations reduces the incidence and severity of these problems too.) α-Adrenergic receptor activation (a) would tend to counteract, not cause or contribute to the vasodilation that is involved in the flush. Calcium channel blockers have no effect on the phenomenon, so we rule out answer b. Similarly, drugs that inhibit angiotensin synthesis or its receptor activation (d), or histamine receptor blockers (e; whether H_1 or H_2), have no effect on the phenomenon.

260. The answer is c. *(Brunton, pp 243-244. Katzung, pp 135-137.)* ISO, PHE, EPI, NE. The correct sequence is isoproterenol, phenylephrine, epinephrine, and norepinephrine. Yes, some responses to these drugs are variable, largely depending on the dose and the speed of administration. Nonetheless, the responses shown are typical.

Isoproterenol, a β_1/β_2 agonist, lowers peripheral resistance (and diastolic blood pressure) via β_2-mediated peripheral vasodilator actions. That fall of diastolic pressure is greater than the rise of systolic pressure (which occurs because of a direct cardiac positive inotropic/β_1-activating effect), so mean pressure falls a bit. The combined reflex response to a fall of mean pressure (albeit slight), plus the drug's direct positive inotropic and chronotropic effects, leads to significant tachycardia.

Phenylephrine, which activates only (and all) α-adrenergic receptors, causes only a vasopressor response that accounts for the changes of pressures and peripheral resistance. These changes activate the baroreceptor reflex, leading to reflex bradycardia. The drug has no β-agonist activity.

Epinephrine, injected in (reasonably) low doses in normal humans, can cause the effects shown here (and certainly no other drug listed as a possible answer could do the same). The fall of peripheral resistance and diastolic pressure reflects predominant β_2-mediated vasodilation; the rise of systolic pressure is a melding of both peripheral vasoconstriction (α) and direct cardiac stimulation (β_1). Heart rate also reflects direct changes (β_1), as there is no appreciable baroreceptor influence because there is no sudden or significant blood pressure change. Responses to epinephrine are arguably more variable than those of any other drugs listed. Clearly, when large doses are given to a hypotensive patient (eg, in anaphylaxis), the predominant and wanted vascular effect is a pressor response, much greater than what we see here.

Norepinephrine, lacking any β_2 activity but being quite effective as an α and β_1 agonist, causes typical responses like those shown here. Peripherally, there is no vasodilation; just constriction. Diastolic, mean, and systolic pressures rise. The rise is sufficient to reflexly slow heart rate; that is, it is sufficient to overcome NE's direct positive chronotropic effects.

261. The answer is d. *(Brunton, pp 832-838. Katzung, pp 181, 199-203.)* Any of the drugs listed in the question would be reasonable for managing essential hypertension, assuming no contraindications and depending on other factors (comorbidities, other medications, etc) that I did not mention in the question. But for this gentleman a calcium channel blocker would be best: we are dealing with the hypertension, a history of hyperuricemia and gout, and a Raynaud-like issue. The latter is mainly due to autonomic hyperreactivity or heightened response of α-adrenergic receptors to vasoconstrictor influences that reduce blood flow and cause blanching and paresthesias. Blocking α-mediated vasoconstriction (eg, with prazosin or labetalol, the former blocking only α_1 receptors, the latter blocking both α and β) would be the most straightforward approach, but I did not give either of these, or other drugs in their classes, as a choice. A calcium channel blocker (dihydropyridine, eg, nifedipine; or a nondihydropyridine such as verapamil or diltiazem) should work just as well, inhibiting not only vascular responsiveness to catecholamines but also to angiotensin II

(A-II).Verapamil (to a lesser extent with diltiazem, and not at all with nifedipine) would also help lower blood pressure by reducing both heart rate and stroke volume.

Since the vasomotor problems mainly involve α-adrenergic receptor activation, not so much heightened responses to A-II, neither an ACE inhibitor nor an ARB (a) would be the best choice. (Their ability to modify adrenergic receptor responses indirectly by reducing levels or effects of A-II are not strong.) Atenolol or metoprolol (c), the so-called cardioselective β-blockers, will probably lower the elevated blood pressure, but they have no beneficial effects to block peripheral vasoconstriction. Propranolol (e; and most other nonselective [β_1/β_2] blockers) wouldn't either. β-Blockers that also block α-receptors, carvedilol or labetalol, would be good choices (but they are not listed in the question), Thiazide (f) or thiazide-like diuretics (chlorthalidone, metolazone, etc) will probably lower blood pressure, and might blunt vascular hyperreactivity (probably secondary to lowered blood Na^+ concentrations). However, these drugs tend to raise plasma uric acid levels; they might benefit both the hypertension and Raynaud, but are likely to aggravate hyperuricemia and perhaps precipitate acute gout.

262. The answer is a. *(Brunton, pp 242, 263-264. Katzung, p 169.)* You should know the answer to this from a basic physiology course. We have mimicked (but not caused) a sudden rise of blood pressure, stretching the baroreceptors and activating the baroreceptor reflex. Consequences of this include a reduction in sympathetic "outflow" from the CNS and a simultaneous unmasking and increase of opposing parasympathetic influences. The increased muscarinic receptor activation breaks the tachycardia, mainly by slowing spontaneous (Phase 4) depolarization of SA nodal cells. Catecholamine release (b) is not a correct choice. In addition to a variety of other reasons, increased epinephrine or norepinephrine release would worsen or at least perpetuate the arrhythmia. The site of massage is well away from the cardiac parasympathetic ganglia, so answer c is incorrect; so is answer e, since venous return would not be occluded by the procedure. The ECG does not show atrial fibrillation being induced (d).

263. The answer is e. *(Brunton, pp 904-911. Katzung, pp 236-237, 244.)* The origin of the arrhythmia is supraventricular (any structure "above" the AV node), and in this case both the expected effects of ACh and of carotid massage suggests the origin is the SA node itself. The His-Purkinje system (b) is distal to the AV node, and would not be affected by vagal tone in response to carotid massage. If you look at the ECG you should be able to rule out the other (and incorrect) answer choices. The ventricular wave form shows no slurring or "hump" that would suggest preactivation of the ventricles by an accessory pathway (answer a; as you might see in Wolff-Parkinson-White syndrome). There is no notching of the QRS that would be consistent with bundle branch block (right or left; answer c). And, since ventricular activation follows atrial activation (P waves), we are not dealing with ventricular ectopy (d).

264. The answer is a. *(Brunton, pp 853, 858. Katzung, p 240.)* Adenosine interacts with G-protein-coupled receptors and increases maximum diastolic membrane potential. When given as a bolus, as described here, the main effects are a transient slowing of sinus (nodal) rate; an increase of AV nodal refractoriness; and a slowing of AV nodal conduction velocity. Also, with this administration route there is no effect on the His-Purkinje system, nor on ventricular myocardial cells per se. Given the lack of ventricular effects, adenosine would not have terminated the arrhythmia if the origin was in the ventricles. Stated otherwise, since the drug does act on the AV node, and it did terminate the original arrhythmia, we must conclude that the arrhythmia originated in the AV node or another supraventricular structure.

Atropine (b), by blocking the electrophysiologic effects of muscarinic receptor activation (eg, in the SA node), would have unmasked opposing sympathetic (β_1) influences and probably worsened (but certainly not stopped) the aberrant electrical activity. Epinephrine (c) or isoproterenol (d) would have done the same, albeit by direct activation of β_1-adrenergic receptors.

We can rule out lidocaine (e) as an acceptable answer in several ways. First, we are dealing with an arrhythmia originating in a supraventricular structure. At usual therapeutic doses lidocaine has no significant effect on SA nodal rate, nor on AV nodal refractory periods. It also has no effects on PR intervals (because it lacks significant effects on AV nodal refractoriness or conduction), QT intervals, or the duration of the QRS. Stated more pragmatically, the drug is not useful for supraventricular arrhythmias (except, perhaps, digoxin-associated atrial arrhythmias). It would not work in the situation described or shown in the ECG.

Renal System and Diuretic Pharmacology

Aldosterone and its antagonists
Antidiuretic hormone and its antagonists
Carbonic anhydrase and its inhibitors
Loop ("high ceiling" or Na-Cl symporter inhibitor) diuretics
Osmotic diuretics
Potassium-sparing diuretics
Thiazides (benzothiadiazides) and thiazide-like diuretics

Questions

265. A hypertensive patient has been on long-term therapy with lisinopril. The drug isn't controlling pressure as well as wanted, so the physician decides to add triamterene as the (only) second drug. What is the most likely potential outcome of adding this diuretic to the ACE inhibitor regimen?

a. Blood pressure would rise abruptly.
b. Blood pressure would fall again once triamterene was added (better BP control), but there's a likelihood that the patient would become hyperkalemic.
c. Cardiac depression, because both drugs depress heart rate and left ventricular contractility.
d. Diabetes insipidus-like syndrome with production of large volumes of dilute urine, plus dilutional hyponatremia.
e. Hypokalemia because of the two drugs' synergistic effects on renal potassium handling.

266. A patient with mild heart failure and edema fails to respond adequately to maximum recommended dosages of chlorthalidone. What is the most likely appropriate and effective next step in terms of restoring the diuretic response?

a. Add hydrochlorothiazide
b. Add metolazone
c. Replace chlorthalidone with furosemide
d. Replace chlorthalidone with hydrochlorothiazide
e. Try increasing the chlorthalidone dose anyway until toxicity develops

267. A patient has unacceptably low cardiac output and intense reflex-mediated sympathetic activation of the peripheral vasculature that is attempting, unsuccessfully, to keep vital organ perfusion pressure sufficiently high. The patient is edematous because of the poor cardiac function and renal compensations for it. Which one of the following drugs should be avoided in this patient because it is most likely to compromise function of the already-failing heart and the circulatory system overall?

a. Amiloride
b. Ethacrynic acid
c. Hydrochlorothiazide
d. Mannitol
e. Spironolactone

268. One of your clinic patients is being treated with spironolactone. Which statement correctly describes a property of this drug?

a. Contraindicated in heart failure, especially if severe
b. Inhibits Na^+ reabsorption in the proximal tubules
c. Interferes with aldosterone synthesis
d. Is a rational choice for a patient with an adrenal cortical tumor
e. Is generally preferred to a thiazide in most patients with essential hypertension

269. A patient taking an oral diuretic for about 6 months presents with elevated fasting and postprandial blood glucose levels. You check the patient's HbA_{1c} and find it is elevated compared with normal baseline values obtained 6 months ago. You suspect the glycemic problems are diuretic-induced. What is the most likely cause?

a. Acetazolamide
b. Amiloride
c. Chlorothiazide
d. Spironolactone
e. Triamterene

270. Chlorthalidone and torsemide are members of different diuretic classes, in terms of mechanisms of action and chemical structure, but they share the ability to cause hypokalemia. Which of the following statements best describes the general and common mechanism by which these drugs cause their effects that lead to net renal potassium loss?

a. Act as aldosterone receptor agonists, thereby favoring K^+ loss
b. Block proximal tubular ATP-dependent secretory pumps for K^+
c. Increase delivery of Na^+ to principal cells in the distal nephron, where tubular Na^+ is exchanged for K^+, which gets eliminated in the urine
d. Stimulate a proximal tubular Na, K-ATPase such that K^+ is actively pumped into the urine
e. Lower distal tubular urine osmolality, thereby favoring passive diffusion of K^+ into the urine

271. A patient was in a recumbent position for a 45-minute oral surgery procedure. When the surgery was completed she stood up quickly and promptly got light-headed and fainted. The cause was hypotension due to hypovolemia from excessive diuresis, attributed to a drug prescribed by her physician and taken for several months. What drug is the most likely cause?

a. Acetazolamide
b. Furosemide
c. Hydrochlorothiazide
d. Spironolactone
e. Triamterene

272. A 52-year-old man presents to your clinic for his first visit with you, after moving from a distant town. His only medications are a statin, aspirin (81 mg/d), and metolazone. The pharmacist who filled his prescriptions explained to the gentleman why he was taking the aspirin and the statin, but merely referred to the metolazone as a "water pill." Thus, you're asked about it. What is the most likely reason why the metolazone was prescribed?

a. Adjunctive management of an adrenal cortical tumor
b. Adjunctive management of hepatic cirrhosis from years of excessive alcohol consumption
c. Hypertension accompanied by a history of gout and diabetes
d. Treatment of essential hypertension
e. Treatment of edema and ascites from heart failure

273. Urinary potassium concentrations are measured before and after several weeks of administering a loop diuretic (typical daily dosages). We find that posttreatment urine K^+ concentrations are substantially lower than those measured at baseline. What is the most likely explanation for this observation?

a. An expected response to the drug.
b. Loop diuretics cause potassium-wasting only in in vitro experimental models.
c. Measurements of posttreatment urine K^+ concentrations were erroneous.
d. The patient has hypoaldosteronism from bilateral adrenalectomy.
e. The patient has significantly impaired renal function.

274. A patient has very high plasma uric acid levels, has had two acute gout attacks in the last 8 months, and is at imminent risk of developing acute uric acid nephropathy. We will treat the patient with proper anti-inflammatory drugs and other agents, but feel that reducing solubility of uric acid in the urine might help ward-off the development of renal problems. What drug is best able to produce this desired renal effect vis-á-vis urate solubility without appreciably increasing systemic risks of the hyperuricemia?

a. Acetazolamide
b. Antidiuretic hormone (ADH; vasopressin)
c. Ethacrynic acid
d. Furosemide
e. Hydrochlorothiazide

275. You have just completed your third-year medicine clerkship, having spent some time in general internal medicine, cardiology, nephrology, and endocrine-metabolism clinics. In each of those venues you have reviewed charts of patients taking eplerenone. What phrase best describes a characteristic or other property of this drug?

a. Facilitates renal sodium and water loss, increases potassium retention
b. Inhibits steroidogenesis
c. Mimics antidiuretic hormone
d. Specifically inhibits aldosterone synthesis
e. Used to counteract glycosuria in patients with Type 1 or 2 diabetes mellitus

276. A 58-year-old man with a history of hypertension and hypercholesterolemia is diagnosed with heart failure. We start therapy with furosemide as one of several medications. Which of the following would you expect to occur along with the increased urine volume caused by this diuretic?

a. Dilute (hypotonic) urine because normal urine concentrating mechanisms are impaired
b. Hypercalcemia due to impaired renal Ca^{2+} excretion
c. Reduced net excretion of Cl^-
d. Metabolic acidosis due to increased renal bicarbonate excretion
e. Reduced plasma urate concentrations because of increased urate excretion

277. A patient post-head trauma is in the neurosurgery unit at your hospital. He has become hypervolemic and hyponatremic from two main causes: (1) trauma probably increased vasopressin release from his posterior pituitary gland; and (2) the staff was not sufficiently careful when administering IV fluids, which further increased blood volume and lowered blood sodium concentrations. This patient also has symptomatic heart failure that would be further compromised by additional rises of blood volume, even if slight or short-lived. He had been on a number of drugs prior to admission. One was an oral potassium supplement to counteract diuretic-induced hypokalemia. Unfortunately, the supplement dose was excessive, and the patient was borderline-hyperkalemic too. What drug would be the most rational to administer, with the goal of normalizing or at least improving blood volume and electrolyte composition and without further compromising the patient's hemodynamic status?

a. Conivaptan
b. Mannitol
c. Metolazone
d. Sodium chloride 0.9% (normal saline)
e. Spironolactone

278. A 60-year-old man has multiple medical problems, including severe hepatic cirrhosis and hepatitis at age 40, and over 30 years of excessive alcohol intake. Three days after a visit to a physician, who prescribed a drug for a condition unrelated to the liver dysfunction, the man is found comatose. He is transported to the emergency department. What drug, prescribed those few days before, most likely induced or contributed to the onset of coma in this man?

a. Acetazolamide
b. Eplerenone
c. Furosemide
d. Hydrochlorothiazide
e. Triamterene

279. After a few weeks on a drug that was prescribed by another physician, a patient reports fine tremors of his fingers, headache and fatigue, and transient GI distress. More worrisome to him is that he is constantly thirsty and urinates copiously and frequently throughout the day and night. A 24-hour urine collection produces nearly 5 L of hypotonic urine. Blood tests show that blood levels of the causative drug are within its therapeutic range. Nonetheless, the clinical picture leads you to hypothesize that the offending drug is causing renal responses quite similar to a syndrome characterized by reduced production or renal response to ADH. Which drug most likely caused or contributed to these signs and symptoms?

a. Diazepam
b. Fluoxetine
c. Haloperidol
d. Lithium
e. Phenytoin

280. Your patient, who lives in Death Valley, California, (altitude 240 ft below sea level) is planning a vacation that includes a short hike to the top of Mount Everest (~29,000 ft above sea level). You're concerned about "altitude sickness." He has no other significant medical conditions, and takes no other drugs that would interact with the drug you will prescribe for his trip. Which drug would you recommend that this adventurer start taking before his trek, and continue until he returns to an altitude much closer to sea level?

a. Acetazolamide
b. Amiloride
c. Bumetanide
d. Furosemide
e. Spironolactone
f. Triamterene

281. A patient with heart failure has been managed with digoxin and furosemide and is doing well by all measures for 3 years. He develops acute rheumatoid arthritis and is placed on rather large doses of a very efficacious nonsteroidal anti-inflammatory drug—one that inhibits both the COX-1 and -2 cyclooxygenase pathways. What is the most likely outcome of adding the NSAID?

a. Hyperchloremic acidosis indicative of acute diuretic toxicity
b. Dramatic increase of furosemide's potassium-sparing effects
c. Edema, weight gain, and other signs/symptoms indicative of reduced diuresis
d. Increased digoxin excretion
e. Reduced digoxin effects because the NSAID competes with digoxin for myocyte receptor-binding sites

282. A patient presents with chronic open angle glaucoma. What "renal" drug, or a drug in the same chemical and pharmacologic class, might be prescribed as an adjunct to lower intraocular pressure and help manage this condition?

a. Acetazolamide
b. Amiloride
c. Furosemide
d. Spironolactone
e. Triamterene

283. A patient with severe infectious disease is being treated with an aminoglycoside antibiotic. Which diuretic should be avoided, if possible, for this patient because of the risk of a serious adverse effect shared by both drugs?

a. Acetazolamide
b. Furosemide
c. Metolazone
d. Spironolactone
e. Triamterene

284. A patient is recently diagnosed with adrenal cortical adenoma. Among the pertinent Cushingoid signs and symptoms are hypertension and weight gain from fluid retention; and hypernatremia and hypokalemia. Which drug would be the most rational to prescribe, alone or adjunctively, to specifically antagonize both the renal and the systemic effects of the hormone excess?

a. Acetazolamide
b. Amiloride
c. Furosemide
d. Metolazone
e. Spironolactone

285. A patient has been referred to your academic medical center because of recent-onset ventricular ectopy, second-degree AV nodal block, chromatopsia, and other extracardiac signs and symptoms of digoxin intoxication. His family doctor, who has been treating him for a host of common medical problems over the last 30 years, had prescribed furosemide and digoxin for this gentleman's heart failure. Blood tests show that digoxin levels are well within a normal range. We believe the problems are diuretic-induced. What did the diuretic most likely do to precipitate the digoxin toxicity?

a. Caused hypercalcemia
b. Caused hypokalemia
c. Caused hyponatremia
d. Displaced digoxin from tissue binding sites
e. Inhibited digoxin's metabolic elimination

286. A 48-year-old man with bilateral diabetic nephropathy develops acute heart failure and additional, and significant, declines of renal function (eg, declines of GFR) as two of several consequences of sepsis. We will administer appropriate antibiotics, vasodilators, and cardiac inotropes, but also need to administer a diuretic to promptly reduce circulating fluid volume and "unload" the failing heart. What drug would be most appropriate in terms of managing the hemodynamic problems for this patient?

a. Acetazolamide
b. Hydrochlorothiazide
c. Mannitol
d. Torsemide
e. Metolazone (or chlorthalidone)

287. Amiloride is a useful drug for managing hypokalemia caused by other drugs. Which of the following phrases best describes the mechanism by which it causes its potassium-sparing effects?

a. Blocks the agonist effects of aldosterone with its renal tubular receptors
b. Blocks distal tubular sodium channels and, ultimately, Na^+-K^+ exchange
c. Hastens metabolic inactivation of aldosterone
d. Stimulates a proximal tubular Na, K-ATPase
e. Suppresses cortisol and aldosterone synthesis and release in the adrenal cortex

288. A patient with severe heart failure is in the ICU. His urine output is dangerously low. We begin an intravenous infusion of dopamine at a usual therapeutic dose and urine output rises quickly and dramatically. What is the most likely mechanism by which the dopamine caused this effect?

a. Blocked β-adrenergic receptors in the juxtaglomerular apparatus, thereby inhibiting renin release and subsequent angiotensin-mediated aldosterone release from the adrenal cortex
b. Directly inhibited a renal Na^+, K^+, $2Cl^-$ cotransporter in the loop of Henle
c. Improved renal blood flow and glomerular filtration
d. Lowered the medullary-to-cortical osmotic gradient, such that normal urine concentrating mechanisms were impaired
e. Reduced the permeability of the ascending limb, loop of Henle, and of the collecting ducts to water

289. A patient who admits to drinking many liters of water each day has had recurrent episodes of symptomatic hyponatremia, and is at great risk of recurrences. Because of another medical problem he now requires administration of a diuretic. Which drug is most likely to precipitate another recurrence of the hyponatremia, whether or not the patient's daily water intake is reduced to a more acceptable level?

a. Bumetanide
b. Ethacrynic acid
c. Furosemide
d. Hydrochlorothiazide
e. Torsemide

290. Consider again the patient described in the previous question. He now presents with diuretic-induced hyponatremia. The condition is symptomatic and severe enough that the excessively low Na^+ concentration needs to be corrected promptly. In addition to cautious intravenous administration of NaCl, adjunctive drug therapy is indicated. Which drug or drug class would be the most rational to use adjunctively, in addition to IV NaCl and stopping the causative diuretic at least temporarily, to help correct sodium concentration?

a. Captopril
b. Furosemide
c. Spironolactone
d. Thiazide-like diuretic (eg, metolazone)
e. Triamterene

291. A patient with essential hypertension is being treated with hydrochlorothiazide and a calcium channel blocker, and is doing well. He also takes atorvastatin for hypercholesterolemia, and aspirin to reduce his risk of an acute coronary syndrome. He is now diagnosed with a seizure disorder. We begin therapy with one of the suitable anticonvulsants that, fortunately, does not alter the metabolism of any of the medications prescribed for his cardiovascular problems. We've also read that systemic administration of acetazolamide may prove to be a useful adjunct to the anticonvulsant therapy: the metabolic acidosis it causes may help suppress seizure development or spread. So, we start acetazolamide therapy too. What is the most likely outcome of adding the acetazolamide?

a. Excessive rises of plasma sodium concentration
b. Hypertensive crisis (antagonism of both antihypertensive drugs)
c. Hypokalemia via synergistic actions with the thiazide
d. Spontaneous bleeding (potentiation of aspirin's actions)
e. Sudden circulating volume expansion, onset of heart failure

292. The table below shows the urinary electrolyte excretion patterns typical of various prototype diuretics. These are qualitative changes, and do not reflect the magnitude of the changes. They show whether excretion of an electrolyte (net amount) is increased or decreased; they do not reflect changes in urine concentrations of these substances.

Drug	Na^+	K^+	Ca^{2+}	Mg^{2+}	Cl^-	HCO_3^-
1.	↑	↑	↓	↑	↑	↑/↓
2.	↑	↑	↑	↑	↑	0
3.	↑	↓	0	0	↑	↑
4.	↑	↑	0	0	↓	↑↑

↑ Increased net loss into urine; ↓ decreased loss into urine; 0 no change; ↑/↓ increased or decreased, largely dependent on dose.

Which drug causes effects most similar, if not identical, to the unknown drug 2, above?

a. Acetazolamide
b. Amiloride
c. Chlorthalidone
d. Furosemide
e. Hydrochlorothiazide

Renal System and Diuretic Pharmacology

Answers

265. The answer is b. *(Brunton, pp 643, 648-649, 800-810. Katzung, pp 181-183, 217, 295-296.)* Lisinopril (a "-pril," and therefore an angiotensin-converting enzyme inhibitor) indirectly reduces aldosterone release from the adrenal cortex by inhibiting angiotensin II (A-II) synthesis. (Remember: A-II is the major physiologic stimulus for aldosterone release.) Normally aldosterone causes renal Na^+ retention and K^+ loss. When there is less aldosterone, the kidneys will now tend to lose Na^+ and retain K^+. Triamterene blocks sodium channels on the luminal face of the principal cells of the nephron. Those sodium channels are responsible for Na^+ and K^+ exchange (some extra Na^+ reclaimed, extra K^+ lost into the urine). In the presence of triamterene (or the similar drug, amiloride) the ion exchange is inhibited and this constitutes the potassium-sparing effects that we use to classify these diuretics. Although aldosterone plays a role in renal handling of Na^+ and K,$^+$ triamterene and amiloride will work in the absence of aldosterone—unlike the potassium-sparing effects of spironolactone or eplerenone, which only work in the presence of aldosterone because its mechanism involves blockade of aldosterone receptors, with no direct effects on principal cell ion exchange.

There is no logical mechanism by which you could envisage an ACE inhibitor/potassium-sparing diuretic causing hypertension (a). Neither an ACE inhibitor nor a K^+-sparing diuretic, alone or together, has direct cardiac-depressant effects (c; unless the drugs were administered at such toxic doses that electrolyte levels changed and affected the heart). Polyuria, a diabetes insipidus-like state (d), and a syndrome of inappropriate ADH secretion (SIADH), do not occur with either of these drugs given alone or with the two combined. As noted above, both drugs exert potassium-sparing effects, and so hypokalemia (e) will not occur.

266. The answer is c. *(Brunton, pp 753, 756-757, 764-765. Katzung, pp 249-250, 254-256.)* Chlorthalidone is a thiazide-like diuretic. If maximum dosages don't yield the desired effects, there is probably little to be gained by switching (c) to another thiazide or thiazide-like agent (eg, hydrochlorothiazide, metolazone, many others). Likewise, and given the relatively "flat" dose-response relationship for these drugs, nothing good is likely to be gained by adding (a, b) yet another agent that works in precisely the same way as the drug that has already proven inadequate. If a maximum recommended dose isn't adequate, giving more of the same or a similar drug won't be better (e). So, in situations such as this, it's time to switch to a drug that is intrinsically more efficacious and works via a different mechanism: a loop diuretic. There is a more prescient question to ask: If our patient had edema and heart failure, why didn't we initiate therapy with a loop diuretic in the first place?

267. The answer is d. *(Brunton, pp 747-748. Katzung, p 263.)* Mannitol is an osmotic diuretic, the prototype of that small class of drugs (glycerin/glycerol is another somewhat noteworthy member of the group) with indications and potential side effects that are quite different from those of "typical" diuretics like the thiazides or loop agents. What happens when you inject (intravenously) this nonmetabolizable sugar, which has a structure similar to that of glucose and the same molecular weight? Initially, and until it is excreted by glomerular filtration, mannitol increases plasma osmolality. That, in turn, osmotically withdraws water from the extracellular space and, ultimately, from the parenchymal cells, and into the interstitium and the blood. If the patient has good renal function, renal blood flow and GFR rise, and the drug is eventually excreted. If he or she has adequate cardiac function, circulating that extra volume (up to a limit) is not a problem.

However, if the patient has sufficient decreased contractility or cardiac output to begin with, or renal perfusion is compromised, the increased blood volume and pressure may be such that the heart simply cannot handle the added workload. Indeed, in a futile attempt to circulate that additional volume and eject it against a higher afterload, the heart may fail acutely.

Amiloride (a), a potassium-wasting diuretic with relatively low efficacy in terms of its ability to increase urine volume, should have no adverse effects in this patient. The same applies to hydrochlorothiazide (c), which is potassium-wasting. Ethacrynic acid (b) is a loop diuretic. It is one of several loop agents we might choose to help "unload" this patient's ventricles, provided the patient isn't hypovolemic already. Spironolactone (e), a potassium-sparing aldosterone antagonist, might ultimately be prescribed for this patient, particularly if his heart failure worsens. Nonetheless, at this time it is not a drug we should avoid.

268. The answer is d. *(Brunton, pp 759-762. Katzung, pp 262, 695, 724.)* Spironolactone is a potassium-sparing diuretic. Its active metabolite blocks aldosterone receptors in the distal nephron (thus answer b is incorrect). Neither spironolactone nor its active metabolite alters aldosterone synthesis (c). The drug is ineffective in the absence of aldosterone. Recall that aldosterone normally causes renal Na^+ retention and K^+ loss. The effects of aldosterone are qualitatively the opposite: Na^+ loss, K^+ retention.

Owing to the ability of spironolactone to counteract the effects of aldosterone, it is particularly suited for patients with primary or secondary hyperaldosteronism (eg, adrenal cortical tumor or hepatic dysfunction, as might occur with long-term/high-dose alcohol consumption, respectively). There is growing evidence that the drug is beneficial in heart failure and probably reduces morbidity in severe heart failure (and so a is incorrect). Although spironolactone has antihypertensive effects, it is not considered to be a first-line choice (e) for most patients with essential hypertension. For those patients a thiazide (most often), an ACE inhibitor, a β-blocker, or a calcium channel blocker, is usually chosen first.

In addition to the potential for causing hyperkalemia (especially if combined with oral potassium supplements, which should not be done) and hyponatremia (overall risk is low if spironolactone is the only diuretic used), spironolactone may cause several other side effects. CNS side effects include lethargy, headache, drowsiness, and mental confusion. Other side effects that are fairly common arise from the drug's androgen receptor-blocking actions: gynecomastia (in men and women) and erectile dysfunction. It may also cause seborrhea, acne, and coarsening of body hair. (Paradoxically, the drug can cause hirsutism in some patients, but it is also used to manage hirsutism in others.)

269. The answer is c. *(Brunton, p 75. Katzung, p 261.)* Thiazides and thiazide-like diuretics (eg, chlorthalidone, metolazone) may elevate blood glucose levels, impair glucose tolerance, and cause frank hyperglycemia.

Several mechanisms have been proposed to explain the effect: decreased release of insulin from the pancreas; increased glycogenolysis and decreased glycogen synthesis; a reduction in the conversion of proinsulin to insulin; and reduced responsiveness of adipocyte and skeletal myocyte insulin receptor response to the hormone (insulin resistance—the most likely mechanism).

(You might recall that diazoxide, mainly used as a parenteral drug for prompt lowering of blood pressure, can be used in its oral dosage form to raise blood glucose levels in some hypoglycemic states. It is, chemically, a thiazide, but is not used as a diuretic.)

Elevations of blood glucose levels, or other manifestations of altered glycemic control, are rarely associated with treatment with acetazolamide (a), amiloride (b), spironolactone (d), or triamterene (e).

270. The answer is c. *(Brunton, pp 742, 749-751, 755. Katzung, pp 260-261.)* Thiazides (and thiazide-like agents such as chlorthalidone and metolazone) and loop diuretics (furosemide, bumetanide, torsemide, ethacrynic acid) increase delivery of Na^+ to the distal nephron because they inhibit reabsorption of Na^+ at more proximal sites. This extra Na^+ reaches the principal cells in the distal nephron, and some of it is taken from the tubular fluid via sodium channels. This reclamation of Na^+ leads to exchange of K^+, which is lost into the urine (ie, potassium "wasting"). In essence, the more Na^+ delivered (and recovered) distally, the more K^+ is eliminated in exchange.

The processes by which these potassium-sparing drugs work do not involve proximal tubular ATP-dependent potassium secretion (b), nor do they involve any direct effect on proximal tubular ATPase (d). In addition, there are no agonist effects on aldosterone receptors (a)—an action that would cause an antidiuretic effect and renal potassium loss. Indeed, no diuretic acts as an aldosterone receptor agonist; spironolactone and eplerenone (not listed here) exert their natriuretic and potassium-sparing effects by blocking aldosterone receptors. Finally, lowering distal tubular osmolality (e) does not occur, nor would such an effect (if it occurred) favor passive diffusion of K^+ into the urine.

271. The answer is b. *(Brunton, pp 752-753. Katzung, pp 257-260.)* One way to simplify answering this question is merely to ask "which diuretic has the greatest ability to cause hypovolemia?" That narrows the choice to furosemide or the other loop diuretics (bumetanide, torsemide, ethacrynic acid). In terms of extra free water loss (and the concomitant risk of hypovolemia) the maximal efficacy of acetazolamide (carbonic anhydrase inhibitor; a) is modest at best, and self-limiting to boot. Hydrochlorothiazide (c) and the two potassium-sparing diuretics listed (spironolactone and triamterene; d, e) also have modest efficacy in terms of the peak diuretic effect, even if unusually large doses were to be given. Note: Hyponatremia reduces the responsiveness of the peripheral vasculature to vasoconstrictors (eg, EPI, NE, and angiotensin II). If I stated that the patient's hypotension were due to diuretic-induced hyponatremia, then the most likely correct answer would be hydrochlorothiazide or another thiazide or thiazide-like diuretic (eg, metolazone); of all the diuretics classes (and most other classes of drugs), they are the most common cause of hyponatremia.

272. The answer is d. *(Brunton, pp 756-757, 764-765. Katzung, p 260.)* Metolazone, although not a thiazide in the chemical sense, is largely (hydrochloro) thiazide-like in terms of its pharmacologic properties and uses, although it has a much longer duration of action than the prototype, hydrochlorothiazide. As far as the "main use" of thiazides goes, that would be essential hypertension (assuming no contraindications), with lesser uses being "mild" and especially transient edema, management of idiopathic hypercalciuria, adjunctive management of nephrogenic diabetes insipidus, and perhaps management of Meniere disease. Thiazides or thiazide-like diuretics would not be rational, nor very efficacious, for drug therapy of an adrenal cortical tumor (a). In that instance, if we are considering only diuretics, the proper drug would be spironolactone or eplerenone, the aldosterone receptor blockers. Likewise, since thiazides can raise circulating urate and glucose levels, they would not be good choices for the patient with hepatic cirrhosis or other diseases characterized by poor liver function (b; here too spironolactone or eplerenone would be the best choice) or gout or diabetes (e). If our goal were to manage severe edema (e) with or without ascites (as in a patient with heart failure), our best choice would be a loop diuretic.

273. The answer is a. *(Brunton, pp 751-753. Katzung, pp 260-261, 264.)* One expected response to therapeutic doses of loop diuretics, which are clearly and correctly classified as potassium-wasting, is a reduction of urinary potassium concentrations. How can this be? Note that the term concentration reflects the amount of a substance (here, potassium) per unit volume; it is not equivalent to "amount" per se. The loop diuretics do increase K^+ excretion: because they work more proximally, they provide an added load of Na^+ delivered to the distal nephron, where sodium channels in the principal cells take up some extra Na^+ in exchange for K^+. Loop diuretics also impair the ability of the kidneys to form a concentrated urine. That is, they promote formation of a large volume of more dilute (less concentrated) urine. The net loss of K^+ (say, on a 24-h basis) is increased, but it's accompanied by a disproportionate increase in free water loss such that urine K^+ concentration (but not total amount lost) is decreased.

274. The answer is a. *(Brunton, pp 743-747. Katzung, pp 252-253, 363.)* Here I asked about reducing the risk of urate nephropathy acutely by increasing uric acid solubility through urinary alkalinization. One key to answering this question correctly is to realize that uric acid becomes more soluble (less likely to precipitate or crystallize) as local pH rises. (Yes, I have asked a question in the renal drugs chapter that requires your knowledge of other areas of pathophysiology and pharmacology.) Recall that normal urine is acidic. We want to alkalinize the urine, and that is precisely what acetazolamide does, by inhibiting carbonic anhydrase in the proximal nephron. Note that acetazolamide is only an adjunct, and in addition to (or instead of) using it, we might also administer sodium bicarbonate which will alkalinize the urine and keep the patient well hydrated to help form large amounts of a dilute urine. Acetazolamide does cause a metabolic acidosis, which would seemingly favor reductions of uric acid solubility in the blood. However, we are keeping our patient well hydrated (helps reduce precipitation); and the volume of blood is far greater than urine volume at any given time, so given the great size of the "blood pool" we have little to worry about in terms of urate precipitation systemically.

Antidiuretic hormone (b) would be illogical. It would reduce urine volume and concentrate solutes such as uric acid in it. Ethacrynic acid (c) and furosemide (d) lead to the formation of copious volumes of dilute urine. In terms of renal problems, that may be beneficial. However, the loop diuretics tend to cause such large amounts of fluid loss via the urine that the concentration of solutes (including uric acid) in the blood may go up.

Hydrochlorothiazide (e) and related drugs tend to form a very concentrated urine by interfering with normal urine-diluting mechanisms in the kidneys. While some of these drugs have some carbonic anhydrase activity, and so alkalinize the urine, these effects are weak in comparison with acetazolamide. The most likely predominant renal effect is the unwanted one: increased risk of urate nephropathy. In addition, thiazides tend to elevate urate levels (by interfering with tubular secretion of urate), and so these drugs are likely to pose additional systemic problems.

275. The answer is a. *(Brunton, 744t, 751, 755-756, 758-759, 761-763. Katzung, pp 262, 695, 724.)* Eplerenone is a relatively new spironolactone-like drug. As such, its main mechanism of action involves blockade of aldosterone receptors (eg, in the nephron). Its main uses are also largely identical to those of spironolactone: heart failure, hypertension (mainly as a potassium-sparing adjunct, and especially when plasma renin levels are elevated. The high plasma renin levels, lead to increased angiotensin II synthesis and aldosterone release from the adrenal cortex). In patients with high aldosterone levels from other causes (eg, adrenal cortical tumor, Cushing disease), an aldosterone receptor blocker would also be a rational choice. The drug has no effect on the synthesis of aldosterone (d) or other steroid hormones (b); its ultimate renal effects are the opposite to those of ADH (at least in terms of free water loss or conservation), so (c) is incorrect. Finally aldosterone antagonists have no direct or clinically useful effects on glucose metabolism or levels, nor on glycosuria (e) and other consequences of hyperglycemia.

276. The answer is a. *(Brunton, p 751. Katzung, pp 252-256, 258-259.)* Recall one of the main mechanisms by which a concentrated urine is formed: a hypertonic milieu in the renal medulla—and a medullary-to-cortical osmotic gradient—osmotically withdraws water (but not solute) from the tubular fluid as it passes through the collecting ducts. What creates that hypertonic medullary-to-cortical gradient? Reabsorption of Na^+ and Cl^- as tubular fluid ascends the loop of Henle, which ultimately increases interstitial osmolality. However, that process of ion resorption is impaired by loop diuretics. That reduces osmolality in the medullary interstitium, thereby reducing the osmotic gradient that enables the tubular fluid to become hypertonic as water is lost in the distal nephron. Thus, in the presence of a loop diuretic the urine remains dilute and hypotonic.

Hypercalcemia (b) is not an expected accompaniment. Loop diuretics (in contrast with thiazides) increase renal Ca^{2+} elimination.

Recall that the main anion excreted (along with Na^+, K^+, etc.) in response to a loop diuretic is chloride, and so net Cl^- excretion goes up (not down; c). Metabolic acidosis from increased bicarbonate excretion (d) doesn't occur. Bicarbonate tends to be reabsorbed. You should recall that hypochloremic alkalosis (also called contraction alkalosis, because blood volume contracts as the result of excessive fluid loss in the urine) is one potential and quite dangerous adverse response caused by loop diuretics.

Loop diuretics do not lower urate concentrations (e). Rather, urate levels tend to rise, in part, because of reduced urate excretion combined with a "concentration" of urate in the blood owing to increased free water loss.

277. The answer is a. *(Brunton, pp 784, 787, 789, 805, 1596-1598, 1603. Katzung, pp 181-183, 264, 297, 692.)* This patient probably has SIADH—a syndrome of inappropriate vasopressin (antidiuretic hormone; ADH) secretion—and the scenario involving hypervolemia and dilutional hyponatremia is a fairly common cause or accompaniment of it. Conivaptan, a relatively new drug, is indicated for managing SIADH. It is a nonpeptide and competitive antagonist of ADH's water-sparing effects in the nephron's collecting duct.

Why not mannitol (b)? Its site of action is the same as conivaptan's, but it increases free water loss through an osmotic, ADH-independent, mechanism. (In fact, a compensatory response to counteract mannitol's effects and conserve water is increased ADH release, but mannitol's effects typically "win out" and diuresis indeed occurs.) Recall that the osmotic mechanism by which mannitol causes diuresis also contributes to increased plasma osmolality and blood volume—at least initially and until sufficient mannitol has been excreted. Heart failure (which this patient had) is a contraindication, or at least an important precaution, to mannitol's use. Even a transient increase of circulating fluid volume, which transiently increases blood pressure, can provide a significant added hemodynamic load on the failing heart. (The risk would be even greater if the patient had poor renal blood flow or function that would slow mannitol's elimination and keep blood osmolality high longer.)

Metolazone (c) is a thiazide-like diuretic. Recall that, as a class, thiazides or related agents have only a modest ability to reduce circulating fluid volume (which would be desirable in SIADH). More importantly, thiazides and thiazide-like agents tend to cause hyponatremia; that's something we don't want to cause or, in this case, worsen. Infusing 0.9% NaCl (d) will not correct sodium concentrations and if too much is infused too quickly it may put additional fluid-overload-related hemodynamic stresses on the failing heart. Spironolactone (e) is irrational. First, it will not correct the excessive free water loss. More important, by antagonizing the renal tubular effects of aldosterone it will increase sodium loss and increase renal potassium retention—precisely the opposite of what we want to do with this patient.

278. The answer is a. *(Brunton, pp 763-767. Katzung, pp 256-258.)* Acetazolamide, the prototypic carbonic anhydrase inhibitor, causes metabolic acidosis as it increases renal bicarbonate excretion, which in turn alkalinizes the urine. Although acetazolamide is infrequently used as a diuretic, it is used more for other conditions including altitude sickness, an adjunct to certain antiepileptic drugs, and (perhaps in this case) for management of glaucoma.

Patients with severe liver dysfunction cannot synthesize urea adequately. As a result, elimination of a variety of endogenous nitrogen-based metabolic waste products becomes dependent on renal excretion of ammonium ion. In normally acidic urine the ammonium ions are eliminated rather efficiently. However, and due to the acetazolamide's urinary-alkalinizing effects, ammonia gas forms in the urine. It then readily diffuses from the urine into the circulation. This causes hyperammonemia, which is the most likely cause of the coma.

Eplerenone (b) and the older related drug, spironolactone, tend not to alter blood or urine pH. Indeed, since patients with severe liver dysfunction (such as this patient, with hepatitis- and alcohol-induced hepatic cirrhosis) tend to have high circulating aldosterone levels, the blockade of aldosterone receptors by eplerenone would probably be beneficial and not likely to account for the coma and related neurologic abnormalities.

Furosemide (c) also is an unlikely explanation. It is likely to facilitate ammonium excretion, and pH-related changes (eg, urinary alkalinization) are not apt to occur. Recall that one manifestation of loop diuretic excess is hypochloremic metabolic alkalosis (also called contraction alkalosis because circulating fluid volume shrinks—contracts). Because the kidneys tend to lose large amounts of chloride, and tend to retain bicarbonate, urinary alkalinization that leads to ammonia production in the urine won't occur.

Some of the thiazides (eg, hydrochlorothiazide; d) and thiazide-like agents (eg, chlorthalidone, metolazone) have carbonic anhydrase activity that could alkalinize the urine. However, this property is generally weak in comparison with acetazolamide or related agents that are more appropriately classified as carbonic anhydrase inhibitors. Triamterene (e; or the related drug amiloride), a potassium-sparing diuretic with actions that are aldosterone-independent (contrast with eplerenone, spironolactone), is not likely to alter urine pH or cause other effects that might precipitate coma in this patient.

279. The answer is d. *(Brunton, pp 429, 485-490. Katzung, pp 500-504.)* Lithium treatment (for bipolar illness) frequently causes polyuria and (as a consequence of excessive renal fluid loss) polydipsia (increased thirst leading to increased fluid intake). The collecting ducts lose the capacity to conserve water via the expected actions of ADH. This amounts to drug-induced nephrogenic diabetes insipidus, dilutional hyponatremia, and SIADH: a syndrome of inappropriate ADH secretion that tries, unsuccessfully, to limit or reduce free water loss from the kidneys. Such findings are not associated with diazepam (a; prototype benzodiazepine anxiolytic); fluoxetine (b; the prototypic SSRI antidepressant); haloperidol (c; butyrophenone antipsychotic); or phenytoin (e; hydantoin anticonvulsant).

280. The answer is a. *(Brunton, pp 391, 743-747. Katzung, pp 254-258.)* The signs and symptoms of altitude sickness are related to the development of respiratory alkalosis: At high altitudes the partial pressure of O_2 in the inspired air is low. The hypoxia triggers hyperventilation, which increases net ventilatory loss of CO_2. Blood pH rises. Acetazolamide inhibits carbonic anhydrase and so increases renal bicarbonate loss. This, in turn, causes a metabolic acidosis that counteracts the ventilatory-induced rise of blood pH. It is the drug of choice for prophylaxis or management of altitude sickness. It is true that some of the thiazide or thiazide-like diuretics inhibit carbonic anhydrase, but the effect is very weak in comparison to that of acetazolamide. None of the other drugs listed would be suitable for this patient and the altitude sickness he is likely to experience.

281. The answer is c. *(Brunton, pp 685-686, 752-753. Katzung, pp 256, 265-267.)* An important element in the renal responses to furosemide is maintenance of adequate renal blood flow. That is, to a degree, prostaglandin-mediated. Prostaglandins dilate the afferent arteriole (to the glomeruli) and increase GFR and urine production.

The NSAIDs, such as the hypothetical one described here, inhibit prostaglandin synthesis. That reduces the desired effects of the loop diuretic, leading to less fluid and salt elimination. Edema, weight gain, and other markers of heart failure may develop as a result. Hyperchloremic alkalosis (a) is incorrect: chronic or acute excessive effects of loop diuretics are characterized by hypochloremic metabolic alkalosis. Regardless, NSAIDs are not likely to potentiate the effects of these diuretics. "Dramatic increases of furosemide's K-sparing effects (b)" is incorrect. Recall that loop diuretics are K-wasting. Digoxin is eliminated by renal excretion. If we accept the notion that loop diuretics may increase excretion of digoxin, then we should accept the likely possibility that NSAID-induced reductions of diuretic action should reduce the glycoside's renal loss, not increase it (d). The NSAIDs do not bind to and inhibit the myocyte Na^+, K^+-ATPase, which is digoxin's cellular receptor (e). Do remember that furosemide (and thiazides) is apt to increase the risk or severity of digoxin toxicity. The mechanism mainly involves diuretic-induced hypokalemia, not changes in circulating fluid volume or urine volume per se.

282. The answer is a. *(Brunton, pp 743-747, 1709-1711, 1723. Katzung, p 257.)* Aqueous humor formation (as well as that of cerebrospinal fluid) involves carbonic anhydrase activity. Reduce aqueous humor synthesis and, all other factors being equal, intraocular pressure goes down. Acetazolamide is, of course, the carbonic anhydrase-inhibiting diuretic.

Note that when a carbonic anhydrase inhibitor is used to manage glaucoma, the drug's renal/diuretic effects, which certainly occur if the drug is given systemically, have nothing to do with the beneficial effects that are due to an ocular (ciliary body) site of action. In fact, those extraocular effects aren't needed for glaucoma control. That is why, when we prescribe a carbonic anhydrase inhibitor for glaucoma, we usually choose a topical ophthalmic carbonic anhydrase inhibitor (eg, dorzolamide or methazolamide).

283. The answer is b. *(Brunton, pp 753, 1162-1163. Katzung, pp 259, 810-811, 813.)* Both the loop diuretics and the aminoglycosides (tobramycin, streptomycin, gentamicin, others) are ototoxic—capable of causing vestibular damage (eg, balance problems) or cochlear damage (tinnitus or sensorineural hearing loss). The ototoxic effects of each drug are enhanced (often significantly) by the other's, and so it is best to avoid use of both these drugs (or other ototoxins) unless the benefits clearly outweigh the risk of perhaps permanent and total hearing loss. (Of course, there are instances in which such combinations are necessary.) There's strong evidence that of all the loop diuretics, the risk of ototoxicity is highest with ethacrynic acid and its parenteral formulation, sodium ethacrynate. Nonetheless, all the other loop diuretics—bumetanide, furosemide, and torsemide—are definitely on the short list of well-documented ototoxic drugs.

Acetazolamide (a), metolazone (c) or other thiazide or thiazide-like diuretics, spironolactone (d), and triamterene (e) are not ototoxic, nor do they potentiate the adverse effects of other ototoxic drugs.

284. The answer is e. *(Brunton, p 762. Katzung, pp 262, 695, 724.)* The most rational choice for specifically antagonizing the consequences of hormone excess—aldosterone being the hormone of most importance in terms of the renal, hemodynamic, and electrolyte problems here—is spironolactone (or eplerenone). Its primary mechanism of action is blockade of aldosterone receptors. Remember that the main renal effects of aldosterone are sodium (and water) retention and increased renal loss of potassium.

Acetazolamide (a), the carbonic anhydrase inhibitor, exerts weak and self-limiting diuretic and natriuretic effects. It is also potassium-wasting, and increased excretion of potassium is what we do not want to do with preexisting hypokalemia. Amiloride (b) would help increase sodium excretion and help normalize potassium levels too. However, it does not provide the "rational" approach to hyperaldosteronism because it does not block aldosterone receptors. Furosemide (c) or another loop diuretic might prove effective in terms of increasing excretion of sodium and reducing that of potassium. Indeed, if the hyperaldosteronism is sufficiently great to cause unacceptable degrees of fluid retention (hypervolemia) and heart failure we may need to administer it. Nonetheless, spironolactone would be a reasonable, rational, and probably necessary element of management. Metolazone (d), a thiazide-like diuretic, would desirably help increase renal sodium excretion and lower blood pressure. Having relatively low efficacy in terms of increased urine production, it may not do much to manage the hypervolemia and the resulting weight gain. More important, metolazone is likely to aggravate the preexisting hypokalemia because it is, of course, a potassium-wasting diuretic.

285. The answer is b. *(Brunton, pp 751, 763, 765-766, 886-889. Katzung, pp 219-221, 259-260.)* While many ionic and other factors can predispose a patient to digoxin toxicity, hypokalemia, as can be caused by a loop diuretic (usually used for edema and/or ascites, including that associated with heart failure) or thiazide diuretic (mainly used for treating essential hypertension), is arguably the most important, if not the most common.

There is a competition between extracellular K^+ and digoxin for binding to digoxin's cellular receptor, the Na^+, K^+-ATPase on the sarcolemma. When circulating (extracellular) K^+ concentration is reduced (ie, when hypokalemia develops), the binding of digoxin is enhanced and so its effects are increased, even without a rise of digoxin concentrations, and usually those increased effects are deleterious, as described here. Hypercalcemia can increase the risk or severity of digoxin toxicity. However, loop diuretics increase renal Ca^{2+} loss, and so hypercalcemia (a) is not a likely explanation. Hyponatremia (c) is not at all likely to have occurred with a loop diuretic, which tends to increase both renal Na^+ and H_2O loss, with the loss of free water being much greater than the loss of Na^+. Thus, hyponatremia can occur. Loop diuretics do not displace digoxin from tissue binding sites (d) or inhibit digoxin's elimination (which involves renal excretion, not metabolism).

Note that in the scenario I described the patient as having been treated by "his family doctor who has been treating him for the last 30 years." This is not at all meant to impugn family doctors or general practitioners. The point is that nowadays, and for a variety of reasons (toxicity being one), digoxin is no longer considered an appropriate drug for managing heart failure, with or without signs or symptoms of congestive failure, until many other reasonable and more suitable options have been tried and the patient's condition has deteriorated to the point that inotropes (digoxin or parenteral agents) are warranted. Recall that our preferred approach for initial therapy of failure involves ACE inhibitors, a β-blocker, and perhaps a loop diuretic. Nonetheless, and unfortunately, some physicians still use the "old way," involving digoxin. It is these patients who are likely to be seen in the hospital when the common problems due to digoxin develop.

286. The answer is d. *(Brunton, pp 749-753. Katzung, pp 265-267.)* This patient needs a diuretic that has a fast onset of action and the ability to rather significantly increase renal excretion of free water to "unload" the heart. Torsemide is very similar in terms of actions and uses to the prototype loop or "high ceiling" diuretic, furosemide, which inhibits a $Na^+/K^+/2Cl^-$ cotransporter in the ascending limb of the loop of Henle. (Note that both furosemide and torsemide end in "-semide"—a tip for name recognition.)

Acetazolamide (a) the prototype carbonic anhydrase inhibitor, would be unsuitable. Its onset of action is slow; its peak effects in terms of increasing free water elimination are low; and its ability to cause metabolic acidosis (secondary to increased renal bicarbonate loss) would not only compromise the patient described in the scenario but also cause loss of the drug's diuretic effects. Hydrochlorothiazide (b) and thiazide-like diuretics (eg, metolazone and chlorthalidone; e) would not be best; their efficacies are low in terms of managing edema; their effects are slow to develop; and only one thiazide, chlorothiazide, can be given parenterally (a point I do not think you need to commit to memory). Mannitol (c), the prototype osmotic diuretic, is given parenterally; it has a relatively prompt onset of action and it can significantly increase fluid elimination via the kidneys. Mannitol's intensity and duration of effects, however, depend on many variables, including baseline renal function. Nonetheless, mannitol initially raises circulating fluid volume—increasing the hemodynamic load on the heart and being particularly problematic in the face of heart failure—and its adverse volume-related effects will be prolonged if GFR is reduced in patients such as the one described in the question.

287. The answer is b. *(Brunton, pp 758-759. Katzung, pp 261-262.)* Amiloride and triamterene block distal tubular Na^+ channels that provide for Na^+ reabsorption in exchange for K^+, which is lost into the urine. This sodium channel, which is the main site of action of amiloride, is on the luminal side of the principal cell membranes. (Principal cells in the nephron are located in the late distal tubule and collecting ducts.) There is an ATPase on the interstitial face of the principal cells (again, these are in the distal nephron, not proximal; d). The ATPase is responsible for the extrusion of potassium into the urine in exchange for extra sodium taken up by the luminal sodium channels, and so it is essential in the overall actions of potassium-sparing diuretics. Nonetheless, the ATPase is not inhibited (or stimulated; d) directly by amiloride.

Amiloride has no direct effects on aldosterone synthesis or metabolism (c), or on aldosterone receptors (a; those receptors are blocked by spironolactone).

288. The answer is c. *(Brunton, pp 248-249. Katzung, pp 216-217, 220-222.)* The often dramatic increases in urine output caused by therapeutic doses of dopamine (so-called "renal doses") are mainly due to improved hemodynamics. The drug, under these conditions, not only improves cardiac contractility and cardiac output (which, in turn, improves renal perfusion), but also dilates the renal arterioles; these effects lead to improved glomerular filtration, and the increased urine volume. Improved hemodynamics will suppress the renin-angiotensin-aldosterone system, which was activated in response to poor renal perfusion. Weak β_1-receptor activation also contributes to this effect (particularly with such drugs as dobutamine). However, dopamine does not block (a) any of the adrenergic receptors.

Dopamine also has renal tubular effects, much like traditional diuretics do, although we often overlook them (perhaps because they are less important than the effects described above). The drug, via its D_1-receptor agonist actions, increases cAMP formation in the proximal tubules and also in the thick ascending limb of the loop of Henle. At the latter site, the result is inhibition of both the Na^+-H^+ exchange mechanism and the Na^+, K^+-ATPase, but not inhibition of water movement (e; recall that the thick ascending limb of the loop of Henle is impermeable to water). Taken together, the renal hemodynamic and tubular actions of dopamine make it particularly useful for managing heart failure that is accompanied by reduced renal function.

Higher doses of dopamine cause positive inotropy via β_1-receptor activation, and cause neuronal NE release. Even higher doses can also activate α_1 receptors in various vascular beds, including renal, leading to vasoconstriction that can raise blood pressure and total peripheral resistance, and can reduce renal blood flow, thereby reducing renal excretory function.

289. The answer is d. *(Brunton, pp 752, 756. Katzung, pp 260-261.)* Thiazide and thiazide-like diuretics should be highest on your list of drugs that are likely to cause hyponatremia. Was it easy to select hydrochlorothiazide as the correct answer because it was the only drug listed that was not a loop diuretic? Were you puzzled because you knew that furosemide is the prototype loop agent, and weren't sure about the classification of bumetanide, ethacrynic acid, or torsemide. Or did you not select the thiazide because you considered its diuretic effects to be mild, or modest, and therefore least likely to cause hyponatremia?

In absolute or relative terms the natriuretic (sodium-wasting) effects of a thiazide can be considered weak (especially in comparison with loop diuretics). They cause relatively slight increases in free water loss in the urine (compared with normal), interfere with normal urine-diluting mechanisms and lead to the formation of a concentrated (in terms of such solutes as sodium) urine. That is, the amount of extra sodium lost is, in a relative sense, much greater than the extra volume lost. This is reflected, in the blood, as not much extra volume loss coupled with proportionally greater declines in the amount of plasma sodium. Remember that hyponatremia means excessively reduced sodium concentration, and concentration is a function of amount per unit volume. The thiazides have caused dilutional hyponatremia.

290. The answer is b. *(Brunton pp 749-753, 784. Katzung, pp 258-259.)* That a loop diuretic (furosemide, bumetanide, torsemide, or perhaps even ethacrynic acid) would be a rational choice for helping to manage diuretic-induced hyponatremia seems irrational, if not plain wrong. After all, these drugs are considered to be the "big guns" of all diuretics, capable of causing almost limitless dose-dependent diuresis—large increases of renal loss of water, sodium, potassium, and other ions. So, what is the explanation?

When I described the actions of a thiazide or thiazide-like diuretics, I said that they impair the kidney's ability to form a normally dilute urine: in a relative sense they cause the loss of more Na^+ than of free water, and so Na^+ concentration in the blood falls (dilutional hyponatremia). The situation is essentially the opposite with loop diuretics. By reducing the medullary-to-cortical interstitial osmotic gradient (the countercurrent multiplier phenomenon) secondary to reduced Na^+ transport out of the urine in the ascending limb of the loop of Henle, they impair the ability of the kidneys to form a normally concentrated urine. In a relative sense, the urine formed in the presence of a loop agent therefore contains more water than sodium, and so the concentration of Na^+ in the blood rises. This tends to correct the hyponatremia. Although loop diuretics are not suitable as the only treatment of hyponatremia, they can be useful adjuncts for some patients.

Captopril (a), the prototype ACE inhibitor, tends to lower or not change blood Na^+ concentrations, but it does not raise them. ACE inhibitors reduce the formation of A-II, which normally stimulates aldosterone release from the adrenal cortex. Aldosterone causes the renal tubules to retain Na^+ and lose K^+. So when aldosterone release is reduced (due to less A-II available), the opposite occurs: Na^+ (and water) elimination rises (but Na^+ concentration tends not to change), and additional K^+ is lost. Spironolactone (c) tends to do many of the same things that an ACE inhibitor does to the kidneys, but it works by blocking renal aldosterone receptors (leading to increased Na^+ loss and K^+ retention) and has no effects on A-II's synthesis or direct effects. Thiazides or related agents (d) are clearly the wrong choice: to reiterate an important point, of all the diuretics, the thiazides and related agents are the most common cause of hyponatremia. Triamterene (and the related drug amiloride) are K^+-sparing diuretics that act by blocking Na^+ channels on the luminal face of the principal cells, thereby inhibiting Na^+ for K^+ exchange, in a manner that is not dependent on aldosterone. They do not raise plasma Na^+ concentrations and are not effective or used for dilutional hyponatremia.

291. The answer is c. *(Brunton, pp 743-746. Katzung, pp 256-257.)* We seldom administer acetazolamide as a diuretic because its effects are "mild;" associated with significant changes of both urine pH (up) and blood pH (down; metabolic acidosis); and self-limiting (once sufficient bicarbonate has been lost from the blood into the urine, refractoriness to further diuresis occurs). More often we administer acetazolamide or other systemic carbonic anhydrase inhibitors for nonrenal/noncardiovascular problems, such as management of altitude sickness or as an adjunct to anticonvulsant therapy as described here. As a result, we may forget that these systemically administered drugs are diuretics, one common property of all the diuretics being increased renal sodium loss (a natriuretic effect; thus, answer a is not correct). We may even forget that carbonic anhydrase inhibitors, given systemically, are potassium-wasting diuretics: they act proximally and deliver extra sodium distally where, at the principal cells of the nephron, some extra Na^+ is taken up in exchange for additional K^+ that gets eliminated in the urine.

In this scenario we have a patient taking a thiazide, which is obviously potassium-wasting and has the potential in its own right to cause hypokalemia. Add a systemic carbonic anhydrase to the regimen and the risks of hypokalemia increase. Acetazolamide does not antagonize the antihypertensive effects of thiazides or calcium channel blockers, nor provoke hypertension or a hypertensive crisis (b). If there were any interactions between the acetazolamide and the aspirin, it would be antagonism, not potentiation (d) of aspirin's antiplatelet effects. Aspirin (salicylate) undergoes renal tubular reabsorption, and that is a pH-dependent effect. Aspirin's reabsorption is reduced (ie, its excretion increases) in an alkaline urine, which is precisely what occurs with acetazolamide. (Recall that alkalinizing the urine is a useful adjunctive measure in treating severe salicylate poisoning, in part because it reduces tubular reabsorption of salicylate.) There is no reason to suspect sudden rises of blood volume, with or without concomitant heart failure from that (e). Indeed, the added diuresis from the acetazolamide may, at least transiently, potentiate the effects of the thiazide on urine volume, blood pressure, or both.

292. The answer is d. *(Brunton, p 744t. Katzung, pp 256-257.)* The profile shown for drug 2 applies to furosemide or another loop diuretic. And so what are the other drugs? Acetazolamide (a) has a profile that best matches drug 4 (note the increased HCO_3^- loss and decreased Cl^- loss). Amiloride's (b) profile fits that of drug 3 (note the reduced renal K^+ loss—this is a potassium-sparing diuretic). Chlorthalidone (c) and hydrochlorothiazide (e) would produce profiles like drug 1 (increased K^+ loss, a decrease of Ca^{2+} excretion, and variable effects on HCO_3^- loss due to variable effects [drug- and dose-dependent] on carbonic anhydrase [CA]). Some of the thiazide and thiazide-like diuretics do have CA-inhibitory actions, but that does not explain the drugs' main mechanisms of action (as applies to acetazolamide), and the CA-inhibitory effects are far weaker than those of acetazolamide.

Rather than rehashing the sites and mechanisms by which the "main" diuretics cause their effects—that's largely been addressed elsewhere above—what follows are some tips for arriving at a correct answer more easily. I'll add some additional comments that may not have been emphasized before.

Note that all the profiles show an increased (qualitative) renal excretion of Na^+. The essence of this is that it reflects the fact that all the common diuretics do that. Indeed, this natriuretic effect (sodium-excreting effect) is part of the working definition of "diuretic."

The next step is to identify which agents increase renal K excretion and which do the opposite, because the main diuretics are either K-sparing or K-wasting. That will narrow your choices nicely. You should be able to place a drug in the proper K-related class instantaneously (with the possible exception of acetazolamide, a K-wasting drug, because we tend to emphasize its CA-inhibitory effects and overlook other important properties; see the answers to Questions 278, 280, and 291 previously).

Once you see that a drug's profile involves increased K^+ loss, you have narrowed your choices to a thiazide or thiazide-like agent (hydrochlorothiazide, chlorthalidone, metolazone, many others), a loop agent, or a CA inhibitor.

Look now at what happens to urinary Ca^{2+} excretion. If it's reduced, it's a thiazide or a related agent (recall we can use these drugs for idiopathic hypercalciuria, an effect that capitalizes on reduced presence of Ca^{2+} in the urine due to reduced renal Ca^{2+} loss). If Ca^{2+} excretion is increased, it's a loop diuretic.

Now how do you identify which agent is a CA inhibitor (ie, acetazolamide)? In addition to looking at Na^+ and K^+, note what happens to HCO_3^- and Cl^-. Acetazolamide causes profound urinary alkalinization from the HCO_3^- loss; so much so that the blood's other major anion, Cl^-, is retained. Just looking at the table you would probably rule out a thiazide (a) as being acetazolamide because I indicate that the effect on that anion is variable (±).

How could you rule out triamterene, since we showed increased HCO_3^- loss with it? (It's a slight effect, by the way, and CA inhibition is not its main nor an important mechanism or outcome, but you can't tell from the table.) Look at the Cl^- profile and you will see that acetazolamide is the only diuretic that lowers Cl^- excretion. That's because, HCO_3^- is lost to such a great degree that Cl^- is conserved.

Respiratory System Pharmacology: Asthma and COPD

Adrenergic agonists
Antimuscarinics
Immunoglobulin antibody
Leukotriene modifiers
Mast cell "stabilizers"
Methylxanthines
Mucolytics
Histamine and histamine receptor blockers

Questions

293. A 27-year-old woman is seen in the outpatient clinic for a routine checkup. She's just moved to your town, and this is the first time you've met her. She has asthma and says she's been using her inhaler (albuterol) three or four times every day as her only therapy. "I breathe a lot easier after I take several puffs," she says. She feels well otherwise. Which of the following statements applies to this patient or her treatment plan?

a. Her treatment plan is inappropriate and needs to be modified
b. If pulmonary function tests performed today are normal, it is likely that the diagnosis is incorrect: she does not have asthma
c. She is likely to enjoy activities, such as skiing and skating, in which she breathes cold, clear air
d. She is most likely to have trouble with her breathing when in a warm, humid atmosphere
e. She is probably slightly bradycardic and hypertensive from the drug's expected actions on the heart and peripheral vasculature

294. Certain adrenergic agonists clearly play a role in managing some patients with asthma, whether for prophylaxis (control medication) or for rescue therapy. Which of the following drugs is classified as an adrenergic agonist, but has no physiologically relevant or clinically useful effects on airway smooth muscle tone?

a. Albuterol
b. Epinephrine
c. Norepinephrine
d. Salmeterol
e. Theophylline

295. A patient with asthma has moderate bronchospasm and wheezing about twice a week. Current medications are inhaled albuterol (mainly for acute symptom control) and inhaled beclomethasone as a "control medication." The patient continues to have occasional and generally mild flare-ups of his asthma. If the physician wishes to make salmeterol part of the treatment plan, how best should it be used for this patient?

a. A replacement for the albuterol
b. A replacement for the corticosteroid
c. An add-on to current medications for additional prophylactic benefits
d. Primary (sole) therapy, replacing both albuterol and the steroid
e. The preferred agent for acute symptom control (rescue therapy)

296. The attending in the outpatient pulmonary clinic states she is going to start omalizumab therapy for a 19-year-old with asthma. What most accurately describes the actions, uses, or adverse effects of this drug?

a. Antibody that binds and therefore inactivates endogenous ACh and histamine.
b. Contraindicated if patient is taking an oral or orally inhaled corticosteroid.
c. Good alternative to albuterol or similar adrenergic bronchodilators for rescue therapy.
d. Immediate- or delayed-onset anaphylactic reactions pose the greatest risk.
e. Novel agent likely to become first-line therapy as a control medication for mild but recurrent asthma.

297. A 19-year-old man moves from a small town to your city and is now your patient. He has a history of asthma, and his previous primary care physician was managing it with oral theophylline. What best summarizes the efficacy or current status of theophylline in particular, or methylxanthines in general, in such patients as this?

a. Dosing is simple and convenient, rarely needs to be adjusted
b. Excellent alternative to an inhaled steroid for "rescue" therapy
c. Is, at best, a second- or third-line agent for long-term asthma control
d. Possesses strong and clinically useful anti-inflammatory activity
e. Sedation is a major side effect, even with therapeutic doses or blood levels

298. An elderly man with chronic obstructive pulmonary disease (COPD) is being managed with several drugs, one of which is inhaled ipratropium. What is the main mechanism that accounts for the beneficial effects of this drug?

a. Blocks receptors upon which an endogenous bronchoconstrictor mediator acts
b. Enhances epinephrine release from the adrenal medulla
c. Inhibits cAMP breakdown via phosphodiesterase inhibition
d. Prevents antigen-antibody reactions that lead to mast cell mediator release
e. Stimulates ventilatory rates (CNS effect in brain's medulla)
f. Suppresses synthesis and release of inflammatory mediators

299. A 16-year-old girl being treated for asthma develops drug-induced skeletal muscle tremors. What is the most likely cause?

a. Albuterol
b. Beclomethasone
c. Cromolyn
d. Ipratropium
e. Montelukast

300. A 26-year-old patient with asthma is being treated with montelukast. What is the main mechanism by which this drug works?

a. Blocks the proinflammatory and bronchoconstrictor effects of certain arachidonic acid metabolites
b. Enhances release of epinephrine from the adrenal (suprarenal) medulla
c. Increases airway β-adrenergic receptor responsiveness to endogenous norepinephrine
d. Inhibits cAMP breakdown via phosphodiesterase inhibition
e. Prevents antigen-antibody reactions that lead to mast cell mediator release
f. Stimulates ventilatory rates (CNS effect in brain's medulla)

301. An elderly man, in obvious respiratory distress due to exacerbation of his emphysema and chronic bronchitis (COPD), presents in the emergency department. One drug ordered by the physician, to be administered by the respiratory therapist, is *N*-acetylcysteine. What is the main action or purpose of this drug?

a. Blocks receptors for the cysteinyl leukotrienes
b. Inhibits metabolic inactivation of epinephrine or β_2 agonists that were administered
c. Inhibits leukotriene synthesis
d. Promptly suppresses airway inflammation
e. Reverses ACh-mediated bronchoconstriction
f. Thins airway mucus secretions for easier removal by suctioning or postural drainage

302. A 23-year-old woman with asthma has what is described as "aspirin (hyper)sensitivity" and experiences severe bronchospasm in response to even small doses of the drug. What is the most likely mechanism by which the aspirin provoked her pulmonary problems?

a. Blocks synthesis of endogenous prostaglandins that have bronchodilator activity
b. Induces formation of antibodies directed against the salicylate on airway mast cells
c. Induces hypersensitivity of H_1 receptors on airway smooth muscles cell
d. Induces hypersensitivity of muscarinic receptors on airway smooth muscles cell
e. Prevents or reduces epinephrine binding to β_2-adrenergic receptors (airways and elsewhere)

303. A young boy is diagnosed with asthma. His primary symptom is frequent cough, not bronchospasm or wheezing. Other asthma medications are started, but until their effects develop fully we wish to suppress the cough without running a risk of suppressing ventilatory drive or causing sedation or other unwanted effects. Which of the following drugs would meet these needs the best?

a. Codeine
b. Dextromethorphan
c. Diphenhydramine
d. Hydrocodone
e. Promethazine

304. A mother brings her 10-year-old son, who has a long-standing history of poorly controlled asthma, to the emergency department. He is in a relatively early stage of what will prove to be a severe asthma attack. Arterial blood gases have not been analyzed yet, but it is obvious that the lad is in great distress. He is panting with great effort at a rate of about 60 breaths/min.

Given the boy's history and the likely diagnosis of acute asthma, the health care team administers all the drugs listed below by the stated routes, and with the purposes noted. The child's condition quickly improves, and the team leaves the boy with his mother while they go to care for other ED patients. Within a couple of minutes the mother comes out of her son's cubicle frantically screaming "he's stopped breathing!" Which of the following drugs most likely precipitated the ventilatory arrest?

a. Albuterol, inhaled, given by nebulizer for prompt bronchodilation
b. Atropine, nebulized and inhaled
c. Midazolam, IV, to normalize ventilatory rate and allay anxiety
d. Methylprednisolone, IV, for prompt suppression of airway inflammation
e. Normal saline, nebulized and inhaled, to hydrate the airway mucosae

305. We prescribe an orally inhaled corticosteroid for a patient with asthma. Previously she was using only a rapidly acting adrenergic bronchodilator for both prophylaxis and for treatment of acute attacks. She used the steroid as directed for 5 days, then stopped taking it. What is the most likely reason why the patient quit using the drug?

a. Disturbing tachycardia and palpitations occurred
b. Relentless diarrhea developed after just 1 day of using the steroid
c. She experienced little or no obvious improvement in breathing
d. The drug caused extreme drowsiness that interfered with daytime activities
e. The drug caused her to retain fluid and gain weight

306. A patient consumes an excessive dose of theophylline and develops toxicity in response to the drug. Which of the following is an expected sign, symptom, or other consequence of this overdose?

a. Bradycardia
b. Drowsiness progressing to sleep and then coma
c. Hepatotoxicity
d. Paradoxical bronchospasm
e. Seizures

307. Acetylcholine esterase inhibitors, muscarinic agonists such as pilocarpine, and β-blockers are among the drugs used to manage patients with glaucoma. They also share properties that are particularly relevant to patients with asthma. Which statement summarizes best what that relevance is?

a. Contraindicated, or pose great risks, for people with asthma
b. Degranulate mast cells, cause drug-mediated allergy
c. Tend to raise intraocular pressure in patients who have both glaucoma and asthma
d. Trigger bronchoconstriction by directly activating H_1-histamine receptors on airway smooth muscle cells
e. Useful for acute asthma, not for ambulatory patients

308. A patient suffering status asthmaticus presents in the emergency department. Blood gases reveal severe respiratory acidosis and hypoxia. Even large parenteral doses of a selective β_2 agonist fail to dilate the airways adequately; rather, they cause dangerous degrees of tachycardia. Which pharmacologic intervention or approach is most likely to control the acute symptoms and restore the bronchodilator efficacy of the adrenergic drug?

a. Add inhaled cromolyn
b. Give a parenteral corticosteroid
c. Give parenteral diphenhydramine
d. Switch to epinephrine
e. Switch to isoproterenol (β_1/β_2 agonist)

309. The FDA has mandated a warning about the increased risk of death in asthma patients taking recommended doses of salmeterol (or other slow-/long-acting adrenergic asthma control medications), alone or in combination with another drug (eg, an inhaled steroid) for too long a period of time. What is the most likely mechanism or phenomenon by which this fatal adverse response, or other severe airway responses, occurs?

a. Anaphylaxis due to gradual formation of antibodies against the drug
b. Hypertensive crisis
c. Inhibited synthesis, release, and anti-inflammatory actions of endogenous cortisol
d. Plugging of the bronchioles with viscous mucus due to the drug's antimuscarinic actions
e. Tolerance of airway smooth muscle cells to the effects of adrenergic bronchodilators

310. A hungry 8-year-old boy is visiting his grandparents' house and sees grandpa sprinkle some powder from a small foil pack onto his applesauce. Grandpa smiles and says "Mmmm, tastes good." The packet contains a theophylline salt that was prescribed for his COPD. Liking applesauce and thinking the drug packets contain candy, the lad opens the applesauce jar, finds grandpa's stash of dozens of theophylline packets, and sprinkles on lots of drug before eating the whole thing. Toxicity ensues. What is this child most likely to experience before anything else significant and untoward develops?

a. Acute urinary retention
b. Bradycardia and hypotension
c. Irritability, other signs/symptoms of CNS stimulation, possibly seizures
d. Ischemic stroke from drug-induced platelet aggregation
e. Ventilatory suppression (centrally mediated) leading to respiratory acidosis and apnea

Respiratory System Pharmacology: Asthma and COPD

Answers

293. The answer is a. *(Brunton, pp 720-721. Katzung, pp 340-344, 351.)* This patient certainly seems to have recurrent episodes of asthma. Even if they are "mild" and ostensibly responsive to an inhaled β_2 agonist, she's not being treated properly. She or her prior prescriber has been overreliant on, and overusing, a medication that only manages symptoms (and not well in her case) and does not address the underlying cause, which is airway inflammation. (Some physicians define overuse of an inhaled adrenergic bronchodilator as using it more than once a day; the NIH says needing to use it more than twice a week is overuse.) Reasonable options for her would be to prescribe an inhaled corticosteroid (beclomethasone, others), since she reports only mild symptoms. (Of course, pulmonary function tests [PFTs] should be done.) If her bouts become more severe or frequent, then an oral steroid (eg, prednisone) might be prescribed for a while, with a proper switch to an inhaled steroid.

PFTs might be reasonably normal (b), but that depends on such factors as when she used her inhaler last, and whether she is simply having a "good day" (eg, no exposure today to allergens). A single normal PFT in a patient who describes frequent need for a bronchodilator does not rule out asthma. (Let's use an analogy that applies to many asthma patients. You are standing right on the edge of a thousand-foot drop-off on the rim of the Grand Canyon. Only a couple of inches from a bad trip down. Take just one little step forward and you're a goner. Same with asthma: you may be "feeling good" with current medications, but just a little provocation of airway inflammation and bronchoconstriction and severe symptoms, possibly necessitating intubation or leading to a fatal attack, can put the patient over the proverbial edge.)

Patients with asthma tend not to do well in cold temperatures (c). Breathing cold air often provokes bronchospasm (probably mediated by increased parasympathetic effects on airway smooth muscle). (Have you ever taken a deep breath when the temperature is near or below zero?) Conversely, asthmatics tend to do well when it is warm and humid. (Ever noticed how many athletes with asthma tend to gravitate to sports that provide a warm, humid environment, eg, swimming?) Finally, β_2 agonists do not cause bradycardia or increases of peripheral resistance. Muscarinic agonists or β-blockers would cause the former, α agonists the latter.

294. The answer is c. *(Brunton, pp 144-145, 127-238, 248. Katzung, pp 88t, 89t, 136-137, 140.)* By way of a brief but essential review of autonomic pharmacology, recall that "adrenergic bronchodilation" requires activation of β_2-adrenergic receptors on airway smooth muscle cells. Norepinephrine is an α and β_1 agonist, with no ability to activate β_2 receptors, and so it has no bronchodilator activity. Albuterol (a), a β_2 agonist, can be considered the prototype of adrenergic bronchodilators used for asthma (prophylaxis/control, but mainly rescue therapy). Epinephrine (b) is a very efficacious bronchodilator, but its use for routine management of asthma is considerably limited due to its ability to cause vasoconstriction (α-agonist activity) and cardiac stimulation (β_1-agonist activity). In terms of pulmonary problems, it is reserved mainly for managing anaphylaxis, but it indeed causes bronchodilation well and promptly. Salmeterol (d) is a β_2 agonist also. Given by inhalation, its bronchodilator effects are slow in onset, but it has a long duration compared with similarly classified drugs such as albuterol. Thus, salmeterol is an efficacious bronchodilator, but not suitable for prompt effects (rescue therapy). Theophylline (e) has modest bronchodilator activity, but it is not an adrenergic agonist. It inhibits phosphodiesterase, and so inhibits metabolic inactivation of cAMP (the "second messenger" formed by adrenergic bronchodilators in airway smooth muscle).

295. The answer is c. *(Brunton, pp 253, 720-721. Katzung, pp 344, 355.)* If we were to decide to use salmeterol in this situation it would be best to consider it as an add-on. Recall that salmeterol, like albuterol, is mainly a β_2 agonist, but salmeterol's onset of action is much slower, its duration of action much longer. The slow onset of salmeterol makes it a useful prophylactic agent for some patients, but renders it completely inappropriate for rescue therapy (a, e). It can be administered separately, or the physician might prescribe one of the proprietary fixed-dose combination products that contain both salmeterol and a steroid (given by oral inhalation). One could reasonably argue that salmeterol is also dangerous if used as the sole intervention for rescue, because serious ventilatory compromise can develop before its bronchodilator effects develop. The patient described needs a corticosteroid. We might increase the dose of the inhaled steroid as a start, or perhaps try a burst of an oral steroid (eg, prednisone) for a while. Regardless, using salmeterol as a replacement for any corticosteroid (b) or for all the other current medications (d) is likely to do little or no good and allow more and more severe asthma attacks; it's simply bad management. Remember: The key to success in asthma therapy long-term requires controlling airway inflammation, and corticosteroids are the key drugs for doing just that.

296. The answer is d. *(Brunton, pp 725-726. Katzung, pp 350, 352-353.)* The most serious adverse response to omalizumab, a monoclonal antibody directed against IgE, is an anaphylactic reaction (often severe, less often fatal). These adverse reactions usually occur after the first dose, and usually within 2 hours of injection. This is one reason why patients should receive the drug only in a "controlled" health care setting and should be under observation for at least 2 hours thereafter. Nonetheless, anaphylaxis or less severe untoward immunologic reactions have been reported after 24 hours or longer, and so the patient should have an epinephrine autoinjector (prescribed or dispensed by the physician) handy for at least several days after an omalizumab dose. The risk of anaphylaxis is also a major reason why the drug should be used only for patients who have severe asthma not adequately controlled with other drugs (adrenergic bronchodilators, leukotriene receptor blockers, corticosteroids).

As noted, the antibody is directed against IgE. The IgE-omalizumab complex then prevents IgE from binding to mast cell and basophil membranes, which otherwise would trigger allergen-mediated cell activation. Omalizumab does not bind other ligands (eg, ACh or histamine; a), nor does it alter the effects of those bronchoconstrictor agonists in any other way. It also has no intrinsic or direct bronchodilator activity.

Owing to the anaphylaxis risk, the drug's slow onset of action, and its lack of bronchodilator activity, omalizumab is not, nor ever will be, first-line therapy for asthma (e), whether mild or severe, frequent or not. It will never be a substitute for a rapidly acting adrenergic bronchodilator for rescue therapy (c). And prior or current use of any of the "traditional" asthma medications does not contraindicate (b) a trial with omalizumab. Indeed, owing to omalizumab's slow onset, continued and otherwise proper corticosteroid therapy to suppress airway inflammation is essential.

297. The answer is c. *(Brunton, pp 727-730. Katzung, pp 345-346, 351.)* Theophylline, the prototype methylxanthine, is an oral bronchodilator that has some beneficial pulmonary effects in patients with asthma or COPD. We don't know precisely how it exerts its bronchodilator activity, at least at concentrations found in human beings (in vitro it inhibits phosphodiesterase, preserving cAMP levels; it also blocks receptors for adenosine, which has bronchoconstrictor activity).

However, there are serious problems with this old drug that relegate it to second or third (or lower) status in therapy; that render it a drug that should be prescribed only by pulmonologists who are quite familiar with the limitations, side effects, and toxicity; and that make its use as primary therapy for asthma usually inappropriate (at best).

Theophylline and other methylxanthines have a very low therapeutic index: it is all too easy (whether because of drug-drug interactions, or simply improper dosing) to have blood levels rise to a range that can cause toxicity (mainly excessive cardiac and CNS stimulation, with the potential for arrhythmias or seizures). Moreover, and because of the problems stated above, frequent blood testing is necessary in order to get, and keep, plasma levels within an acceptable therapeutic range and hopefully avoid subtherapeutic or toxic blood levels. The drug depends on hepatic P450 status for its elimination, and that makes elimination very easily influenced by liver dysfunction or other interacting drugs that can either induce or inhibit its metabolism.

Most important is the fact that theophylline has no anti-inflammatory activity; as I said, if we are treating asthma long-term, the "secret to success" is controlling airway inflammation. For our foundation we use corticosteroids to suppress inflammation.

If we were dealing with COPD and the goal is bronchodilation (it is), such drugs as ipratropium (inhaled antimuscarinic) are not only more efficacious than a methylxanthine or an adrenergic bronchodilator, but also associated with fewer dosing problems, monitoring needs, and side effects. In COPD the pathophysiology involves not only bronchoconstriction but also goblet cell hyperplasia, leading to increased mucus production. Such drugs as ipratropium are, therefore, usually a first choice and usually improve symptoms and pulmonary function tests the most.

298. The answer is a. *(Brunton, pp 189-190, 194-196, 730-732. Katzung, pp 347, 351.)* You should be able to deduce quickly (if not simply know outright) that ipratropium is an atropine-like drug—an antimuscarinic that blocks the bronchoconstrictor effect of ACh on airway smooth muscle. It is a quaternary, inhaled antimuscarinic: that is, it acts locally in the airways, and very little of the "always charged" molecule diffuses into the circulation to cause systemic effects. Ipratropium has no effects on the adrenal medulla (b), on mast cells (d) or other elements of the inflammatory response (f), or in the CNS (e). Ipratropium is approved for managing COPD, but is often used for some asthma patients. The drug has a rapid onset of action. However, some studies indicate that it is not as efficacious a bronchodilator as β_2 agonists, and so it is not a suitable agent for rescue therapy. Finally, the bronchodilator effects of ipratropium and β agonists are synergistic (same effect, different mechanisms), and so there's some logic to using them both.

299. The answer is a. *(Brunton, pp 719-721, 252-253. Katzung, p 344.)* Of the drugs listed in the question, skeletal muscle tremor is a side effect most often associated with β_2-adrenergic agonists—albuterol and others. It is almost always a dose-dependent phenomenon.

Note: Some physicians titrate the dose of adrenergic bronchodilators upward, stopping when tremors develop and equating the blood level associated with that dose as being therapeutic with respect to controlling the pulmonary disease. The wisdom of that is questionable; proper dosage adjustments or other therapy changes should be based on pulmonary symptom relief (subjective assessment) in general and, ideally, quantitative pulmonary function tests.

None of the other drugs listed is associated with skeletal muscle tremor. Beclomethasone (b) is an inhaled corticosteroid; cromolyn (c), also inhaled for asthma, reduces mast cell degranulation; ipratropium (d) is an inhaled antimuscarinic indicated for COPD; montelukast (e) is a leukotriene receptor blocker that is also indicated for asthma prophylaxis.

300. The answer is a. *(Brunton, pp 722-724. Katzung, pp 344-350, 352.)* Montelukast (and a related drug, zafirlukast) blocks receptors for leukotrienes (LTs). (When you see "leuk" or "luk" as part of these drugs' generic names, think leukotrienes or leukotriene modifiers, and think of drugs for asthma.)

Recall that the LTs are proinflammatory and bronchoconstrictor mediators formed as part of normal arachidonic acid metabolism via the 5′-lipoxygenase pathway. (The other main part of arachidonic acid metabolism, involving cyclooxygenases, forms various prostaglandins and thromboxane A_2.) LTs also participate in recruiting eosinophils to the inflamed regions (recall that local eosinophilia is often an accompaniment of asthma), thereby blunting the local inflammatory processes in yet another way.

These LT receptor blockers are indicated for prophylaxis (control therapy) only, and should not be used in lieu of corticosteroids (oral or orally inhaled) when corticosteroids are suitable (which is most of the time). They will do virtually no good in a short enough time if they were administered to suppress ongoing bronchoconstriction (eg, for rescue therapy), mainly because they are too slow-acting. And, although this class of drugs is among the newest approved for asthma in many years, they are not panaceas for all asthma patients, and for some patients their efficacy appears to be no better than placebo.

Note: Montelukast has at least two advantages over zafirlukast. It does not inhibit the hepatic P450 system to cause drug-drug interactions, particularly with such other drugs as theophylline or warfarin. The risk of hepatotoxicity also seems substantially lower with montelukast.

The LT modifiers do not enhance epinephrine release from the adrenal medulla (suprarenal medulla; b); increase β-adrenergic receptor responsiveness (c; note that norepinephrine, mentioned in the question, has no bronchodilator/β_2 activity); inhibit phosphodiesterase (d); or interfere with mast cell function or mast cell responsiveness to antigens (e).

301. The answer is f. *(Brunton, pp 694-695. Katzung, p 1019.)* You should know *N*-acetylcysteine as an antidote for acetaminophen poisoning. When used for that purpose, it is given orally or intravenously. The sulfhydryl groups that are part of the molecule are important, as they react with the toxic acetaminophen metabolite and spare glutathione-depleted hepatocytes from oxidative attack. *N*-acetylcysteine is also a mucolytic (mucus-thinning) drug, given by inhalation in a nebulized solution or by intratracheal instillation, to reduce the viscosity of airway mucus that can then be removed easily by coughing, postural drainage and chest percussion, or by airway suctioning. Here, too, the mechanism is based on its –SH-rich composition. *N*-acetylcysteine lacks other airway effects such as bronchodilation or suppression or inflammation.

302. The answer is a. *(Brunton, pp 683-689. Katzung, pp 320, 322.)* Aspirin, the prototype of the nonsteroidal anti-inflammatory drugs (NSAIDs), inhibits cyclooxygenases (COX-1 and -2) and the "arachidonic acid cascade." One outcome of that is inhibited synthesis of PGE_2. The PGE_2 (along with circulating epinephrine) is a physiologically important endogenous bronchodilator that is particularly important to maintain airway patency (dilation) for most asthmatics. Inhibit this synthesis, with aspirin or another nonselective cyclooxygenase inhibitor/NSAID, and bronchoconstriction or bronchospasm may ensue in that population of asthmatics who often are exquisitely sensitive to these drugs. This aspirin hypersensitivity phenomenon is relatively uncommon in children with asthma, but more prevalent in adults. Estimates are that it affects between 10% and 25% of adult asthmatics with so-called "triad asthma": asthma plus nasal polyps and chronic urticaria.

Virtually all other NSAIDs that nonselectively inhibit cyclooxygenases may cross-react, although the incidence of severe pulmonary reactions seems the highest with aspirin itself. Selective COX-2 inhibitors (eg, celecoxib) pose less of a problem because they are less likely to inhibit synthesis of bronchodilator prostaglandins, which are formed by the COX-1 pathway, but they are not absolutely free from the potential problem. If one needs a drug to manage fever or mild pain in an asthmatic, acetaminophen is preferred: it does not cross-react, and owing to negligible effects on prostaglandin synthesis via cyclooxygenase-dependent pathways it is not classified as an NSAID.

303. The answer is b. *(Brunton, pp 122, 578-579. Katzung, p 547.)* Dextromethorphan is a centrally acting antitussive drug that is about as efficacious a cough-suppressant as codeine. It is thought to suppress the vagal afferent neural pathway involved in the cough reflex. However, unlike codeine (c) and hydrocodone (d; another useful antitussive in some cases), dextromethorphan is not an opioid and lacks analgesic effects or the potential for ventilatory suppression or abuse.

Diphenhydramine (c) and promethazine (e) also have antitussive action. However, they too can cause generalized CNS and ventilatory depression. They also exert significant antimuscarinic effects, but neither is a preferred or even frequently used drug for cough suppression in most patients. Although the atropine-like effects of these drugs may be beneficial in terms of inhibiting ACh-mediated bronchoconstriction in a patient with asthma, they may also cause thickening of airway mucus, favoring plugging of the airways with viscous mucus deposits that cannot be removed normally by mucociliary transport or coughing. That is, the benefits of bronchodilation may be outweighed by the risks of mucus plugging in some asthma patients.

304. The answer is c. *(Brunton, pp 361-362, 407. Katzung pp 340-341.)* The term asthma derives from a Greek word that means, literally, "to pant." In severe asthma attacks such as the one I describe here, the hyperpnea precedes the likely development of ventilatory depression and, in some cases, ventilatory arrest. This panting is a sometimes successful yet sometimes inadequate physiologic response elicited to increase ventilatory oxygen uptake and eliminate excess CO_2, although it may be insufficient to raise arterial O_2 saturation adequately and more than sufficient to induce metabolic alkalosis from excess CO_2 loss. Nonetheless, it is a "protective" ventilatory response, and breathing too quickly, even inefficiently, is better than not breathing at all. This leads to the admonition: Never give a drug that can depress ventilatory drive to an asthma patient unless he or she has a protected airway and ventilation can be controlled and supported mechanically. IV midazolam (or the IV administration of virtually any other benzodiazepine, opioid, or barbiturate) will allay anxiety, but will also tend to suppress ventilatory drive and hasten the onset of ventilatory arrest. In the scenario described here, midazolam is the wrong drug to give.

Albuterol (a) or a similar β_2-agonist bronchodilator, whether given by inhalation or parenterally, would not be expected to worsen the boy's ventilatory status. They should not be the only drugs relied on, but they would be appropriate adjunctive treatments, as would be all the rest for the stated purposes. As an important aside, you may recall that atropine (b) and other drugs with antimuscarinic activity have bronchodilator activity, and also tend to make airway mucus secretions more viscous, leading to airway mucus plugging. In the context of this scenario, with the administration of other drugs that I listed and the availability of airway suctioning devices as needed, the mucus-thickening effects of an antimuscarinic should not be a problem with which we cannot easily deal by way of airway suctioning and the administration of mucus-thinning (mucolytic) drugs. Glucocorticoids

(d) and nebulized saline would be valuable, if not essential, adjuncts to this boy's therapy.

305. The answer is c. *(Brunton, pp 721-722, 1598-1599, 1603-1604. Katzung, pp 347-348, 351-352.)* It usually takes a couple of weeks of inhaled corticosteroid use "as directed" to suppress airway inflammation and the resulting bronchoconstriction well enough that the patient can sense clinical improvement (fewer or milder asthma symptoms). Unless the patient is forewarned about this slow onset, and urged to remain compliant, they are likely to believe the drug is ineffective and therefore not worth taking. Clearly, inhaled corticosteroids do not cause the obvious "rush"—the prompt, dramatic, and unmistakable symptom relief that typically occurs with adrenergic bronchodilators. Nonetheless, given adequate time, the inhaled steroids often prove to be the key to effective long-term control of asthma. Inhaled corticosteroids act locally; little enters the systemic circulation; such side effects as fluid retention, weight gain (e), and hyperglycemia, that are typical with systemic steroids (eg, prednisone), rarely occur or become problematic. Inhaled steroids do not cause cardiac stimulation (a), diarrhea (b), or drowsiness (d).

306. The answer is e. *(Brunton, pp 728-730. Katzung, pp 345-347.)* Theophylline, a methylxanthine, is a caffeine-like drug that is becoming outmoded as therapy for asthma in most adolescents and adults. A low margin of safety, extreme dependence on adequate liver function for metabolism, susceptibility to numerous clinically significant drug interactions, and a lack of airway anti-inflammatory activity, are among the reasons why it should probably not be prescribed by any physician other than a pulmonologist who is familiar with the limitations and problems with this class of drugs. Without proper dosage adjustments and monitoring, it is all too easy, and common, for blood levels to fall into subtherapeutic ranges or, as we see here, into toxic ranges. The earliest signs and symptoms of excess involve CNS stimulation (jitteriness, tremors, difficulty sleeping, anxiety). As blood levels rise the CNS is increasingly stimulated. Seizures may occur, and when they do the inability to breathe during the seizures is the main cause of death. Thus, answer b is incorrect.

Theophylline tends to cause tachycardia, increases of cardiac contractility and, potentially, tachyarrhythmias. This occurs mainly because methylxanthines inhibit phosphodiesterase, which normally metabolically inactivates cAMP, the levels of which are increased in smooth and cardiac muscles by β-adrenergic agonists. Bradycardia (a) is not at all likely. Theophylline is not hepatotoxic (c); it does not cause paradoxical bronchospasm (d), even when plasma levels are very high or truly toxic.

307. The answer is a. *(Brunton, pp 187-188, 193-194, 208-209. Katzung, pp 101-103, 105.)* By now you should be able to recall the classifications and actions of the drugs listed in this question. Acetylcholinesterase inhibitors and such muscarinic agonists as pilocarpine are sometimes used as topical miotics for managing glaucoma (mainly angle-closure/narrow angle forms of the disease). Certain topical β-blockers are used for open-angle glaucoma, probably working by inhibiting aqueous humor production. However, all these drugs (and others in these classes, used systemically for a host of other common medical conditions) are contraindicated for asthma patients—even if they are used topically on the eye(s). An important element in the pathophysiology of asthma is airway smooth-muscle hyperresponsiveness to various bronchoconstrictor stimuli, and muscarinic receptor activation is clearly a phenomenon that leads to often intense bronchoconstriction.

You may recall that the choline ester, methacholine, is used to help diagnose asthma when the diagnosis is otherwise questionable. The basis of this "methacholine challenge" centers on the concept of airway hyperreactivity (in this case, to muscarinic agonists) in asthmatics. Very low doses of methacholine are given, by inhalation, while pulmonary function tests are recorded. Asthmatics experience significant (sometimes dangerous) bronchoconstrictor responses to methacholine doses that are far lower than those that would provoke even slight pulmonary function test changes in nonasthmatics.

Recall that ACh esterase inhibitors cause what amounts to a "buildup" of ACh at the cholinergic neuroeffector junction, leading to heightened muscarinic receptor activation. These cholinesterase inhibitors, whether used for glaucoma or such other conditions as myasthenia gravis, can have lethal effects in some asthma patients. (Note, too, that cholinesterase inhibitors are found in some insecticides, so there is an extra and significant risk to the asthma patient in agricultural or gardening/lawn care settings.) Muscarinic agonists, whether those used for glaucoma or for stimulating the gut or urinary tract (eg, bethanechol for functional urinary retention), may prove lethal too. Finally, asthmatics tend to be extremely dependent on the bronchodilator actions of circulating epinephrine. Block the β_2 receptors that mediate that effect and the outcome can be disastrous. Even the so-called "cardioselective" β-blockers (atenolol, metoprolol) can cause serious problems for some asthmatics. That is because their ability to block β_1 receptors is relative and dose-dependent, not absolute: they may pose no pulmonary problems for persons without asthma, but may be deadly in those who do.

308. The answer is b. *(Brunton, p 722. Katzung, pp 342-344, 351.)* When pulmonary function deteriorates so much that respiratory acidosis ensues (because sufficient amounts of CO_2 aren't being eliminated by ventilation) and severe hypoxia develops (because of inadequate oxygen transfer), acute tolerance (in essence, desensitization) develops to the bronchodilator effects of drugs with β_2-agonist activity—all of them, including isoproterenol (e). If this point is forgotten, repeated administration of a β_2 agonist will lead to increasing degrees of cardiac stimulation (rate, contractility, automaticity, conduction) because under these conditions they lose their selectivity for β_2 receptors and also begin activating β_1 receptors very effectively. (They become isoproterenol-like in their profiles.)

Even epinephrine (d) won't work as well as a bronchodilator under these conditions, and repeated injections of it will do little more than cause further cardiac stimulation plus vasoconstriction via β_1 activation. Through mechanisms that are not quite clear, administering suitable doses of a parenteral steroid under these conditions of acidosis and hypoxia "restores" a substantial degree of airway responsiveness to β agonists. Giving a steroid (plus oxygen, which helps correct the underlying blood gas and pH changes) is essential.

Giving diphenhydramine (c), even though it blocks the bronchoconstrictor effects of both ACh and histamine, will not do much good for the acute and life-threatening signs and symptoms. Giving cromolyn (a) will prove largely worthless and certainly not lifesaving.

309. The answer is e. *(Brunton, pp 720-721. Katzung, pp 344, 351.)* Long-term, more or less round-the-clock exposure of β_2-adrenergic receptors to an agonist eventually causes those receptors to lose sensitivity to those very drugs. The loss of responsiveness to usual bronchodilator actions—that is, airway smooth muscle tolerance—affects not only responses to salmeterol or the pharmacokinetically similar drug, formoterol, but also to albuterol or similar rapidly acting adrenergic bronchodilators typically used for rescue therapy.

Of course, for most drugs overcoming tolerance and restoring effects to a certain intensity can be achieved by increasing the dose, the dose frequency, or both. This is precisely what asthma patients who are poorly managed do, especially with their rapidly acting rescue inhalers (albuterol, etc): four or more puffs at a time, many times each 24 hours. Thus, the "solution" to the tolerance, higher and more frequent doses, actually becomes the cause. And so the usual outcome of excessive or excessively prolonged adrenergic bronchodilator use is a faster onset and progression of tolerance and a greater degree of tolerance. That is, increasing dose and/or frequency only makes matters worse over the long-run.

So, patients taking one or two β_2 agonists month after month gradually get less and less bronchodilation and symptom relief over time; their breathing difficulty becomes worse; and should severe bronchoconstriction occur, usual or even relatively high doses of a rapidly acting (rescue) bronchodilator will fail to work well, if at all. Usually this will be assessed, clinically, by diminishing improvement of FEV1 in response to a rapidly acting adrenergic bronchodilator (eg, albuterol). Thus, the patient gets in severe ventilatory distress or may even die. Thus, what might be called "antiasthma" drugs can actually lead to asthma-related fatalities under some conditions.

Answer a is incorrect; antibodies against salmeterol or other adrenergic bronchodilators do not develop. Answer b is not acceptable. Although high doses of a so-called "selective β_2 agonist" may increase blood pressure (at high blood levels selectivity for β_2 receptors is lost and β_1 receptors can be activated, raising blood pressure via increases of both heart rate and left ventricular contractility), a significant rise of pressure is very unlikely; hypertensive crisis will not occur. Salmeterol or other adrenergic bronchodilators have no direct or major effects on cortisol synthesis, release, or actions (c); nor do they have antimuscarinic effects, whether on mucus viscosity, airway smooth muscle tone, or any other processes mediated by muscarinic (cholinergic) receptors.

310. The answer is c. *(Brunton, pp 727-729. Katzung, pp 345-346.)* Theophylline (or the related drug aminophylline) is classified as a methylxanthine, just like the caffeine and other methylxanthines in your favorite coffee, tea, cola, or chocolates. So to answer this question, simply imagine what is likely to happen if you consumed, say, eight cups of strong caffeinated coffee in a short time. You're typically wide awake (if not "hyper"), tachycardic, urinating (from cardiac-mediated increased renal perfusion and GFR), and tremorous.

Methylxanthines are CNS stimulants, not just bronchodilators or cardiac stimulants. In overdoses, irritability or increased alertness and wakefulness develop first. As blood levels rise, ultimately seizures occur, and that is one of the major things we would see if this child took a sufficient overdose. Methylxanthines don't cause urinary retention (a); as noted above, increased GFR will lead to more urine production and more frequent diuresis. Bradycardia and hypotension (b) are the opposite of what is apt to occur in the cardiovascular system. Methylxanthines do not induce platelet aggregation (they weakly inhibit it via a cAMP-dependent mechanism) nor ischemic stroke because of it. If anything, rises of blood pressure from excessive cardiac stimulation might (rarely) cause hemorrhagic stroke. Methylxanthines, of course, stimulate central ventilatory control mechanisms, tending to cause hyperpnea. (Caffeine has been used as a ventilatory stimulant, mainly in newborns.) That, in turn, would likely cause respiratory alkalosis, not acidosis (e). Apnea is not likely.

Autacoids and Anti-Inflammatory Pharmacology

Acetaminophen
Arachidonic acid metabolism
Ergot alkaloids
Histamine and its antagonists
Leukotriene synthesis inhibitors and receptor blockers
Mast cell "stabilizers"
Nonsteroidal anti-inflammatory drugs (eicosanoid synthesis inhibitors)
Prostaglandins and related eicosanoids
Purine metabolism, hyperuricemia, gout
Serotonin agonists and antagonists

Questions

311. Febuxostat was recently approved for use by the FDA. It is the first new drug in its class in four decades. It is indicated for managing hyperuricemia, including that which is drug-induced, but is not indicated for administration during an acute gout attack. Its basic mechanism of action is inhibition of purine degradation at the formation of hypoxanthine (HX), preventing further metabolism of HX to xanthine and uric acid. It should not be administered to patients receiving purine antimetabolites (eg, mercaptopurine, thioguanine, for certain cancers) because the metabolic inactivation of those drugs will be inhibited and toxicity may occur. Based on the description given, what drug is most similar to febuxostat?

a. Allopurinol
b. Aspirin
c. Colchicine
d. Indomethacin
e. Probenecid

312. A patient receives a drug that inhibits the lipoxygenase pathway of arachidonic acid metabolism. What naturally occurring metabolite(s) will be produced in lesser amounts in response to this drug?

a. Leukotrienes
b. Prostacyclin (PGI_2)
c. Prostaglandins
d. Thromboxanes
e. Uric acid

313. A patient has mild cutaneous and systemic manifestations of an allergic response. Before you prescribe a short course of diphenhydramine for symptom relief, you should realize that this drug has one mechanism of action resembling, causes many side effects similar to, and shares many contraindications with, an "autonomic" drug with which you should be very familiar. What is that drug?

a. Atropine
b. Bethanechol
c. Norepinephrine
d. Phentolamine
e. Physostigmine
f. Propranolol

314. A patient presents with a history of frequent and severe migraine headaches. When we give one of the more commonly used drugs for abortive therapy, sumatriptan, upon which of the following "local control substances" is it mainly acting?

a. Histamine
b. $PGF_{2\alpha}$
c. Prostacyclin
d. Serotonin
e. Thromboxane A_2 (TXA_2)

315. A male patient with severe arthritis will be placed on long-term therapy with indomethacin. We recognize the risk of NSAID-induced gastrointestinal ulceration, and want to prescribe another drug for ulcer prophylaxis. Which drug would you most likely choose as an add-on to the indomethacin?

a. Celecoxib
b. Cimetidine
c. Diclofenac
d. Diphenhydramine
e. Misoprostol

316. Aspirin causes significant bronchoconstriction and bronchospasm in a patient who was subsequently identified as being "aspirin-sensitive." Which mechanism summarizes best why or how aspirin provoked the respiratory problems in this patient?

a. Drug-mediated hypersensitivity of H_1 receptors on airway smooth muscles
b. Drug-mediated hypersensitivity of muscarinic receptors on airway smooth muscles
c. Enhanced formation of antibodies directed against the salicylate on airway mast cells
d. Inhibited synthesis of endogenous prostaglandins that have bronchodilator activity
e. Reduced (blocked) epinephrine binding to β_2-adrenergic receptors on airway smooth-muscle cells

317. A child takes what comes close to being a lethal dose of acetaminophen. What is the most likely pathology, that ultimately can lead to death, involved in this drug overdose?

a. Acute nephropathy
b. AV conduction disturbances, heart block
c. Liver failure
d. Status asthmaticus
e. Status epilepticus

318. A patient with asymptomatic hyperuricemia is started on probenecid. In a couple of days he develops acute gout. What is the mechanism by which probenecid triggered this acute gouty arthritic episode?

a. Accelerated synthesis of uric acid by the probenecid
b. Coprecipitation of probenecid and urate in the joints
c. Idiosyncratic response
d. Probenecid-induced systemic acidosis, favoring uric acid crystallization
e. Reduced renal excretion of uric acid

319. Epidemiologic data published in the early 1980s found a probable relationship between aspirin and a serious adverse response when the drug was administered to children with influenza, chickenpox, and other viral illnesses. Although no causal relationship between aspirin, viral illness, and this adverse effect was proven, you still caution the parents or caregivers of children to avoid giving any aspirin or aspirin-containing product when there is even a remote possibility that a child's illness might involve a virus. Avoidance of aspirin is necessary to avoid which specific adverse response?

a. Asthma
b. Cardiomyopathy
c. Renal failure
d. Reye syndrome
e. Thrombocytopenia and related bleeding disorders

320. Such drugs as methotrexate, hydroxychloroquine, or penicillamine are often turned to for managing rheumatoid arthritis that is not controlled adequately with "traditional" NSAIDs (eg, aspirin, ibuprofen, or indomethacin). Which statement most accurately summarizes how these drugs differ from a typical NSAID?

a. Activate the immune system to neutralize inflammatory mediators
b. Are primary therapies for gouty arthritis
c. Are remarkably free from serious toxicities
d. Provide much quicker relief of arthritis signs, symptoms
e. Slow, stop, possibly reverse joint pathology in rheumatoid arthritis

321. For quite a while the "coxibs" (selective COX-2 inhibitors) were prescribed in preference to nonselective COX inhibitors for managing such conditions as rheumatoid arthritis. Now we have basically one drug in this class, celecoxib. Which statement best describes an action or property of this COX-2 inhibitor?

a. Associated with a lower risk of gastric or duodenal ulceration
b. Cures arthritis, rather than just give symptom relief
c. Effectively inhibits uric acid synthesis
d. Has a lower risk of adverse or fatal cardiac events
e. Has significantly faster onset of action

322. Glucocorticoids are widely used for a host of inflammatory reactions and the diseases they cause. In terms of inflammatory responses and underlying metabolic reactions, which enzyme or process is the main target of these drugs when they are given at pharmacologic (supraphysiologic) doses?

a. Cyclooxygenases (COX-1 and -2)
b. Histidine decarboxylase
c. 5′-Lipoxygenase
d. Phospholipase A_2
e. Xanthine oxidase

323. Bradykinin plays important roles in local responses to tissue damage and a variety of inflammatory processes. It also has vasodilator activity. Which statement is correct about this endogenous peptide?

a. Captopril inhibits its metabolic inactivation
b. Drugs that are metabolized to, or generate, nitric oxide counteract bradykinin's vascular effects
c. Increased blood pressure is the predominant cardiovascular response
d. Newer histamine H_1 blockers (eg, fexofenadine; "second-generation" antihistamine) also competitively block bradykinin receptors
e. The main renal responses to endogenous bradykinin are arteriolar constriction and reduced glomerular filtration rate (GFR)

324. A newborn has oxygenation and hemodynamic problems because of a patent ductus arteriosus. Which drug usually would be administered in an attempt to close the lesion?

a. Cimetidine
b. Diphenhydramine
c. Indomethacin
d. Misoprostol
e. Prostaglandin E_1 (PGE_1; alprostadil)

325. A 29-year-old woman develops frequent, debilitating migraine headaches. Sumatriptan is prescribed for abortive therapy. Not long after taking the drug she is rushed to the hospital. Her vital signs are unstable, and she has muscle rigidity, myoclonus, generalized CNS irritability and altered consciousness, and shivering. You learn that for several months she had been taking another drug with which the triptan interacted. Which of the following add-on drugs most likely caused these acute and serious problems?

a. Acetaminophen
b. Codeine
c. Diazepam
d. Fluoxetine
e. Phenytoin

326. A patient suffers badly from a variety of upper respiratory responses during "hay fever" (seasonal allergy) seasons, and their asthma is provoked. We prescribe orally inhaled nedocromil for prophylaxis. What is the main mechanism by which nedocromil causes its desired effects?

a. Competitively blocks histamine H_1 receptors, thereby blocking bronchoconstriction
b. Decongests mucous membranes via a local vasoconstrictor action
c. Directly binds antigens, preventing them from interacting with mast cell antibodies
d. Inhibits mediator release from immunologically sensitized mast cells
e. Inhibits synthesis of histamine and leukotrienes

327. A patient has been taking doses of aspirin that are too high for several weeks. Low-grade aspirin toxicity (salicylism) develops. What sign or symptom would be consistent with salicylism and the high salicylate levels that caused it (assume the patient is taking no other drugs)?

a. Constipation
b. Cough
c. Hypertension
d. Myopia
e. Tinnitus

328. Aspirin generally should be avoided as an anti-inflammatory, analgesic, or antipyretic drug by patients with hyperuricemia or gout. That is because it counteracts the effects of one important drug the hyperuricemic patient may be taking. Which drug has its desired uric acid-related effects reduced or eliminated by this prototypic NSAID?

a. Acetaminophen
b. Allopurinol
c. Colchicine
d. Indomethacin
e. Probenecid

329. Misoprostol, an analog of PGE_1, is sometimes used adjunctively to stimulate gastric mucus production and help reduce the incidence of gastric ulcers associated with long-term or high-dose NSAID therapy for arthritis. What is the other main use for this drug?

a. Closure of a patent ductus arteriosus in newborns
b. Contraception in women who should not receive estrogens or progestins
c. Induction of abortion in conjunction with mifepristone (RU486)
d. Prophylaxis of asthma in lieu of a corticosteroid
e. Suppression of uterine contractility in women with premature labor

330. A patient who was transported by ambulance to the emergency department took a potentially lethal overdose of aspirin. What drug would be a helpful, if not life-saving, adjunct to manage this severe aspirin poisoning?

a. Acetaminophen
b. Amphetamines (eg, dextroamphetamine)
c. *N*-Acetylcysteine
d. Phenobarbital
e. Sodium bicarbonate

331. We look at data that summarize the actions of two prototypic histamine receptor blockers: diphenhydramine as the exemplar of the older antihistamines (competitive histamine receptor antagonists); and fexofenadine as a representative agent of the "second-generation" antihistamines. Which statement correctly describes, compares, or contrasts these drugs or the pharmacologic groups to which they belong?

a. Diphenhydramine and other drugs in its class (ethanolamines) tend to cause drowsiness more often than fexofenadine and related second-generation antihistamines
b. Diphenhydramine is preferred for patients with prostate hypertrophy or angle-closure glaucoma, whereas fexofenadine and related drugs are contraindicated
c. Diphenhydramine overdoses tend to cause bradycardia, whereas fexofenadine overdoses tend to cause significant increases of heart rate
d. Fexofenadine and related second-generation histamine antagonists have intrinsic bronchodilator activity which makes them suitable as primary/sole therapy for people with asthma
e. Fexofenadine and drugs in its class have better efficacy in terms of suppressing histamine-mediated gastric acid secretion

332. A patient has been taking one of the drugs listed below for about 4 months and is experiencing the desired therapeutic effects from it. The physician now prescribes indomethacin to treat a particularly severe flare-up of rheumatoid arthritis. Within a matter of days the therapeutic effects of the first drug wane dramatically, its actions antagonized by the indomethacin. Which drug was affected by the indomethacin?

a. Allopurinol, given for prophylaxis of hyperuricemia
b. Captopril, given for essential hypertension
c. Fexofenadine, given for managing seasonal allergy signs and symptoms
d. Sumatriptan, given for abortive therapy of migraine headaches
e. Warfarin, given for prophylaxis of venous thrombosis

333. A patient takes an acute, massive overdose of aspirin that, without proper intervention, will probably be fatal. What would you expect to occur in the advanced (late) stages of aspirin (salicylate) poisoning?

a. Hypothermia
b. Metabolic alkalosis
c. Respiratory alkalosis
d. Respiratory plus metabolic acidosis
e. Ventilatory stimulation

334. A patient presents in the emergency department with an overdose of a drug. The physician knows what the drug is, and so orders appropriate "symptomatic and supportive care," plus multiple doses of *N*-acetylcysteine. Upon which drug did the patient overdose?

a. Acetaminophen
b. Aspirin
c. Colchicine
d. Diphenhydramine
e. Loratadine
f. Methotrexate

335. A patient has acute gout. The physician initially thinks about prescribing just one or two oral doses of colchicine, 12 hours apart, but then decides otherwise. What is the main and most common reason for avoiding colchicine, even with a very short oral course, and prescribing another drug for the acute gout instead?

a. Bone marrow suppression.
b. Bronchospasm.
c. GI distress that is almost as bad as the acute gout discomfort.
d. Hepatotoxicity.
e. One or two oral doses seldom relieve gout pain.
f. Refractoriness/tolerance with just a dose or two.

336. A patient with hyperuricemia is placed on an "antigout" drug. Before starting the drug you measure the total uric acid (amount, not concentration) in a 24-hour urine sample and then do the same several weeks after continued drug therapy at therapeutic doses. The posttreatment sample shows a significant reduction in urate content. There were no new pathologies developing during therapy, and the patient's daily purine intake did not change at all. What drug most likely accounted for these findings?

a. Acetaminophen
b. Allopurinol
c. Colchicine
d. Indomethacin
e. Probenecid

337. We administer sodium bicarbonate to a patient who has severe hyperuricemia and is at great risk of developing urate stones in his urinary tract. What is the basis for using the bicarbonate?

a. Causes an antidiuretic effect, reduces urate content of the urine
b. Causes metabolic alkalosis that inhibits catalytic activity of xanthine oxidase
c. Counteracts metabolic acidosis that is characteristic of severe hyperuricemia
d. Lowers urate elimination by lowering GFR
e. Reduces solubility of urate in the urine

338. A patient with annoying hay fever (seasonal allergy) symptoms (mainly rhinorrhea) goes to the store, intent on purchasing an oral medication to make them more comfortable. They see the prices for loratadine and related second-generation antihistamines and are shocked about how high they are. Nearby on the shelf they see store-brand allergy relief pills that are much less expensive, the cheapest ones having diphenhydramine as the sole active ingredient. If they were to take full therapeutic doses of the diphenhydramine, based on label directions, which effects or side effects are they most likely to experience as an additional price to be paid for their allergy relief?

a. Bradycardia
b. Diarrhea
c. Drowsiness, somnolence
d. "Heartburn" from increased gastric acid secretion
e. Urinary frequency

339. Your patient has rheumatoid arthritis that has been refractory to diclofenac, ibuprofen, indomethacin, and sulindac. In addition, she has experienced significant GI distress, and several GI bleeds, following attempts to get better anti-inflammatory effects by raising the doses. We start her on therapy with etanercept. What is the most likely mechanism by which etanercept suppresses the signs, symptoms, or underlying pathophysiology of rheumatoid arthritis?

a. Inhibits eicosanoid synthesis by inhibiting phospholipase A_2
b. Inhibits leukocyte migration by blocking microtubular formation
c. Neutralizes circulating tumor necrosis factor (TNF-α)
d. Selectively and effectively inhibits COX-2
e. Stimulates collagen and mucopolysaccharide synthesis in the joints

Autacoid and Anti-Inflammatory Pharmacology

Answers

311. The answer is a. *(Brunton, pp 708-709, 1016, 1414. Katzung, pp 638-639.)* The description of febuxostat in the question—actions, uses, drug interactions and more—applies directly to allopurinol, which is classified as a xanthine oxidase inhibitor and has been available for decades. As you should recall, allopurinol (and now febuxostat) is indicated for managing hyperuricemia, whether idiopathic, associated with certain diseases (including many malignancies), or drug-induced (eg, by thiazide or loop diuretics, and cancer chemotherapeutic agents). Aspirin (b) has no effects on purine metabolism in general or specifically on xanthine oxidase. At all but very high dosages it can raise plasma uric acid (and xanthine) levels by inhibiting tubular secretion of uric acid, and is generally contraindicated for patients with hyperuricemia or gout. Colchicine (b) is an anti-inflammatory drug used for acute gout, or for prophylaxis, but it has no effect on endogenous purine metabolism or the metabolism of purine antimetabolites such as mercaptopurine. Indomethacin (d) is an NSAID that has many indications, including treating inflammation secondary to gout, but once again it shares none of the other properties noted in the question. Probenecid (e) can be considered the prototype uricosuric drug. It is indicated for prophylaxis, but not for treatment, of gout. Therapeutic blood levels of probenecid lower plasma uric acid levels by blocking tubular reabsorption of urate.

312. The answer is a. *(Brunton, pp 655-657. Katzung, pp 313-316, 625f.)* The arachidonic acid (AA) "cascade" begins with AA synthesis from membrane phospholipids by phospholipase A_2. Once arachidonic acid is formed, the metabolic pathways diverge into the lipoxygenase pathway (that forms cysteinyl leukotrienes [LTs]) and the cyclooxygenase pathways that synthesize prostaglandins, prostacyclin, thromboxane A_2, and several other eicosanoids. One important intermediate early on in the lipoxygenase pathway is LTA_4.

From that we get LTB_4, which mainly regulates chemotaxis (cytokine activity) and activates phagocytosis in white blood cells. Also derived from LTB_4 are, sequentially, LTC_4, LTD_4, and LTE_4 (cysteinyl leukotrienes, historically and collectively called SRS-A, for slow-reacting substance of anaphylaxis), which cause mainly bronchoconstriction. Leukotriene synthesis can be inhibited by zileuton (no longer used clinically), a 5′-lipoxygenase inhibitor. The leukotriene receptors can be blocked by montelukast and zafirlukast, which are used prophylactically (control meds) to suppress airway inflammation and bronchoconstriction in asthma. They should not be used in lieu of corticosteroids (oral or inhaled) when control of airway inflammation is necessary.

Prostaglandins (c), including prostacyclin (b), and thromboxane A_2 (d) are synthesized via the cyclooxygenase pathways. Uric acid (e) is synthesized by what is generally referred to as the ATP degradation pathway, in which the final two steps in the pathway (conversion of hypoxanthine to xanthine, and conversion of xanthine to uric acid) are catalyzed by xanthine oxidase.

313. The answer is a. *(Brunton, pp 637-640, 642, 1004. Katzung, pp 275-279.)* Diphenhydramine, an older or "first-generation" antihistamine, is a competitive antagonist of histamine's effects on H_1 receptors, and also strongly blocks muscarinic cholinergic receptors. Other older H_1 blockers (but none of the second-generation H_1 blockers, such as fexofenadine) possess this atropine-like effect, often to a lesser degree than diphenhydramine. (If you wished to argue that because diphenhydramine was more like scopolamine, because it causes not only anticholinergic effects but also a considerable degree of sedation, you would be correct.) Thus, common side effects related to antimuscarinic activity include dry mouth, photophobia, and cycloplegia (paralysis of accommodation). Key contraindications include prostatic hypertrophy, bowel or bladder obstruction or hypomotility, tachycardia, and narrow-angle (angle-closure) glaucoma.

To refresh your memory about the other drugs listed, bethanechol (b) is a muscarinic agonist; norepinephrine (c) is an effective agonist for β_1- and α-adrenergic receptors; phentolamine (d) is a nonselective α-blocker; physostigmine (e) is an acetylcholinesterase inhibitor; and propranolol (f) is, of course, the prototypic nonselective β-adrenergic blocker.

314. The answer is d. *(Brunton, pp 300t, 305-308, 334. Katzung, pp 282-285.)* Acute migraine therapy often involves giving a drug that mimics the effects of endogenous serotonin (5-hydroxytryptamine), thereby reversing the cerebrovasodilation that contributes significantly to migraine signs and symptoms. A good example is sumatriptan (member of a small group of drugs called triptans). These are $5\text{-HT}_{1B/2D}$ receptor agonists. Histamine (a), and to a lesser extent prostacyclin (PGI_2, answer c), are vasodilators, too, but they don't seem to have appreciable roles in migraine, nor are they targets of antimigraine drug activity. Activation of β_2-adrenergic receptors in the cerebral vasculature also leads to vasodilation and migraine symptoms. β-Adrenergic blockers (particularly propranolol) are useful for some migraineurs, but only for prophylaxis, not for abortive therapy.

315. The answer is e. *(Brunton, pp 665, 973, 979. Katzung, pp 315, 325, 327, 1076.)* Misoprostol is a long-acting synthetic analog of PGE_1, and its only use (outside of reproductive medicine) is prophylaxis of NSAID-induced gastric ulcers. Its main effects are suppression of gastric acid secretion (modest); and, more importantly, enhanced gastric mucus production (a so-called mucotropic or cytoprotective effect). The need for the drug arises, of course, because such drugs as indomethacin (and most other COX-nonselective inhibitors) inhibit PGE_1 synthesis (as well as that of other prostaglandins, prostacyclin, and thromboxane A_2).

Although cimetidine (b) might help reduce gastric acid secretion (via H_2 blockade) and diphenhydramine (c) may too (via antimuscarinic effects), their antisecretory effects (with respect to gastric acid) are weak, and they don't increase formation of the stomach's protective mucus.

Celecoxib (a), a COX-2 selective NSAID, is associated with a lower risk or incidence of GI ulcers than more traditional COX-1/-2 NSAIDs, including indomethacin (or diclofenac, ibuprofen, many others). However, adding a COX-2 inhibitor would be irrational in terms of reducing ulcer risk. Diclofenac (c) is an NSAID that, when used long-term (eg, as an alternative to indomethacin or any of the other reasonable options), may cause ulcers just as indomethacin may. A fixed-dose combination product containing diclofenac and misoprostol is available, the latter drug being used to reduce the risk of ulcers caused by the former.

316. The answer is d. *(Brunton, pp 664, 683, 685, 689-690. Katzung, pp 624-625.)* Inhibited synthesis of prostaglandins that are bronchodilators (mainly PGE_2) is thought to be responsible for severe or fatal responses to aspirin in some asthmatics. Note that aspirin inhibits the synthesis of $PGF_{2\alpha}$

and of TXA_2, both of which are bronchoconstrictors. As a result, one would predict reduced bronchoconstriction with aspirin. However, in those patients with aspirin-sensitive asthma (indeed, in many asthmatics overall), the adverse effects arising from inhibited PGE_2 synthesis tend to predominate, and so aspirin and other efficacious NSAIDs are generally contraindicated.

Aspirin does not cause increased responsiveness of airway smooth muscle cells to the bronchoconstrictor effects of histamine (a) or muscarinic agonists (b). It does not elicit antibody formation (c) or have any effect on the interaction between β_2 agonists and their cellular receptors (e).

317. The answer is c. *(Brunton, pp 83, 694, 1741. Katzung, pp 635-636, 1020.)* The primary cause of death from acetaminophen overdoses is hepatic necrosis. Indeed, acetaminophen is the most common cause of liver failure in the United States. And contrary to what might seem intuitive, most of those cases are not due to acute overdoses taken as part of a suicide attempt. Rather, they are inadvertent overdoses, often taken over months or years, that for a time may be asymptomatic but eventually lead to cumulative liver damage and clinical manifestations of hepatic failure. While many of those cases involve exceeding recommended dosages for a period of time, some data strongly suggest that even limiting individual doses to what is recommended on the product label may cause harm. There are many likely factors that contribute to the problem, but two are worth mentioning. First, the drug is available OTC, and as applies to virtually all OTC drugs there is the perception that such medications are invariably safe. The other main reason—which applies to acetaminophen more so than to other OTC drugs—is its presence as the sole agent or major ingredient in a host of products, several of which may be taken at the same time, and the consumer simply doesn't realize that he or she is taking multiple doses of the same active and potentially toxic medicine.

Acetaminophen's main toxic metabolite is *N*-acetyl-benzoqinoneimine (don't memorize that chemical name!). It reacts with sulfhydryl groups that are constituents of key macromolecules and metabolic cofactors (eg, glutathione) in the liver. If acetaminophen doses are low, glutathione conjugates the metabolite. With toxic doses, however, glutathione is depleted and other –SH groups on hepatocyte proteins are attacked and irreversibly altered. Concomitant with overall hepatic damage we find, eventually, profound hypoglycemia (as the liver's stores of glycogen are depleted) and coagulopathies (as hepatic clotting factor synthesis stops and the patient begins bleeding spontaneously).

Nephropathy (a) is not a primary or important consequence of acetaminophen toxicity. If AV conduction disturbances, heart block, or other cardiac electrophysiologic anomalies (b) occur, they are secondary to hepatic dysfunction. Status asthmaticus (d) and acute seizures (e) are not likely or direct consequences of acetaminophen poisoning.

Note: Since I don't think you'll find this information in a textbook you are likely to be using, permit me to summarize the main events or "stages" (they're arbitrary) of what otherwise would be a lethal dose of acetaminophen.

APPROXIMATE (AND ARBITRARY) "STAGES" OF ULTIMATELY FATAL ACETAMINOPHEN POISONING

Time After Acute Ingestion	Major Events, Signs, Symptoms	Comments
First 24 h or so	Nausea, vomiting, cramping, possibly severe.	If a serious or lethal overdose is even suspected, this is the time to begin therapy with the antidote, *N*-acetylcysteine.
End of first 24-h period	Subjective relief; lessening of initial signs and symptoms.	The apparent and sometimes significant "relief" can mislead patient or physician into thinking everything is OK, the patient did not ingest a toxic (let alone lethal) dose. This is what makes acetaminophen poisoning so insidious.
24-48 h	Initial symptoms return; abdominal distress becomes more diffuse and severe; coagulopathies, falls of blood glucose, apparent.	Hepatotoxic metabolite continues to be formed; liver damaged by rising levels of liver enzymes (AST, ALT, etc). Hepatic coagulation factor synthesis, activation, impaired. Liver glycogen becomes depleted. Hepatotoxicity often irreversible by now, and *N*-acetylcysteine administration at this time probably too late.
3rd-5th day	Appearance of jaundice, oliguria, hematuria, hemorrhage, hypoglycemic coma, death.	

A typical lethal dose for an otherwise-healthy child, taken all at once, is around 12 g. For otherwise healthy adults it is around 25 g. Various illnesses and consuming other drugs (including aspirin) can dramatically lower the dose sufficient to cause serious or lethal toxicity. A "standard strength" acetaminophen tablet contains 300 mg. "Extra strength" tablets can contain up to 1 g—and these probably will be pulled from the market (perhaps by the time you read this) by the FDA because of renewed concerns over liver damage.

318. The answer is e. *(Brunton, pp 710-711. Katzung, pp 637-638.)* It has been said that the initial phase of uricosuric therapy is the most worrisome. Probenecid is a uricosuric drug (one that increases renal elimination of uric acid) but that effect is highly dose- (blood concentration) dependent. Desired uricosuric actions depend on having therapeutic probenecid blood levels that are sufficient to inhibit active tubular reabsorption of urate. However, at subtherapeutic blood levels the main effect is inhibition of tubular secretion of urate which reduces net urate excretion and raises plasma urate levels (sometimes to the point of causing clinical gout). It is only once probenecid levels are therapeutic that the desired effects to inhibit tubular urate reabsorption (ie, increase excretion) predominate. Thus, and intuitively, once a patient starts probenecid therapy, drug levels must pass through that stage in which urate excretion will actually go down, plasma urate levels up. Similar problems can occur if, for example, the patient frequently skips doses in order to "stretch their pills" for a longer time, eg, to reduce the expense of more frequent prescription refills. In this case, the longer interval between doses may allow trough blood concentrations of the drug to fall to the point where more urate is retained (from inhibited tubular secretion) than is excreted.

Some texts suggest using a short course of colchicine or another (nonaspirin) NSAID that is indicated for gout when probenecid therapy is started. That is for prophylaxis of acute gout that might occur. Although this may be acceptable, other guidelines are perhaps more important: (1) do not administer a uricosuric during a gout attack; (2) if the patient has had a gout attack recently, suppress the inflammation for 2 to 3 months with a suitable anti-inflammatory and consider starting a uricosuric only after that symptom-free interval; and (3) do not use uricosurics for patients with "severe hyperuricemia" and/or poor renal function. Giving them to such a patient is associated with a great risk of potentially severe renal tubular damage as the uricosuric shifts large amounts of uric acid from the blood (the relatively large blood volume keeps urate relatively "dilute") into a small volume of normally acidic urine, which concentrates urate and lowers its solubility via pH-dependent mechanisms.

319. The answer is d. *(Brunton, pp 682, 687.)* Before the warning was issued, well over 500 children with any viral illness (influenza, chickenpox, for example) and who received aspirin, (even in usual recommended pediatric doses at the time) developed Reye syndrome. It is characterized by encephalopathy and fatty liver degeneration. The mortality rate ranged from about 20% to 30%, and many more patients developed permanent and serious CNS and/or liver dysfunction. Nowadays there are fewer than five cases of Reye syndrome per year as a result of the aspirin/viral illness "interaction." The reason? We've basically stopped administering aspirin to children who have a virus or even a possibility of it. (Note: The age range for which aspirin should not be administered in the presence of viral illness is debatable; some suggest the risk of Reye syndrome lessens dramatically by the age of 12 years, but many experts suggest that the risk may persist up to 18-20 years of age.)

Asthma (a) is the most common cause of hospitalizations in children, and many patients have their asthma provoked or worsened by aspirin or other NSAIDs. However, the potential asthma-NSAID problems are unrelated to the presence or absence of viral illnesses. There is no evidence of a linkage between aspirin and cardiomyopathies (b). Long-term, high-dose administration of NSAIDs (other than aspirin) may cause renal dysfunction or failure (c). Here, too, there is no linkage with viral illness, and the kidney problems are not at all limited to the pediatric population. Aspirin obviously has antiplatelet-aggregatory effects, but whether the patient is a child or older, thrombocytopenia (e) is not a concern.

320. The answer is e. *(Brunton, pp 690, 706, 1336. Katzung, pp 631-632, 944-946, 975, 1090-1091.)* Methotrexate, gold salts, and penicillamine are members of a diverse group of drugs called DMARDs (disease-modifying antirheumatic drugs) or SAARDs (slow-acting antirheumatic drugs). The former term derives from the ability of these drugs to slow, stop, or in some cases reverse joint damage associated with rheumatoid arthritis (RA). They do more than merely mask or relieve RA symptoms, which is mainly what the traditional NSAIDs do. The second acronym derives from the fact that it may take a month (or a couple more) for meaningful symptom relief to develop; they are not at all quick-acting drugs. Their actions probably are due to suppression of immune responses that contribute to the etiology of RA.

Their toxicities can be serious, which is one reason why, until not long ago, these agents were considered third-line or even last resort treatments for refractory rheumatoid disease. (Methotrexate is now being used much earlier, and safely, for RA, now that we know better how to use it and monitor for serious toxicities; see the chapter, "Cancer Chemotherapy and Immunosuppressants.") Most of these drugs can cause serious blood dyscrasias; in addition, penicillamine can cause renal and pulmonary toxicity; hydroxychloroquine is associated with vision impairments/retinopathy.

321. The answer is a. *(Brunton, pp 657-658, 671, 681, 684, 702-705. Katzung, pp 313-315, 626.)* Celecoxib, by virtue of selective COX-2 inhibition, does not interfere as much with synthesis of PGE_2, which normally suppresses a component of gastric acid secretion and stimulates gastric mucus production. Overall, then, the risks of gastric and duodenal ulcers are reduced. The selectivity also means that COX-2 inhibitors do not interfere with the production of other eicosanoids, such as TXA_2. That is both good and bad, clinically. On the good side, this means that COX-2 inhibitors don't cause antiplatelet effects and increase the risk of excessive or spontaneous bleeding. On the other hand, this lack of effect renders them unsuitable for causing desired antiplatelet-aggregatory effects, as might be wanted when we administer aspirin. This may explain the finding that some COX-2 inhibitors have been associated with (cause?) a higher risk of sudden cardiac death (d) in vulnerable patients, and why some have been pulled off the market (and are subjects of considerable litigation).

COX-2 inhibitors, like the nonselective alternatives, aren't cures for arthritis (b); they alleviate signs and symptoms but seem to have no demonstrable impact on the underlying pathophysiology. They have no effect on uric acid metabolism (c) or excretion. Their onsets of action are clearly not faster (e) than those of a typical NSAID.

322. The answer is d. *(Brunton, pp 721-722, 1407, 1594-1596, 1599-1600. Katzung, pp 313-316, 321, 635-636.)* Anti-inflammatory doses of glucocorticosteroids inhibit phospholipase A_2 activity. In doing so, they inhibit arachidonic acid synthesis and, therefore, synthesis of all subsequent products of the cyclooxygenase and lipoxygenase pathways, both of which originate with arachidonic acid. This action of glucocorticoids is indirect because their initial or direct effect is induced synthesis of annexins (previously called lipocortins), which are the moieties that directly inhibit PLA_2 activity. Glucocorticoids have no intrinsic or direct inhibitory effects on later steps in AA metabolism, that is, no direct effects on cyclooxygenase or lipoxygenase activity.

Cyclooxygenases (a) are inhibited by NSAIDs such as aspirin (nonselective COX-1 and -2 inhibitors) or the "coxibs" (celecoxib), which relatively selectively inhibit COX-2. We have no clinically useful inhibitors of histamine synthesis (which involves histidine decarboxylase activity; b). As noted elsewhere, zileuton inhibits 5′-lipoxygenase (c) and the subsequent formation of leukotrienes. Allopurinol inhibits the synthesis of xanthine and uric acid by inhibiting xanthine oxidase (e).

323. The answer is a. *(Brunton, pp 646, 648-649, 800-801. Katzung, pp 295-296.)* Bradykinin is metabolized to biologically inactive peptides by an enzyme that has three names: angiotensin-converting enzyme (ACE; recall that the prototype ACE inhibitor is captopril), bradykininase, and kininase II. The name that is used depends on the substrate. When the substrate is angiotensin I, the enzyme is called ACE. When the substrate is bradykinin we call it either bradykininase or, less often, kininase II.

Bradykinin, whether injected experimentally or derived from endogenous sources (kininogens cleaved by specific proteases called kallikreins), exerts significant vasodilator effects that can lower systolic and diastolic blood pressures. Although this may not be an important pressure-regulating mechanism in normotensive individuals, it probably is in many (most?) patients with essential hypertension. Clearly, bradykinin does not increase blood pressure (c) or constrict the renal vasculature (e).

Recall that ACE inhibitors lower blood pressure in many hypertensive patients. One mechanism involves "preserving" bradykinin by inhibiting its enzymatic inactivation. Bradykinin also causes prerenal arteriolar vasodilation and increases GFR, leading to diuretic effects.

The peptide's vascular effects are mediated by endothelial cell–derived nitric oxide, and they are enhanced (not counteracted; b) by other drugs that cause vasodilation by a nitric oxide–related mechanism.

Bradykinin receptor blockers prevent the peptide's vasodilator effects. However, no currently approved drugs, including the so-called second-generation antihistamines such as fexofenadine (d), exert that effect.

324. The answer is c. *(Brunton, p 695. Katzung, p 627.)* The ductus arteriosus in a neonate may remain patent largely because of the vasodilator effects of endogenous PGE_1, formed via the cyclooxygenase pathway. When the goal is to close a patent ductus after birth we generally use the very efficacious prostaglandin synthesis (COX-1/-2) inhibitor, indomethacin. (Conversely, there are times when surgical procedures are required on a congenitally anomalous heart in newborns, and we want to keep the ductus open until surgery. In that case, alprostadil [PGE_1, answer e] may be administered.)

Misoprostol (d) is a prostaglandin analog. Giving it to a newborn with a patent ductus is likely to keep the lesion open, not close it. None of the H_2 blockers (eg, cimetidine, a) nor H_1 blockers (diphenhydramine, b, and many others) have any important effects on prostaglandin synthesis, nor are they used either to close a patent ductus arteriosus or to keep it open for subsequent surgery.

325. The answer is d. *(Brunton, pp 305-308, 334, 450. Katzung, pp 282-284, 526, 1021.)* This patient has what is almost certainly the serotonin syndrome. The triptan "adds" serotonin to serotoninergic synapse, and serotonin's neuronal reuptake will be blocked by fluoxetine (or sertraline, others), which is classified as a selective serotonin reuptake inhibitor (SSRI) antidepressant. When sumatriptan (or other triptans used for migraine) is added, rapid accumulation of serotonin and/or the triptan in brain synapses can occur.

The other drugs listed (acetaminophen, a; codeine, b; diazepam, c; and phenytoin, e) are not likely to interact with serotoninergic drugs.

326. The answer is d. *(Brunton, pp 726-727. Katzung, pp 348-349.)* The precise mechanism by which nedocromil or the related drug cromolyn works is not known, but the most likely explanation is "stabilization" of immunologically sensitized mast cells. This may involve calcium channel blockade: Calcium entry into mast cells is a critical step in their immunologically mediated activation. There is no direct or indirect interaction with antigens (c) or mast cell antibodies, but the drug does suppress the release of preformed mast cell mediators. Nedocromil and cromolyn have no histamine receptor-blocking activity (a), nor vasoconstrictor or other decongestant effects (b). They do not inhibit synthesis of histamine, leukotrienes, or other vasodepressor, bronchoconstrictor, or inflammatory mediators in mast cells or elsewhere.

327. The answer is e. *(Brunton, p 691. Katzung, pp 624, 1021.)* Tinnitus, along with a feeling of dizziness or lightheadedness, GI upset (including nausea and some pain or other discomfort, and diarrhea more so than constipation), and such visual changes as blurred or diplopia (but not myopia, d), all are part of a low-grade aspirin "toxicity" syndrome called salicylism. It is not necessarily worrisome (provided the physician intentionally prescribed the drug at dosages likely to produce the syndrome), dangerous, or indicative of imminent and severe toxicity. Indeed, some patients experience one or more signs or symptoms of salicylism in response to high (antiarthritic) doses of aspirin.

Constipation (a) or hypertension (c) is not causally associated with salicylate administration, regardless of the dose. Cough (b) may occur, but that is only likely to occur in patients who have "aspirin-sensitive" asthma, and for those patients bronchoconstriction is a more likely response than cough.

328. The answer is e. *(Brunton, pp 673-693, 707. Katzung, pp 637-638, 1148t.)* Probenecid (and the related drug, sulfinpyrazone) are classified as uricosurics: A sufficiently high (therapeutic) doses they enhance the renal elimination of uric acid by inhibiting tubular reabsorption of filtered urate. Aspirin significantly impairs the uricosurics' actions.

Important note: Aspirin (given alone) has blood level–dependent effects on urate elimination by the kidneys. At "low doses," perhaps up to about 1 g/d, it selectively inhibits tubular secretion of urate and so can raise plasma urate levels. At doses much higher than that (including doses sometimes prescribed for arthritis other than gout), the predominant effect (and the net or overall effect) is uricosuria due to blockade of tubular reabsorption of urate (this effect is greater than the drug's inhibitory effect on tubular secretion of urate). Nonetheless, aspirin is not used as a uricosuric drug because the doses/blood levels needed to increase urate elimination are sufficiently high that they cause significant side effects (eg, salicylism; see Question 327) that don't arise with the traditional uriciosurics such as probenecid.

Acetaminophen (a) has no appreciable or clinically useful effects on uric acid elimination or synthesis. Allopurinol (b; and the new related drug febuxostat) inhibits uric acid synthesis, but its xanthine oxidase-inhibitory effects are not altered by aspirin. However, since allopurinol is used to lower plasma urate levels it is largely irrational to use aspirin at the same time. The same applies to colchicine (c) and indomethacin (d), both of which are used for in acute gout and neither of which has its main biochemical effects (suppression of inflammation) impaired by aspirin.

329. The answer is c. *(Brunton, pp 665, 973. Kaztung, pp 315, 325-327, 1029t, 1076.)* In addition to misoprostol's use as a cytoprotective/mucotropic drug for some patients taking NSAIDs, it is also used as an adjunct to mifepristone to induce therapeutic abortion. This capitalizes on the prostaglandin analog's strong uterine-stimulating effects (thus, answer e is incorrect). The drug is sometimes used to maintain patency of an open ductus arteriosus, not to close it (a). It is not a contraceptive in the typical sense, such as we would associate with estrogen-progestin oral contraceptives. Given misoprostol's drug's abortifacient effects, it is contraindicated for women who are pregnant or wish to become pregnant (b). Misoprostol has bronchodilator activity, but it is relatively weak and the drug is not suitable as a substitute for corticosteroids (d) or other typical asthma medications.

330. The answer is e. *(Brunton, pp 686-689, 691-692. Katzung, p 1021.)* Adjunctive use of sodium bicarbonate (IV) can be an important adjunct to managing severe salicylate poisoning for two main reasons: (1) it helps raise blood pH, which as stated earlier is profoundly reduced from metabolic plus respiratory acidosis; (2) it alkalinizes the urine, which (via a pH-dependent mechanism, *a la* Henderson-Hasselbach) converts more aspirin molecules into the ionized form in the renal tubules, thereby reducing tubular reabsorption of a substance we want to eliminate from the body as quickly as possible.

Acetaminophen (a), even though it is usually an effective antipyretic, is not good for managing fever of severe aspirin poisoning. It would add yet another drug that might complicate an already problematic clinical picture, and ordinary (and ordinarily safe) doses aren't likely to do much to lower temperature quickly or sufficiently. (Thus, we use physical means to lower body temperature.) *N*-Acetylcysteine (c), the antidote for acetaminophen poisoning, does nothing for salicylate poisoning. Amphetamines (b) might seem rational for managing ventilatory depression that characterizes late stages of severe aspirin poisoning. However, a more likely outcome of giving an amphetamine is simply to hasten the onset of seizures. Phenobarbital (d), or other CNS depressants, would aggravate an already bad state of CNS/ventilatory depression. (However, if seizures develop they must be managed—eg, with IV lorazepam and phenytoin, even though they cause CNS depression. Without them, the patient may quickly die from status epilepticus.)

Just as I provided a table (answer to Question 317) to summarize the general sequence of events in acetaminophen toxicity, I'll provide one here for aspirin overdoses. Again, the "stages" I present are arbitrary, but they should be helpful—knowing what is likely to come next as toxicity progresses helps you prepare for what you'll probably need to do next.

Note that the average lethal dose for an otherwise healthy child is around 5 to 8 g, taken all at once. For adults, it is around 10 to 30 g. "Usual strength" aspirin tablets—those used for aches, pains, mild inflammation, and fever—contain 325 mg of the drug. "Heart dose" aspirin tablets contain 81 mg. Higher doses may be prescribed for arthritis—several grams a day—and although these usually are not sufficient to cause death they are likely to cause side effects that often are disturbing enough that the physician will prescribe another antiarthritic drug instead of plain, cheap aspirin. Ulcers in the GI tract may also occur.

Final note: While treating aspirin poisoning may sound difficult, ask a physician or nurse who has had to deal with it many times. They are likely to tell you that it's a "piece of cake"—and more often successful—than dealing with acetaminophen poisoning.

APPROXIMATE (AND ARBITRARY) "STAGES" OF ASPIRIN (SALICYLATE) TOXICITY

"Phases" or "Stages"	Major Events, Signs, Symptoms	Comments
1 (Salicylism)	GI upset (pain, sometimes with nausea and vomiting); tinnitus; headache; dizziness, drowsiness, confusion; blurred vision; paresthesias. Hyperpnea leads to respiratory alkalosis.	These signs and symptoms caused by excessive aspirin (salicylate) blood levels constitute a syndrome called salicylism. May develop acutely or over time. May be worrisome (eg, if the aspirin doses were not recommended by a physician, eg, for arthritis) or not (salicylism occurs commonly in patients taking high doses that might be prescribed for arthritis). Respiratory alkalosis occurs because of medullary stimulating effects associated with these doses: the patient "blows-off" CO_2; impaired platelet aggregation (TXA_2 synthesis suppressed).

(Continued)

APPROXIMATE (AND ARBITRARY) "STAGES" OF ASPIRIN (SALICYLATE) TOXICITY (CONTINUED)

"Phases" or "Stages"	Major Events, Signs, Symptoms	Comments
2 (Compensated respiratory alkalosis)	Persistence of signs, symptoms of salicylism.	Kidneys compensate for respiratory alkalosis by increasing elimination of HCO_3 (and Na^+). Not serious at this point. Patients taking high doses of aspirin, such as those that might be prescribed for arthritis, can be in a rather perpetual stage of compensated respiratory alkalosis; antithrombotic effect persists but blood levels of salicylate may be sufficient to inhibit prostacyclin (PGI_2) synthesis, leading to platelet adhesion to endothelium, lessening of prostaglandin-mediated vasodilation.
3 (True salicylate poisoning; respiratory + metabolic acidosis)	Initial symptoms worsen; GI bleeding may occur; fluid and electrolyte imbalances from loss via GI tract (emesis, diarrhea), urine, skin ventilation becomes depressed; body temperature rises, diaphoresis more apparent in attempt to lower body temperature; blood electrolyte abnormalities develop; hematocrit rises.	Respiratory acidosis: high circulating salicylate levels now cause medullary depression. This leads to rise of arterial pCO_2 and fall of blood pH. Metabolic acidosis: high salicylate levels in blood lower pH; mitochondrial oxidative phosphorylation uncoupled, little/no ATP formed, abundant metabolic heat generated causes fever, then seizures. Suppressed oxidative ATP synthesis leads to increased glycolysis: lactic acid accumulates causing further and profound lowering of blood pH.

APPROXIMATE (AND ARBITRARY) "STAGES" OF ASPIRIN (SALICYLATE) TOXICITY (CONTINUED)		
"Phases" or "Stages"	Major Events, Signs, Symptoms	Comments
4 (Lethality)	Body temperature >104°F not uncommon; seizures; dehydration, shock from fluid/electrolyte loss from GI tract, skin; bleeding; ventilatory, circulatory collapse, coma, death.	No antidote, so symptomatic/supportive care required, including: ventilatory, cardiovascular support; correction of clotting abnormalities; transfusions (whole blood, platelets, etc; note that as long as some salicylate remains in bloodstream, antiplatelet effects will still impair function of transfused platelets); correction of fluids and electrolytes with IV solutions of proper composition accompanied by osmotic diuresis; IV bicarbonate helps correct the acidosis, alkalinizes urine and inhibits salicylate reabsorption (increases excretion); lower elevated body temperature with physical means (ice packs, hypothermia blanket, etc; antipyretics may complicate clinical picture, are not likely to be effective anyway); anticonvulsants as needed.

331. The answer is a. *(Brunton, pp 639-640. Katzung, pp 275-279.)* One of the main advantages of the first-generation antihistamines (fexofenadine, loratadine, others) over the older (second-generation) H_1 antagonists such as diphenhydramine is a relative lack of CNS depressant (sedating) effects when administered at usual recommended doses. The implication of this difference is that the newer agents are much less likely to cause daytime drowsiness or other problems that might interfere with daytime activities requiring alertness. Sedation is a particular problem with diphenhydramine, doxylamine, and other members of the ethanolamine class of first-generation antihistamines, yet it also provides a clinically useful effect based on this action: they are useful as OTC (diphenhydramine, doxylamine) and prescription (diphenhydramine) sleep-aids.

Diphenhydramine, and to a large degree all the other first-generation antihistamines, tend to cause appreciable muscarinic receptor-blocking (atropinelike) effects, and so they are unsuitable or potentially dangerous for patients with such atropine-related comorbidities as prostatic hypertrophy, hypomotility disorders of the urinary or GI tracts, tachycardia, or angle-closure glaucoma (so answer b is not correct). Owing to antimuscarinic effects, diphenhydramine overdoses are more likely to cause tachycardia (by blocking parasympathetic-ACh-muscarinic receptor influences on the SA node) than bradycardia (c). The second-generation antihistamines do block histamine-related bronchoconstriction, but in the absence of histamine they have no intrinsic bronchodilator activity. More important is the fact that these drugs play no role as primary therapy for asthma. They may be preferred to older antihistamines (largely because they lack the antimuscarinic-related mucus-thickening effects of such drugs as diphenhydramine), but they should be used only as adjuncts to more appropriate asthma drugs such as inhaled corticosteroids (to suppress airway inflammation) and inhaled β-adrenergic drugs for control or rescue therapy.

None of the H_1 blockers—first- or second-generation agents—have H_2-blocking activity that is necessary to suppress histamine-mediated acid secretion by gastric parietal cells.

332. The answer is b. *(Brunton, pp 123, 695, 851. Katzung, pp 183, 1147, 1149.)* A major component of the antihypertensive actions of captopril and other ACE inhibitors is prostaglandin-dependent. That element of drug action is antagonized by indomethacin due to its great efficacy to inhibit prostaglandin synthesis. Other drugs with actions that may be inhibited by prostaglandin synthesis inhibitors such as indomethacin include the thiazide and loop diuretics and (allegedly) many if not most of the β-blockers. The actions of none of the other drugs listed are antagonized by indomethacin. I should note, however, that giving indomethacin to a patient taking warfarin or any of the antiplatelet drugs (used for prophylaxis of arterial thrombosis) is risky. One of the major toxicities of the NSAIDs is gastric mucosal damage and the risk of GI bleeds. In the presence of anticoagulants or antiplatelet drugs the risk of a serious GI bleed, perhaps progressing to hemorrhage, goes up markedly. The anticoagulants' effects certainly are not inhibited by the NSAID.

333. The answer is d. *(Brunton, pp 686, 691-692. Katzung, pp 624, 1021.)* Late, severe aspirin poisoning is characterized by a combination of respiratory and metabolic acidosis. In early stages of aspirin poisoning (or even with high "therapeutic" doses of the drug), ventilatory stimulation occurs. That induces a respiratory alkalosis (c; net CO_2 loss, relative HCO_3 retention). The kidneys compensate for this by increasing HCO_3 excretion to help normalize blood pH and causing what has been called "compensated respiratory alkalosis." As plasma levels of aspirin rise, however, blood pH falls precipitously. Part of that is due to the accumulation of acidic salicylic acid in the blood, and part is due to inhibited oxidative phosphorylation that shifts metabolism from oxidative to glycolytic (with lactic acid being the key end product). No longer synthesizing ATP effectively, the mitochondria generate metabolic heat, which contributes to fever (not hypothermia; a). Ventilatory failure (not stimulation; e) ensues, leading to respiratory acidosis (from CO_2 retention) along with the metabolic acidosis. Cardiovascular collapse and seizures eventually cause death. Note that hepatotoxicity is not a component of this: that is the main cause of morbidity and mortality with acetaminophen poisoning. Review the table in the answer to Question 330 if you wish.

334. The answer is a. *(Brunton, 83, 694-695, 1741. Katzung, pp 635-636, 1020.)* Acetaminophen's main toxic metabolite is *N*-acetyl-benzoqinoneimine. It reacts with sulfhydryl groups (particularly with glutathione) in hepatocytes, ultimately leading to hepatic necrosis when acetaminophen levels are sufficiently high. *N*-acetylcysteine is rich in –SH groups. It therefore reacts with the imine, hopefully sparing endogenous sulfhydryl compounds from further attack and, hopefully, allowing time for the hepatocytes to recover from the biochemical stress. This foul-smelling antidote must be given early after acetaminophen poisoning occurs or is likely (it is usually given orally), and it must be given repeatedly. It is a preventative against hepatotoxicity, not a reversing agent. As an aside, various nomograms are available to give some reasonable information about whether a particular acetaminophen dose (more precisely, blood level) is likely to be hepatotoxic or not. They plot plasma acetaminophen levels as a function of time after drug ingestion (yielding, basically, an elimination rate or half-life). If the patient's acetaminophen level at a specified time following drug ingestion is above the line, hepatotoxicity is probable. Such a finding, however, does not mean that *N*-acetylcysteine administration will be without benefit and so should not be done. (See the explanation for Question 317 for more information, and a look at this issue from a somewhat different perspective.)

All of the other drugs listed can exert toxic effects (often serious) with overdoses, but *N*-acetylcysteine is not an appropriate or effective antidote for any of them.

335. The answer is c. *(Brunton, pp 707-708. Katzung, pp 636-637.)* The main reason why many physicians are shunning oral colchicine for acute gout is that many patients develop horrible GI discomfort, vomiting, diarrhea, and the like. For some, the "cure" is almost as bad as the disorder for which the drug is given. This GI distress can be alleviated somewhat by giving colchicine IV, but more serious systemic responses can develop if the IV dose is too great or too many IV doses are given in a short period of time. (These are among the reasons why IV formulations of colchicine are no longer available.) Indomethacin seems to have become one of the preferred colchicine alternatives for anti-inflammatory therapy of acute gout or for prophylaxis of recurrences. (And clearly indomethacin is not without side effects or toxicities; the risks and discomforts are simply more acceptable, for some patients, with it.)

But when colchicine does work in acute gout, relief may be dramatic and occur literally "overnight" with just a dose or two. The likely mechanism of action involves impaired microtubular assembly or function in leukocytes, which limits their migration to the area of crystal deposition and so limits their ability to amplify the inflammatory reaction.

Bone marrow suppression can occur, but that is mainly with long-term, high-dose oral or parenteral colchicine administration (the latter of which must be avoided). The same applies to frank gastric damage (with the possibility of gastric bleeding or hemorrhage) and to blood dyscrasias (bone marrow toxicity).

336. The answer is b. *(Brunton, pp 708-709. Katzung, pp 638-639.)* You may think that reductions in urate content in a 24-hour urine sample would be bad for the hyperuricemic patient, but that is because you probably automatically (and incorrectly) equate lower urine urate concentrations with increased plasma urate. Not necessarily so. Allopurinol inhibits uric acid synthesis by inhibiting xanthine oxidase: less uric acid made, less to be excreted in the urine, and less to be detected there. This is one manifestation of allopurinol "at work." Acetaminophen (a) has no effects on uric acid synthesis, excretion, or solubility. Colchicine (c) is sometimes used for prophylaxis or treatment of gout, but its actions derive from its anti-inflammatory action and, probably, suppression of neutrophil chemotaxis by interfering with microtubular function. It has no effects on urate synthesis or elimination. The same applies to indomethacin (d): anti-inflammatory actions, but no effects per se on uric acid. Probenecid (e) is a uricosuric drug that acts by inhibiting tubular reabsorption of urate when plasma levels of the drug are therapeutic. As a result, the more likely outcome of this drug is an increase of urate concentrations in a urine sample. Probenecid does not affect uric acid synthesis.

337. The answer is e. *(Brunton, pp 708-709, 974-975. Katzung, p 636.)* The use of sodium bicarbonate (unless otherwise contraindicated) for prophylaxis of urate stone formation in the renal tubules is based on the fact that uric acid (sodium urate) is poorly soluble in body fluids and solubility is greatly influenced by local pH. When local pH falls, more urate crystallizes (ie, the K_{SP} falls). Considering that urine pH is normally lower than blood (or synovial fluid) pH, and since relatively large amounts of urate are excreted in the urine (even in the absence of a uricosuric drug, eg, probenecid), there is a greater tendency for urate to crystallize in the urinary tract. Conversely, as urine pH rises (as occurs with sodium bicarbonate administration), urate is more soluble (for a given concentration) and less likely to precipitate. This pH related phenomenon also contributes to the "vicious cycle" that starts when an acute gout attack in a joint occurs.

An additional body load of sodium bicarbonate will induce, through normal renal compensatory processes, a diuretic (not antidiuretic; answer a) effect; this should also increase the amount of urate that is lost into the urine. Although sodium bicarbonate raises blood pH, that has no clinically relevant effect on formation of xanthine and uric acid by xanthine oxidase (b). There is no metabolic acidosis that is characteristic of severe hyperuricemia (c). Sodium bicarbonate does not lower GFR and/or urate elimination (d).

338. The answer is c. *(Brunton, pp 422, 637-640, 642. Katzung, pp 275-278.)* Diphenhydramine, a member of the ethanolamine class of H_1 antagonists and arguably the prototype of all the older ("first-generation") antihistamines, possesses two main properties in addition to effective competitive blockade of H_1 receptors: sedation (c), in part due to the drug's lipophilicity; and muscarinic (cholinergic) receptor blockade that is also competitive. Both effects occur commonly, and can be quite intense. The CNS depressant effects of diphenhydramine are such that this drug is the main (if not only) active ingredient in OTC sleep aids, helping one drift off to sleep even in the absence of allergy signs and symptoms and probably in a way that is unrelated to the drug's peripheral H_1-blocking activity.

The antimuscarinic (atropine-like) effects would be manifest by such side effects as tachycardia (not bradycardia; a); constipation (not diarrhea; b); a suppression of ACh-induced gastric acid secretion (not the opposite; d); and a tendency for urinary retention (not frequency; e). The strong antimuscarinic effects of diphenhydramine earn it the same precautions and contraindications we normally apply to atropine itself, including prostatic hypertrophy and angle-closure glaucoma. Other side effects include xerostomia, blurred vision, paralysis of accommodation, and inhibition of sweating. Diphenhydramine toxicity manifests in ways that are markedly similar to what occurs with atropine poisoning, and is managed in the same way, including the use of physostigmine (ACh esterase inhibitor with actions in both the peripheral and central nervous systems) for severe or life-threatening toxicity.

As an important aside, loratadine, desloratadine, fexofenadine, and related newer (second-generation) H_1 blockers (piperidine class) are associated with much less CNS depression (they are advertised as "nonsedating"—usually with a disclaimer, in fine print, "when taken as directed"). Unlike diphenhydramine and most of the older H_1 blockers, the newer agents cause no antimuscarinic effects and have no atropine-related precautions or contraindications.

339. The answer is c. *(Brunton, pp 1017, 1419. Katzung, pp 633-634.)* Etanercept (and the related drug infliximab) binds to and neutralizes TNF-α, which is one of the primary pathophysiologic mediators in rheumatoid arthritis and Crohn disease. It functions, then, as an antibody. Etanercept has no effect on eicosanoid synthesis (a, d) or leukocyte migration (b). It does not stimulate collagen, mucopolysaccharide, or synovial fluid synthesis (e).

Gastrointestinal and Urinary Tract Pharmacology, Nutrition (Vitamins)

Acid secretion inhibitors (H_2 blockers, proton pump inhibitors, others)
Antacids
Antidiarrheals
Drugs affecting GI or urinary tract musculature
Emetics, antiemetics
Gallstone-dissolving drugs
Gastric mucotropic/cytoprotective protective drugs
Inflammatory bowel disease drugs
Laxatives, cathartics
Pancreatic enzyme replacement
Vitamins

Questions

340. A patient has severe gastroesophageal reflux disease (GERD). Immediate, albeit temporary, symptom relief will be provided by an OTC combination antacid product taken as needed. However, the long-term goal is to suppress gastric acid secretion as completely as possible so symptoms do not recur and the irritated tissues can heal. Which of the following drugs is best suited to achieve that goal, and is likely to pose the lowest risk of causing disturbing or otherwise unwanted side effects?

a. Atropine
b. Calcium carbonate
c. Cimetidine
d. Esomeprazole
e. Misoprostol

341. A patient with multiple medical problems is taking several drugs, including theophylline, warfarin, quinidine, and phenytoin. Despite the likelihood of interactions, dosages of each were adjusted carefully so their plasma concentrations and effects are acceptable. However, the patient suffers some GI distress and starts taking a drug provided by one of his "well-intentioned" friends. He presents with excessive or toxic effects from all his other medications and blood tests reveal that plasma concentrations of all the prescribed drugs are high. Which of the following drugs did the patient most likely self-prescribe and take?

a. Antacid (typical magnesium-aluminum combination)
b. Cimetidine
c. Famotidine
d. Nizatidine
e. Ranitidine

342. We have two patients. One requires suppression of emesis from an anticancer drug that causes a high incidence and severity of vomiting (a highly emetogenic drug). Another patient has severe diabetic gastroparesis and gastroesophageal reflux. Which one of the following drugs would be most suitable for both indications?

a. Diphenoxylate
b. Dronabinol
c. Loperamide
d. Metoclopramide
e. Ondansetron

343. A patient with multiple GI complaints is receiving ursodeoxycholic acid (ursodiol) as part of his drug regimen. What is the most likely purpose for which this drug is being given?

a. Dissolving cholesterol stones in the bile ducts
b. Enhancing intestinal digestion and absorption of dietary fats
c. Helping to reverse malabsorption of fat-soluble vitamins from the diet
d. Stimulating gastric acid secretion in achlorhydria
e. Suppressing steatorrhea and its consequences

344. A patient who has been a high-dose alcohol abuser for many years presents with hepatic portal-systemic encephalopathy. Which drug, given in relatively high doses, would be most suitable for the relief of some of the signs and symptoms of the encephalopathy and the likely underlying biochemical anomalies?

a. Diphenoxylate
b. Esomeprazole
c. Lactulose
d. Loperamide
e. Ondansetron

345. Fat-soluble vitamins, compared with their water-soluble counterparts, generally have a greater potential toxicity to the user when taken in excess. What property of those vitamins—A, D, E, and K—is the main reason for this finding?

a. Administered in larger doses
b. Avidly stored by the body
c. Capable of dissolving membrane phospholipids
d. Involved in more essential metabolic pathways
e. Metabolized much more slowly

346. A patient is transported from a distant hospital to your surgical service by air ambulance. He had abdominal surgery and in the postoperative care unit he received a drug that was clearly not indicated. The drug caused intense contraction of the detrusor and trigone muscles of his bladder. The first dose failed to cause emptying of the bladder, so a second dose was given. However, and unknown to his prior care team, he has a mass that rather significantly obstructs his urethra, and has structural weakening in a portion of his bladder. Upon administration of the drug he first suffered retrograde urine flow that caused renal damage. Soon thereafter his bladder wall ruptured. Which drug or drug class most likely caused these adverse effects?

a. Albuterol
b. Atropine or a similar antimuscarinic
c. Bethanechol
d. Furosemide
e. Propranolol or a similar β-blocker

347. A patient presents with malaise and her skin and mucous membranes appear pale. Among the key findings from blood work are hypochromic, microcytic red cells; reduced red cell count/hematocrit; reduced reticulocyte count; and reduced total hemoglobin content. Which of the following drugs would be indicated, based on the presentation?

a. Cyanocobalamin (vitamin B_{12})
b. Folic acid
c. Iron
d. Vitamin C
e. Vitamin D

348. A patient will start taking one of the drugs listed below. As you hand them the prescription you advise them not to take supplemental vitamin B_6 (pyridoxine), whether alone or as part of a multivitamin supplement, because the vitamin is likely to counteract a desired effect of the prescribed drug. To which of the following drugs does this advice apply?

a. Captopril for heart failure or hypertension
b. Haloperidol for Tourette syndrome
c. Levodopa/carbidopa for Parkinson disease
d. Niacin for hypertriglyceridemia
e. Phenytoin for epilepsy

349. You have a patient who has been consuming extraordinarily large amounts of alcohol for several years, and is generally malnourished. He goes into acute alcohol withdrawal and manifests nystagmus, bizarre ocular movements, and confusion (Wernicke encephalopathy). Although this patient's alcohol consumption pattern has been accompanied by poor nutrient intake overall, you need to manage the encephalopathy. Which of the following drugs is most appropriate for this use?

a. α-Tocopherol (vitamin E)
b. Cyanocobalamin (vitamin B_{12})
c. Folic acid
d. Phytonadione (vitamin K)
e. Thiamine (vitamin B_1)

350. A patient with tuberculosis is being treated with isoniazid. She develops paresthesias, muscle aches, and unsteadiness. Which of the following vitamins needs to be given in supplemental doses in order to reverse these symptoms—or used from the outset to prevent them in high-risk patients?

a. Vitamin A
b. Vitamin B_1 (thiamine)
c. Vitamin B_6 (pyridoxine)
d. Vitamin C
e. Vitamin K

351. An opioid abuser, seeking something to self-administer for subjective responses, gets a large amount of diphenoxylate, an antidiarrheal drug, and consumes it all at once. He is not likely to do this again because he has consumed a combination product that contains not only the diphenoxylate but also another drug that causes a host of unpleasant systemic responses. What is the other drug found in combination with the diphenoxylate?

a. Apomorphine
b. Atropine
c. Ipecac
d. Magnesium sulfate
e. Naltrexone

352. During a regular checkup, your patient states "You know, doc, sometimes after eating I get heartburn . . . you know, acid-indigestion." Since the symptoms seem to be mild and infrequent, you suggest an empiric trial of an OTC antacid for prompt symptom relief, plus an oral anti-acid-secretory drug for long-term control. You recommend several antacid brands for the patient to try, all of which are combination products that contain a magnesium (Mg) salt and an aluminum (Al) salt. What is main rationale or reason why the vast majority of these products contain these two particular drug salts?

a. Al salts counteract the gastric mucosal-irritating effects of Mg salts
b. Al salts require activation by an Mg-dependent enzyme in order to inhibit the parietal cell proton pumps
c. Mg salts cause a diuresis that helps reduce systemic accumulation of the Al salt by increasing renal Al excretion
d. Mg salts potentiate the ability of Al salts to inhibit gastric acid secretion
e. Mg salts tend to cause a laxative effect (increased gut motility) that counteracts the tendency of an Al salt to cause constipation

353. On your first day on a general medicine clerkship you encounter a patient who is taking a proton pump inhibitor plus bismuth, metronidazole, and tetracycline. What is the most likely condition for which this drug combination is being used?

a. Antibiotic-associated pseudomembranous colitis
b. Irritable bowel syndrome
c. Refractory or recurrent, and severe, gastric ulcers secondary to *Helicobacter pylori*
d. "Traveler's diarrhea," severe, *Escherichia coli*—induced, from drinking contaminated water
e. Ulcers that occurred in response to long-term, high-dose traditional nonsteroidal anti-inflammatory drug (NSAID) therapy for arthritis

354. You just confirmed that your patient is pregnant, and emphasize to her to avoid taking supplements of a vitamin, especially in high doses, because it is highly teratogenic. For the same reason you also want to avoid administering during pregnancy any drugs that are derivatives of this nutrient. To which one of the following vitamins does this precaution apply?

a. A
b. B_{12}
c. C
d. E
e. Folic acid

355. A patient has undiagnosed multiple gastric ulcers. Shortly after consuming a large meal and large amounts of alcohol he experiences significant GI distress. He takes an OTC heartburn remedy purchased at a local supermarket. Within a minute or two he develops what he will later describe as a "bad bloated feeling." Several of the ulcers have begun to bleed and he experiences searing pain.

The patient becomes profoundly hypotensive from upper GI blood loss and is transported to the hospital. Endoscopy confirms multiple bleeds; the endoscopist remarks that it appears as if the lesions had been literally stretched apart, causing additional tissue damage that led to the hemorrhage. Which drug or product did the patient most likely take?

a. An aluminum salt
b. An aluminum-magnesium combination antacid product
c. Magnesium hydroxide
d. Ranitidine
e. Sodium bicarbonate

356. A patient has steatorrhea secondary to cystic fibrosis. Which of the following drugs usually is considered the most reasonable and usually effective drug for managing the fatty stools?

a. Atorvastatin (or any other HMG Co-A-reductase inhibitor)
b. Cimetidine (or an alternative, eg, famotidine)
c. Bile salts
d. Metoclopramide
e. Pancrelipase

357. A 26-year-old woman is losing most of her hearing. She works as a fashion model for clothing and jewelry designers, and several cosmetics companies, and given her occupation she is concerned about getting hearing aids that were strongly recommended by her ENT doctor. She consults web-based "support groups" for people with hearing loss and reads claims that nicotinic acid (niacin) can improve cochlear blood flow and reverse or at least halt further hearing loss. She goes to the health food store and purchases the nutrient. Believing that if the recommended dose of niacin is good, taking much higher doses would be even better: "after all, it's just a vitamin," she reasons. Which side effect(s) is this young woman most likely to experience shortly after starting to consume high doses of this vitamin?

a. Bradycardia
b. Facial flushing and pruritus
c. Hypercholesterolemia, hypertriglyceridemia
d. Hypoglycemia
e. Photophobia due to intense mydriasis

358. Several brand name and store brand "pink medications," administered orally and available without prescription, are widely used to help alleviate occasional and short-lived nausea and vomiting, diarrhea, and other mild GI distress. They are also recommended for prophylaxis of "traveler's diarrhea," which typically is caused by ingestion of foods or beverages contaminated with *E coli*. These products contain bismuth subsalicylate, and because of the presence of an aspirin-like compound (salicylate) they should not be taken by or administered to certain patients. Which patient-related factor or comorbidity contraindicates use of this drug or product?

a. Essential hypertension
b. Flu, chickenpox, or other viral illness in a child or adolescent
c. Hot flashes and other signs/symptoms of menopause
d. Prostatic hypertrophy or glaucoma in elderly men
e. Rheumatoid or osteoarthritis
f. Severe seasonal allergy signs and symptoms

359. A patient being cared for by the gastroenterology service is being treated with sulfasalazine. What is the most likely purpose for which it is being given?

a. Antibiotic-associated pseudomembranous colitis
b. *Escherichia coli*-induced diarrhea
c. Gastric *H pylori* infections
d. Inflammatory bowel disease
e. NSAID-induced gastric ulcer prophylaxis

360. A patient with renal failure is undergoing periodic hemodialysis while awaiting a transplant. Between dialysis sessions you want to reduce the body's phosphate load by reducing dietary phosphate absorption and removing, via the gastrointestinal tract, some phosphate already in the blood. Which drug would be most suitable for this purpose?

a. Aluminum hydroxide
b. Bismuth subsalicylate
c. Magnesium hydroxide/oxide
d. Sodium bicarbonate
e. Sucralfate

361. A patient has severe irritable bowel syndrome characterized by frequent and profuse diarrhea. She has not responded to first-line therapies and is started on alosetron. What is the most worrisome adverse effect associated with this drug?

a. Cardiac arrhythmias (serious, eg, ventricular fibrillation)
b. Constipation, bowel impaction, ischemic colitis
c. Parkinsonian extrapyramidal reactions
d. Pulmonary fibrosis
e. Renal failure

362. A patient undergoing cancer chemotherapy gets ondansetron for prophylaxis of drug-induced nausea and vomiting. Which statement best describes this drug's main mechanism of action in this setting?

a. Activates μ-type opioid receptors in the chemoreceptor trigger zone
b. Blocks central serotonin (5-HT_3) receptors
c. Blocks dopamine receptors
d. Blocks histamine H_1 receptors in the brainstem and inner ear
e. Suppresses gastric motility and acid secretion via muscarinic blockade

Gastrointestinal and Urinary Tract Pharmacology, Nutrition (Vitamins)

Answers

340. The answer is d. *(Brunton, pp 967-971. Katzung, pp 1071-1075.)* Esomeprazole and related drugs (eg, lansoprazole, omeprazole, pantoprazole, rabeprazole) inhibit the parietal cell H^+-K^+ATPase—the "proton pump"—that is the "final common pathway" for acid secretion triggered by all the major stimuli of gastric acid secretion. As a result, they are the most efficacious, causing near complete anti–acid-secretory activity.

Recall some of the main agonists that provoke acid secretion. One is gastrin, for which we have no clinically useful antagonists. Histamine, arising from enterochromaffin-like (ECL) cells, activates H_2 receptors. Histamine's effects can be blocked by cimetidine (c) or other H_2 blockers (famotidine, nizatidine, ranitidine). Acetylcholine increases gastric acid secretion by activating muscarinic receptors on both ECL cells and parietal cells. Its effects can be blocked by atropine (a), propantheline, pirenzepine (widely taught in medical schools for many years, but never approved for use in the United States), and several other drugs with antimuscarinic activity. However, blocking only the histaminergic influences or only the cholinergic influences—or even blocking both types of receptors—only partially inhibits acid secretion: just those mediated by histamine and ACh, respectively. One additional disadvantage of using muscarinic blockade to suppress acid secretion, aside from the fact that inhibition of secretion is not complete, is the prevalence of often disturbing and usually unwanted atropine-like side effects elsewhere, for example, on the eyes, heart, urinary tract, and exocrine gland secretions.

Calcium carbonate (b) is widely used as an antacid (neutralizes already-secreted HCl), but it is almost always self-prescribed and purchased OTC. Interestingly, although calcium carbonate neutralizes gastric acid, calcium ion enhances parietal cell acid secretion.

Misoprostol (e) is unique in several ways. One is that this prostaglandin analog mimics the effects of endogenous prostaglandins (mainly PGE_2) to inhibit acid secretion. Overall, however, misoprostol's anti-acid-secretory effects are relatively weak. It is used for GI disorders (reductions in the risk of ulceration caused by traditional nonsteroidal anti-inflammatory drug therapy) mainly because it stimulates gastric mucosal mucus formation (called a mucotropic or gastric cytoprotective effect).

Ultimately, however, regardless of whether gastrin, ACh, or histamine is present, parietal cell acid secretion ultimately "funnels through" the proton pump. Block the receptors for any of the mediators noted above and you will suppress acid caused only by that mediator—but that is only a fraction of total acid secretion. Block the proton pump and acid secretion will be inhibited nearly fully, no matter which one or more agonists are present "upstream."

Calcium carbonate (b), as well as aluminum and magnesium salts and sodium bicarbonate, are the main antacids. They have no inhibitory effects on acid secretion. Instead, they neutralize acid that has already been secreted (and aluminum salts also adsorb pepsins). Calcium and aluminum salts tend to cause constipation, and magnesium salts, diarrhea/ laxation. Sodium bicarbonate, the use of which as an antacid is seldom justified, tends to cause no changes of gut motility. However, the significant sodium absorption poses problems for many patients (eg, those with or at risk of hypertension, heart failure, edema), and bicarbonate absorption causes metabolic alkalosis. Magnesium salts, which are also absorbed, pose a risk of hypermagnesemia in patients with impaired or otherwise inadequate renal function.

341. The answer is b. *(Brunton, pp 971-973. Katzung, pp 65t, 596t, 1069-1071, 1143t.)* Cimetidine differs significantly from the other H_2 blockers, famotidine, nizatidine, and ranitidine, in that it is a very effective inhibitor of the hepatic mixed function oxidase (P450) drug-metabolizing enzyme systems. (Cimetidine inhibits CYP 1A2, 2C9, 2D6, and 3A4.) The other H_2 blockers (famotidine, c; nizatidine, d; ranitidine, e) have no significant P450 effects, nor do they cause side effects as frequent or as problematic as those caused by cimetidine, especially at higher doses. The outcome of P450 inhibition, of course, is reduced hepatic clearance of the interactants, leading to excessive plasma concentrations and effects if their dosages are not reduced properly. The examples cited in the question—phenytoin, warfarin, quinidine, and theophylline—are among the most important interactants with cimetidine. They, and other interactants such as lidocaine, have rather low margins of safety, so even slight increases in plasma levels (reductions of metabolic clearance) may be enough to cause toxicity. Given the fact that the alternative H_2 blockers don't inhibit the P450 system, there's no good reason for prescribing cimetidine to patients on multiple drug therapy (and in this case, the patient should have been warned about self-medicating with it).

Antacids tend to adsorb other drugs in the gut at or around the same time, and inhibit their absorption (rate, extent, or both). If this patient had taken an antacid with his other medicines, we would see reduced blood levels and effects—not increases as described in the question.

Note: Not long after the newer H_2 blockers came on the market, and we knew they caused fewer side effects than cimetidine and certainly did not inhibit various CYP enzymes to cause drug-drug interactions, I asked a gastroenterologist why cimetidine would ever be prescribed. She couldn't think of a valid reason except cost. And now, as costs for the alternatives have come down, even that's not a consideration. Finally, it is important to remember: Cimetidine is still available OTC, and patients who should not be taking it (mainly because of interactions with other drugs they may be taking) can still use this drug without your OK or even your knowledge.

342. The answer is d. *(Brunton, pp 343, 467, 985-986. Katzung, pp 1078, 1086.)* Metoclopramide has clinically useful antiemetic and prokinetic actions and would be suitable for either of the patients described in the question. The antiemetic effect arises from blockade of dopamine D_2 (and, probably, serotonin) receptors in the brain's chemoreceptor trigger zone (CTZ). The drug is indicated for not only chemotherapy-induced nausea and vomiting, but also that which may occur with radiation therapy, postoperatively, or in response to opioid analgesics or emetogenic toxins. Note that there are increasing reports that metoclopramide can cause parkinsonian signs and symptoms, and even tardive dyskinesias. This should not be a surprise, given the drug's central dopamine receptor blocking actions.

The enhanced gastric and upper intestinal motility probably reflects an enhancement of the expected effects of ACh on muscarinic receptors found on longitudinal smooth muscle in the GI tract. Metoclopramide raises the lower esophageal sphincter tone and relaxes the pyloric sphincter, which hastens gastric emptying. This helps explain its beneficial effects in both gastroparesis and GERD.

Diphenoxylate (a) is an oral opioid indicated only for managing diarrhea. Typical antidiarrheal doses inhibit bowel motility well but cause no central opioid-like effects (ventilatory depression, analgesia, euphoria, etc). However, the commercial product contains atropine for two main purposes: (1) the atropine contributes, albeit comparatively weakly, to the antidiarrheal effects; and (2) should someone take excessive doses of the combination to get a morphine-like "high," the unpleasant antimuscarinic effects hopefully would stifle further attempts. Dronabinol (b) is a cannabinoid, and a psychoactive chemical in marijuana. It is used to suppress chemotherapy-induced nausea and vomiting. The drug has no role in managing gastroparesis or GERD. Loperamide (c) is an antidiarrheal that is available OTC. Although it is a meperidine analog, it lacks opioid- or meperidine-like systemic or central effects at usual doses. It probably works not only by suppressing bowel motility and fluid secretion into the intestines. Ondansetron (e), like dronabinol, is used to manage emetogenic drug-induced symptoms. It is a serotonin receptor (5-HT_3) blocker that acts mainly in the CTZ and on vagal efferents to parts of the upper GI tract.

343. The answer is a. *(Brunton, p 1007. Katzung, p 1049.)* Ursodeoxycholic acid (ursodiol), one of several naturally occurring bile acids, is effective in some patients with gallstones. Its main initial action is reduced hepatic cholesterol synthesis. That, in turn, lowers the cholesterol content in the bile, which favors the dissolution of cholesterol stones that have formed already and reduces the incidence of new stone formation.

Ursodeoxycholic acid tends to inhibit (not enhance; answer b) intestinal fat digestion and absorption, and may contribute to (not reverse; answer c) impaired absorption of vitamins A, D, E, and K. The drug does not stimulate gastric acid secretion (d) and is not indicated for managing achlorhydria. Steatorrhea may develop in response to ursodeoxycholic acid; the incidence of fatty stools is not reduced (e) by the drug.

344. The answer is c. *(Brunton, pp 992-993. Katzung p 1079.)* Lactulose is a synthetic nonabsorbable disaccharide (galactose-fructose). In moderate doses it acts as an osmotic laxative. In higher doses it binds intestinal ammonia and other toxins that accumulate in the intestine in the face of severe liver dysfunction. These toxins, and perhaps more so the ammonia, contribute to the signs and symptoms of encephalopathy. None of the other drugs listed provide this benefit.

Diphenoxylate (a; more in the answer to Question 342) and loperamide (c) are opioid-like antidiarrheal drugs. Esomeprazole (b) is a proton pump inhibitor used to suppress gastric acid secretion. And ondansetron (e), a 5-HT_3 antagonist, is mainly used to manage nausea and vomiting in response to chemotherapy.

345. The answer is b. *(Brunton, pp 763-764.)* Fat-soluble vitamins, especially A and D (the others being vitamins E and K), can be stored in massive amounts and, hence, have a potential for serious toxicities. (However, this abundant storage means that relatively brief periods of inadequate intake are not likely to cause clinical signs and symptoms of deficiency.) Water-soluble vitamins are easily excreted by the kidneys and accumulation to toxic levels is much less common. However, inadequate dietary intake will lead to manifestations of deficiency relatively faster.

On average, most people consume excessive amounts (a) of fat-soluble vitamins no more often than they do water-soluble ones. Even very large doses of fat-soluble vitamins that might be consumed will not alter membrane structure or function (c), although such effects can be demonstrated in certain in vitro settings that bear little relevance to intact humans. Differences involving greater or more roles in overall cell metabolism (d), or rates of the metabolism of the vitamins themselves (e), are not reasonable explanations for the relatively greater toxic potential of vitamins A, D, E, and K.

346. The answer is c. *(Brunton, pp 183-184, 188-189, 985. Katzung, pp 97-98.)* Bethanechol is a muscarinic agonist that is used to manage functional urinary retention—that is, urinary retention or a significant inability to void caused by some functional defect in the bladder musculature. It is contraindicated for patients with bladder walls that are damaged or unable to respond safely to drugs that stimulate the bladder musculature, and patients with mechanical obstruction of the urethra (from, say, prostatism or a prostatic cancer). This was what caused the bethanechol-induced problems for this patient.

Albuterol (a), predominantly a β_2 agonist used for its bronchodilator effects, has no significant effects on the healthy or damaged bladder: β-receptors just aren't there. Atropine (b) or other antimuscarinics will weaken contraction of the trigone and detrusor, and stimulate contraction of the bladder sphincter, causing just the opposite of what I described. Furosemide

(d) and other loop diuretics (torsemide, bumetanide, ethacrynic acid) obviously increase the need to urinate and the volume of urine that is excreted. However, the bladder activation that ensues is mediated by reflexes triggered by a full bladder. There is no direct stimulation or inhibition of bladder musculature. Finally, just as β agonists have no appreciable effect on bladder musculature, neither do drugs that block β-adrenergic receptors (e).

347. The answer is c. *(Brunton, pp 1442-1450. Katzung, pp 570-573, 1024.)* The description contains many of the characteristics of "iron-deficiency anemia." Oral iron salts (eg, ferrous sulfate, gluconate, or fumarate) are usually the first choice for management (after ruling out such causes as blood loss). Changes of gut motility (sometimes diarrhea, sometimes constipation), nausea, and heartburn are common complaints with oral iron salts, but using the oral drugs is often preferable to, just as effective as, and safer than using parenteral iron products such as iron-dextran (risk of anaphylaxis) or other iron complexes, which typically involve erythropoietin administration adjunctively.

Megaloblastic anemia (in contrast with the microcytic anemia I described here) would be treated differently. If it is caused by vitamin B_{12} deficiency (vitamin malabsorption due to deficiency of intrinsic factor; answer a), we would treat with cyanocobalamin. The other cause, folate deficiency (inadequate dietary intake) is managed with oral folic acid (b). Deficiencies of vitamin C or D (answers d, e, respectively) don't typically cause anemias.

348. The answer is c. *(Brunton, pp 530, 533-534. Katzung, pp 142, 470-474, 1146t.)* Recall that DOPA decarboxylase, an enzyme whose activity is dependent on pyridoxine, is responsible for metabolizing orally administered levodopa to dopamine in the gut; and that only unmetabolized levodopa crosses the blood-brain barrier to be efficacious in relieving parkinsonian signs and symptoms. Recall, too, that levodopa is often administered with carbidopa, a drug that inhibits the peripheral decarboxylase, sparing levodopa for entry into the brain. Carbidopa's actions are antagonized by pyridoxine, and so administering supplemental B_6 will reduce the bioavailability of levodopa and counteract its antiparkinson effectiveness. None of the other drugs listed, whether used for the stated purpose or others, has its effects antagonized by pyridoxine: captopril or other ACE inhibitors (a); haloperidol or any of the other antipsychotic drugs (b); niacin (nicotinic acid; d); or phenytoin (e) or other anticonvulsants.

Note: If you seem to recall something about phenytoin and vitamin or other nutrient supplements, you're on the right track. Phenytoin and several other anticonvulsants administered during pregnancy pose a risk of embryopathy or teratogenesis to the fetus. These risks can be reduced by ensuring adequate maternal intake of folic acid during pregnancy. And, newborns of mothers taking phenytoin and several other anticonvulsants during pregnancy are at risk of excessive bleeding (or other bleeding disorders) at birth. Those problems are related to vitamin K, and the risk is reduced by administering vitamin K to the mother before delivery and giving an injection of vitamin K to the newborn.

349. The answer is e. *(Brunton, pp 594, 598. Katzung, pp 824f, 825.)* Thiamine administered parenterally before or at the same time as administering glucose is used for Wernicke encephalopathy. It dramatically ameliorates the signs and symptoms. Thiamine must be given if glucose is to be given. Thiamine serves as a cofactor for many enzymatic reactions, including those involved in carbohydrate metabolism. If glucose is administered in a thiamine-deficient state, what little vitamin is left in the circulation will be depleted, aberrant glucose metabolism will continue, and the pathology (particularly neurologic) likely will be worsened.

Thiamine deficiency is also responsible for Korsakoff psychosis (or Korsakoff amnestic syndrome), another accompaniment of severe, long-term alcohol consumption (especially without adequately nutritional diets). Unfortunately, the signs and symptoms of Korsakoff (short-term memory problems, a tendency to fabricate, polyneuropathies) are not reversible.

Vitamin E (a) is not indicated for Wernicke encephalopathy. Supplements of that fat-soluble vitamin are often used (misused?) by the lay public for the vitamin's "antioxidant" and "antiaging" effects. Cyanocobalamin (B_{12}; b) is often used for macrocytic anemias that involve deficiencies of intrinsic factor (see Question 347). Folic acid (c) supplements have a variety of uses, including reducing the risk of teratogenic or similar effects in pregnant women, especially if they are taking certain antiepileptic drugs. The most common use of phytonadione (vitamin K; d) is to help reverse excessive anticoagulant effects of warfarin.

350. The answer is c. *(Brunton, pp 1102, 1206-1207. Katzung, p 784.)* Pyridoxine deficiencies tend to develop during isoniazid therapy because the antimycobacterial drug interferes with metabolic activation of the vitamin.

The treatment or prophylaxis for at-risk patients is to administer relatively large doses of B_6. There are no isoniazid-related issues with vitamins A (a), B_1 (thiamine, b), C (d), or K (e).

351. The answer is b. *(Brunton, pp 194-195, 570. Katzung, pp 546, 1081, 1099.)* Diphenoxylate tablet contains a small amount of atropine—usually not enough to cause side effects when the proper dose of the product is consumed, but clearly able to cause all the typical and unpleasant antimuscarinic side effects of which you should be aware (see Chapter 2) when excessive doses are taken. This pharmaceutical manufacturing "trick" discourages diphenoxylate abuse. (Also see the answer for Question 342.)

Apomorphine (a) and ipecac (c) are dopaminergic emetics (for parenteral and oral administration, respectively) that are used in some poisonings where inducing emesis is desired and safe. Magnesium sulfate ("Epson salt"—clearly a foul-tasting substance; answer d) is occasionally and usually inappropriately used as a laxative or cathartic. Naltrexone (e) is an opioid antagonist (μ and κ receptors, naloxone-like, but given orally).

352. The answer is e. *(Brunton, pp 974-975. Katzung, pp 1069, 1079.)* Magnesium salts (eg, oxide/hydroxide, as found in ordinary milk of magnesia and magnesium citrate (more commonly known as citrate of magnesia), when used alone, tend to cause a laxative effect. (Indeed, at dosages higher than those used for acid neutralization, magnesium salts are used for their laxative or stronger [cathartic] effects.) Aluminum (or calcium) antacids, given alone, tend to cause constipation. Combining a magnesium salt with an aluminum salt (and/or calcium antacid) thereby provides an often successful approach to minimizing antacid-induced changes of net gut motility: the net inhibitory effects of the aluminum or calcium salts on overall gut motility is counteracted by the opposite effects of the magnesium salt.

Magnesium salts, in usual antacid dosages, generally are not irritating to the gastric mucosa, and should it occur aluminum salts will not counteract that effect (thus answer a is incorrect). Likewise, aluminum salts act by simple physicochemical means, neutralizing some acid and adsorbing pepsins. They do not require activation by any enzymes and do not inhibit gastric acid secretion (and so b and d are incorrect). Likewise, answer c is incorrect. Although magnesium salts are readily absorbed and cause a slight diuresis in patients with normal renal function, any such effect has no impact on the elimination of aluminum salts: aluminum-containing antacids are called nonsystemic antacids because they are not absorbed, and they are eliminated solely via the GI tract.

353. The answer is c. *(Brunton, pp 967, 976-980, 1104. Katzung, pp 1073-1074.)* Several professional organizations, including the American College of Gastroenterology, have guidelines for managing severe, refractory, or recurrent duodenal and/or gastric ulcers in which *H pylori* clearly play an important pathophysiologic role. Although several regimens have been suggested, all of them include an anti–acid-secretory drug (usually a proton pump inhibitor, sometimes an H_2 blocker), two or three antimicrobials (eg, amoxicillin, clarithromycin, or tetracycline, usually with metronidazole), and bismuth. In many cases, this so-called eradicative therapy can cause a clinical cure and prevent recurrences after about 8 weeks of treatment. (The treatment is expensive, but pales in comparison with the financial and personal costs of treating recurrent episodes or potentially serious complications such as GI bleeding or hemorrhage, either pharmacologically or surgically.)

Antibiotic-associated pseudomembranous colitis (a) is typically managed with vancomycin or metronidazole, along with discontinuation of the causative agent (usually clindamycin). Dietary modifications (especially increased dietary fiber intake) and various drugs that alter gut motility (laxatives in constipation-predominant IBS; opioid, opioid-like, or serotonin antagonist antidiarrheals when diarrhea predominates) are often chosen to help manage irritable bowel syndrome (b). Doxycycline and/or bismuth salts are often used to prevent or treat *E coli*-mediated diarrhea (d). If the goal is to prevent NSAID-induced gastric ulcers (e), misoprostol or a proton pump inhibitor (eg, esomeprazole) are common choices.

354. The answer is a. *(Brunton, pp 1685-1687. Katzung, p 1028t.)* Pregnant women should not take more than a 25% increase in the normal recommended daily dietary intake of vitamin A, because it is highly teratogenic, especially in the first trimester. Note that the vitamin A derivative isotretinoin, which is indicated for systemic therapy of refractory and severe acne vulgaris (nodulocystic acne), is contraindicated (pregnancy class X). Although the systemic toxicity of a related drug, tretinoin (topical agent for mild-to-moderate acne), is far lower than with systemic isotretinoin, it too should be avoided during pregnancy.

Supplemental use of vitamins B_{12} (b), C (c), and E (d) is not contraindicated during pregnancy, but of course excessive dosages should be avoided. Supplemental doses of folic acid (e) are often recommended during pregnancy, and are deemed important if the mother is taking certain drugs (eg, phenytoin, valproic acid, and several other antiepileptic agents) that either cause folate deficiencies or in other ways increase maternal folic acid requirements that might lead to teratogenic effects in the fetus.

355. The answer is e. *(Brunton, pp 974-975. Katzung, p 1069.)* You've all done the experiment: mix vinegar and baking soda (sodium bicarbonate) and one product is CO_2. This gas is formed when sodium bicarbonate—still used as a lay remedy for "heartburn" (esophageal reflux) and other acid-related GI disturbances—reacts with HCl in the stomach.

Normally intragastric pressure is kept in check when the gastroesophageal sphincter opens. However, when pressure can't be relieved quickly enough, or adequately, the stomach distends like a balloon. In the presence of ulcers the lesions are stretched mechanically, favoring further damage that can lead to acute bleeding. Even in the absence of ulcers, any weakness of the gastric wall can lead to rupture. (Reports about a very similar situation, published in the lay press many years ago and laced with more than a little hyperbole, stated that "[the man's] stomach exploded after a big night on the town" soon after ingesting baking soda for relief.)

None of the other antacids listed, whether alone or in combination, lead to production of CO_2 or any other gas that might lead to the outcome described here. Aluminum salts (a) seldom are used alone for neutralizing gastric acid, but are used occasionally to reduce circulating phosphate levels in such patients as those with renal failure. Used alone, aluminum salts tend to cause constipation. Aluminum-magnesium combination products (b) are the most commonly prescribed or self-prescribed antacids. The rationale for this combination, aside from overall efficacy, is that the laxative effects of the magnesium salts (c) are counteracted by the constipating effects of the aluminum salts. (Calcium salts, particularly calcium carbonate, also have antacid effects and, when used alone tend to cause constipation.) You will find more information about the aluminum and magnesium salts in the explanation to Question 352.

Ranitidine (d) is an H_2 blocker that modestly suppresses gastric acid secretion (that component mediated by histamine), and that lacks any direct physical or chemical interactions with already-secreted acid. The other H_2 blockers are famotidine, nizatidine, and the lesser-used cimetidine.

356. The answer is e. *(Brunton, pp 1005-1006. Katzung, p 1093.)* Pancrelipase is an alcoholic extract of hog pancreas that contains lipase, trypsin, and amylase. (The related drug, pancreatin, is similar.) The goal in using it here is not so much to control the symptom, diarrhea, but do so by attacking the cause, which is endogenous pancreatic enzyme deficiency (lipases, amylase, chymotrypsin, and trypsin) that leads to impaired fat digestion and absorption.

None of the other drugs mentioned (a statin, a; an H_2 blocker, b; bile salts, c; metoclopramide, d) have actions that would be as effective (if effective at all) or specific as pancrelipase. Antidiarrheals, for example, would only treat the symptoms, not the underlying cause.

Note: You may find pancrelipase administered with antacids, or an acid secretion inhibitor (H_2 blocker or proton pump inhibitor). The purpose of combined therapy is not related to preventing adverse effects of acid on the gastric mucosa, but rather to raise gastric pH and prevent the pancrelipase from being hydrolyzed and inactivated by acid.

357. The answer is b. *(Brunton, pp 683-684, 946-956. Katzung, pp 613-614, 617.)* Niacin (nicotinic acid, vitamin B_3) is mainly used therapeutically for dyslipidemias. The drug often is quite effective in lowering elevated total and LDL cholesterol, raising HDL cholesterol, and lowering elevated triglycerides. (Thus, answer c is incorrect.) One of the main limitations to using this "nutrient," however, is the prevalence of severe facial flushing and pruritus, and GI distress that the patient will often describe as heartburn or acid-indigestion. Although these side effects are potentially severe and disturbing, and a major cause of noncompliance, they are dose-dependent and tolerance develops after a couple of weeks of continued therapy. They occur no matter the reason for which the drug is taken, whether for documented favorable effects on lipid profiles, or based on many anecdotal and largely unsubstantiated reports that they improve cochlear blood flow and slow, or otherwise reduce, hearing loss.

These niacin-induced side effects can be minimized by keeping dosages relatively low; by using sustained-release (slow-release) formulations; and by pretreatment with aspirin (which suggests that prostaglandins play some role in the unwanted responses). Whether prostaglandin-mediated or not, vasodilation appears to be involved, and that is more likely to trigger reflex tachycardia than bradycardia (a). Therapeutic doses of niacin, regardless of the purpose for which it is given, tend to cause hyperglycemia, not hypoglycemia (d). The rises of blood glucose levels may be dramatic, and may involve the phenomenon of insulin resistance in parenchymal cells such as adipocytes and skeletal muscle. Nonetheless, the drug should not be administered to patients with diabetes mellitus unless dosages of other antidiabetic drugs are adjusted, if necessary, to account for the problem. Photophobia (e) usually arises in response to α-adrenergic agonists or muscarinic receptor blockers. Niacin affects neither of these receptors, and is not associated with photophobia for any other reason.

358. The answer is b. *(Brunton, pp 682, 687. Katzung, pp 1076-1077.)* Bismuth salts such as the subsalicylate (best known, perhaps, as the brand-name product Pepto-Bismol) exert antibiotic activity against *H pylori* and probably *E coli* also. They are commonly prescribed for the eradicative therapy of *H pylori*-induced refractory gastric ulcers, along with an antibiotic and metronidazole. The salicylate in this formulation contraindicates its use in children with influenza or any other viral illness, owing to the risk of Reye syndrome. It is somewhat controversial what the term "children" means in this Reye-related context. The risk clearly applies to children in their adolescent (and earlier) years of age, but it may also extend to people younger than about 21 years of age. This is important to know, since children experiencing such viral illnesses as influenza, chickenpox, or even a common cold, may report that their "tummy hurts" and they may experience diarrhea for a variety of reasons. The "pink meds" described in the question are quite well known to many parents. Since they are available OTC (that automatically conveys the notion that they are "safe" and effective), the unknowing caregiver might give the child precisely the wrong drug. Warnings against the use of these bismuth-containing medications are printed on the labels of these products, but as you probably know by now many people don't (or can't) read product labels.

The salicylate component also poses risks in other situations for which a salicylate should be avoided. Aspirin-sensitive asthma is a prime example.

Bismuth salts (or the salicylate moiety specifically) lack significant effects on blood pressure or the effects of antihypertensive drugs (a). There are no well-documented beneficial or adverse effects on signs and symptoms typically associated with menopause (c). Likewise, there are no known desired or unwanted effects on prostate, urinary tract, or ocular function or disease (d), whether in older men or not; no effects on arthritic disease (the salicylate in bismuth subsalicylate is apparently sufficient to warrant the Reye syndrome warning, but not sufficient to favorably influence inflammatory diseases such as arthritis); nor affect signs and symptoms of seasonal (or other) allergic responses (f).

Bismuth salts have no H_2-blocking or muscarinic receptor-blocking activity. In the absence of any contraindications, bismuth subsalicylate may be useful for managing some cases of diarrhea, such as "traveler's diarrhea" that often is caused by *E coli*.

359. The answer is d. *(Brunton, pp 691, 1009, 1012-1014. Katzung, pp 632-633.)* Sulfasalazine, which is a combination of sulfapyridine and 5-aminosalicylic acid (5-ASA) linked covalently (azo bond), is quite effective for managing inflammatory bowel disease (eg, ulcerative colitis and Crohn disease). Some of the sulfasalazine is absorbed, and a portion of that is excreted unchanged back into the colon. Colonic bacteria split the azo linkage, releasing the two drugs. The 5-ASA is responsible for local anti-inflammatory activity (suppression of inflammatory mediators, but how is not well understood) and symptom relief. The sulfapyridine is primarily responsible for side effects associated with this "two drugs in one" combination: nausea, vomiting, and headaches (dose-dependent); sulfonamide allergic reactions in "sulfa-sensitive" patients; and rare but potentially fatal blood reactions including immune-mediated hemolysis and aplastic anemia.

A related drug, mesalamine, contains only the active 5-ASA. Lacking any sulfapyridine, the side effects and adverse responses are very low compared with sulfasalazine. An even neater strategy applies to olsalazine: the drug is comprised of two azo-linked 5-ASA molecules; the bond is cleaved by gut bacteria, releasing two 5-ASA molecules for every molecule of olsalazine administered.

Sulfasalazine is not indicated for antibiotic-induced superinfections/pseudomembranous colitis (a); for *E coli*-induced diarrhea (b); for *H pylori* infections of the GI tract (c); or for prophylaxis of ulcers caused by traditional NSAIDs (e; misoprostol is the drug used for that purpose).

360. The answer is a. *(Brunton, pp 975, 1656. Katzung, p 1069.)* Aluminum salts (other than the phosphate) used therapeutically have a high affinity for phosphate. The aluminum salts bind phosphate in the gut and prevent its absorption quite well. They also induce a blood-to-gut phosphorus gradient that favors elimination of circulating phosphate. (Used inappropriately, aluminum salts other than the phosphate may cause hypophosphatemia: sustained, high-dose use of aluminum-containing antacids is one of the most common causes of hypophosphatemia.) None of the other drugs listed (bismuth subsalicylate, b; magnesium salts, c; sodium bicarbonate, d; sucralfate, e) are effective in or used for reducing phosphate absorption or lowering plasma phosphate levels.

A special note about magnesium salts is warranted, particularly in the context of the scenario described in the question. If I were to ask which is the *least* suitable drug for this dialysis patient, a magnesium salt would be the correct answer. Magnesium salts are systemic: that is, magnesium ions are readily absorbed into the systemic circulation, and normal renal function is a prerequisite for avoiding hypermagnesemia unless the dose of the magnesium is quite small and administration is infrequent. As a result, and regardless of whether a magnesium salt is administered alone or in combination with another antacid (eg, aluminum), giving it to a patient with renal disease can pose significant dangers. Indeed, even modest declines of renal excretory function, regardless of the cause and including that normally associated with older age, weigh against or actually contraindicate use of any magnesium salt as either an antacid or laxative. Similar renal concerns apply to the other systemic antacids: calcium (Ca^{2+} is readily absorbed and when calcium carbonate is administered, Cl^- is eventually formed and absorbed); and sodium bicarbonate (both Na^+ and HCO_3^- are readily absorbed).

361. The answer is b. *(Brunton, pp 999-1003. Katzung, pp 1082-1083.)* Constipation is the most common and most worrisome adverse response to alosetron. This drug's mechanism of desired action involves selective blockade of serotonin receptors (5-HT_3) in the gut; the main outcomes include slowing of colonic transport time, increased sodium and water reabsorption from the colon, and reduced secretion of water and electrolytes into the colon.

Although constipation might be viewed as a trivial, minor, or merely annoying complaint with most drugs, with alosetron it is worrisome. It may progress to fecal impaction, bowel perforation or obstruction, and ischemic colitis. Fatalities have occurred. These risks are such that the drug was pulled from the market in early 2000 and reapproved 2 years later with a limited indication (prolonged, severe diarrhea associated with irritable bowel syndrome in women); strong warnings in the package insert; and a comprehensive risk-management/-avoidance program that includes a requirement for (among other things) a special "sign-off" by both the prescriber and the patient that they understand, acknowledge, and can identify the risks and agree to treatment anyway.

Serious cardiac arrhythmias (a), extrapyramidal reactions (c), pulmonary fibrosis (d), or renal failure (e) are not the most likely or most worrisome adverse effects associated with alosetron.

362. The answer is b. *(Brunton, pp 1000-1003. Katzung, p 295.)* The antiemetic effects of ondansetron—a drug that is widely and effectively used to manage nausea and emesis associated with chemotherapy or surgery—is mainly due to blockade of 5-HT_3 receptors in the brain's chemoreceptor trigger zone (CTZ) and, probably, in the solitary tract nucleus and in the stomach and small intestine.

Activation of μ-opioid receptors in the CTZ (a) is what causes the nausea and emesis that is so common with such drugs as morphine and other opioid analgesics.

Blockade of central dopamine receptors (c), particularly D_2 receptors in the CTZ, is the main mechanism by which phenothiazines (eg, chlorpromazine, prochlorperazine) cause their antinausea/antiemetic effects. They are useful and effective for some patients with chemotherapy-induced nausea and vomiting, but better suited for prophylaxis of these symptoms due to other causes or for prophylaxis of motion sickness. Central antimuscarinic and antihistaminic actions may contribute to the overall effects.

Blockade of H_1-histamine receptors (d) in the brain stem and vestibular apparatus of the inner ear accounts for the main mechanism of action of such drugs as cyclizine, diphenhydramine (and its derivative, dimenhydrinate), and hydroxyzine. Antimuscarinic effects of these antihistamines may contribute to the overall effect. They are best suited for motion sickness prophylaxis, as opposed to treating it; less effective as "general antiemetics;" and not very effective or well tolerated at usual full therapeutic doses for chemotherapy-induced symptoms.

Antimuscarinic agents (e; scopolamine can be considered the prototype in terms of motion sickness or emesis control) do not exert their effects via actions on the GI musculature, although suppression of ACh-mediated GI motility and tone certainly occurs. Rather, their effects occur in the central nervous system.

Endocrine Pharmacology, Uterine Stimulants and Relaxants

- Anabolic steroids, testosterone, related drugs
- Calcium-regulating drugs, including parathyroid hormone and vitamin D
- Corticosteroids
- Diabetes mellitus and hypoglycemia
- Diagnosis, management, of adrenal dysfunction
- Erectile dysfunction
- Estrogens, progestins, contraceptives, fertility agents
- Thyroid disorders

Questions

363. A 20-year-old woman, otherwise healthy, presents with irregular and occasionally missed menstrual periods, oily facial skin and acne, and slight hirsutism. She was a competitive runner during high school, and now is in training for a triathlon. She is not taking any medications other than an estrogen-progesterone oral contraceptive. A pelvic ultrasound evaluation reveals numerous immature ovarian follicles (generally but incorrectly referred to as cysts). The diagnosis is polycystic ovarian syndrome. Which of the following drugs would be the most rational initial therapy to prescribe to help provide symptom relief without compromising the woman's ability to conceive?

a. Estrogen (dose higher than in her oral contraceptive)
b. Ketoconazole
c. Metformin
d. Prednisone (or a similar oral glucocorticoid)
e. Testosterone

364. A patient with a previously undiagnosed thyroid cancer presents with thyrotoxicosis. One drug that is administered as part of early management, and may be lifesaving, is propranolol. Which of the following best summarizes why we give this drug, or what we want it to do?

a. Block parenchymal cell receptors for thyroid hormones
b. Block thyroid hormone release by a direct effect on the gland
c. Inhibit thyroid hormone synthesis
d. Lessen dangerous cardiovascular signs and symptoms of thyroid hormone excess
e. Lower TSH levels

Questions 365 and 366

The next two questions (365 and 366) apply to a 44-year-old businessman who was just diagnosed with Type 2 diabetes mellitus. His HbA_{1c} is now 8.5%, equivalent to an estimated average plasma glucose (eAG) of about 200 mg/dL. He also has essential hypertension for which he is taking an ACE inhibitor; it maintains his resting blood pressure at around 130/90 mm Hg—no greater than 130/80 is a preferred target for patients with diabetes. You prescribed an exercise and diet plan, but this gentleman wouldn't be compliant. He habitually has a morning cup of black coffee, gets in his car, and drives until late afternoon visiting his clients. He says he rarely stops and eats in between. He is what many physicians would call a "meal skipper."

His evening meals are large and contain an excess of calories from fats and carbohydrates, and very little dietary fiber. He also likes to snack before bedtime. Not surprisingly, his plasma glucose levels swing widely from quite low (65-75 mg/dL) before his evening meal to very high (sometimes as high as 250-300 mg/dL) postprandial levels.

365. You would like to get this man's HbA_{1c} down to a maximum of 7.5%. Knowing his poor eating habits, you are rightly concerned about the diabetes drug you prescribe causing or worsening hypoglycemia that you've documented after what amounts to 18-hour daily fasts. Which drug poses the greatest relative risk of causing or exacerbating his hypoglycemia, even though it may help keep peak glucose concentrations at a more acceptable level?

a. Acarbose
b. Glyburide
c. Metformin
d. Pioglitazone
e. Repaglinide

366. You are contemplating prescribing metformin for this gentleman. If you do, which effect, typically associated with this drug compared with other oral antidiabetic medications, is most likely to occur?

a. Further suppression of appetite
b. Induction or worsening of essential hypertension
c. Lactic acidosis
d. Onset of heart failure
e. Rises of HDL cholesterol and triglyceride levels

367. A woman deemed at high risk of postmenopausal osteoporosis is started on alendronate. What is this representative bisphosphonate's main mechanism of action?

a. Activates vitamin D
b. Directly forms hydroxyapatite crystals in bone
c. Provides supplemental calcium in the diet
d. Provides supplemental phosphate, which indirectly elevates plasma Ca^{2+}
e. Reduces the number and activity of osteoclasts in bone

368. Some patients who are taking high doses of a bisphosphonate for Paget disease of the bone develop an endocrine/metabolic disorder. Which of the following would that be?

a. Cushing syndrome
b. Diabetes insipidus
c. Diabetes mellitus
d. Hyperparathyroidism
e. Hyperthyroidism

369. Metyrapone is useful in testing hyper- or hypofunction of certain endocrine conditions or biological processes those glands normally control. When we administer this drug for diagnostic purposes, which structure or function are we most likely assessing?

a. α Cells of pancreatic islets
b. β Cells of pancreatic islets
c. Leydig cells of the testes
d. Pituitary-adrenal axis
e. Thyroid gland's response to TSH

370. A 60-year-old man on long-term therapy with a drug develops hypertension, hyperglycemia, and decreased bone density. Blood tests indicate anemia. Some of his stool samples initially were positive for occult blood, and then the stool developed a "coffee-grounds" appearance. Which of the following is most likely responsible for the patient's symptoms?

a. Beclomethasone
b. Hydrochlorothiazide
c. Metformin
d. Pamidronate
e. Prednisone

371. A woman with atrial fibrillation is being treated long-term with amiodarone (and warfarin). This antiarrhythmic can cause biochemical changes and clinical signs and symptoms that resemble those associated with which of the following endocrine disorders?

a. Addisonian crisis
b. Cushing syndrome
c. Diabetes insipidus
d. Diabetes mellitus
e. Hypothyroidism
f. Ovarian hyperstimulation syndrome

372. A 22-year-old woman has been sexually assaulted and she wishes to have the pregnancy terminated by pharmacologic means. What is generally the most appropriate drug, assuming no contraindications?

a. Ergonovine (or methylergonovine)
b. Mifepristone
c. Raloxifene
d. Tamoxifen
e. Terbutaline

373. A patient has hyperthyroidism from a thyroid cancer, and the medical team concludes that oral radioiodine (sodium iodide 131 [^{131}I]) is the preferred treatment. The dosage is calculated correctly, and the drug is administered. What statement about this approach is also correct?

a. A β-adrenergic blocker should not be used for symptom control if or when ^{131}I is used.
b. Hyperthyroidism symptoms resolve almost completely within 24 to 48 hours after dosing with ^{131}I.
c. Many patients treated with ^{131}I develop metastatic nonthyroid cancers in response to the drug.
d. Oral antithyroid drugs should be administered up to and including the day of ^{131}I administration.
e. There is a high incidence of delayed hypothyroidism after using ^{131}I for eradication of a thyroid tumor, and so thyroid hormone supplements may be needed later on.

374. A patient has an inoperable pancreatic islet cell carcinoma and is chronically hypoglycemic. Which drug would be most likely chosen for relatively long-term oral therapy that attempts to raise blood glucose levels into a more acceptable range?

a. Atenolol (or metoprolol)
b. Diazoxide
c. Glucagon
d. Octreotide (somatostatin analog)
e. Oxytocin

375. A 50-year-old woman at very high risk of breast cancer is given tamoxifen for prophylaxis. What is the main mechanism or effect of this drug?

a. Blocks estrogen receptors in breast tissue
b. Blocks estrogen receptors in the endometrium
c. Increases the risk of osteoporosis
d. Raises plasma LDL cholesterol and total cholesterol, lowers HDL
e. Reduces the risk of thromboembolic disorders

376. A 50-year-old woman is recently diagnosed with Type 2 diabetes mellitus. Exercise and diet do not provide adequate glycemic control, so drug therapy needs to start. The physician contemplates prescribing metformin. Which of the following statements about this drug is correct?

a. Beneficial and unwanted actions are unaffected by liver function status.
b. Lactic acidosis occurs frequently, but it is seldom serious.
c. Metformin-induced hypoglycemia seldom occurs.
d. Useful for Type 1 diabetes also.
e. Weight gain is a common and unwanted side effect.

377. A 76-year-old man complains of progressive difficulty starting his urine stream and having to get up several times during each night to urinate. Rectal examination reveals a generally enlarged, smooth-surfaced prostate. Prostate-specific antigen (PSA) titers are elevated. Finasteride treatment is started and eventually urine flow increases and prostate size decreases. Which of the following phrases best summarizes the mechanism by which finasteride caused symptom relief?

a. Blocks α-adrenergic receptors
b. Blocks testosterone receptors
c. Inhibits dihydrotestosterone synthesis
d. Inhibits testosterone synthesis
e. Lowers plasma testosterone levels by increasing its renal clearance

378. A stubborn patient with Type 2 diabetes mellitus is notoriously noncompliant with medication and diet recommendations. However, he thinks he's smart enough to fool the physician into thinking otherwise: he takes his medication and eliminates nearly all carbohydrate intake for a few days before each clinic visit, knowing he will get a finger stick for a spot check of plasma glucose levels. What measurement would be the simplest, most cost-effective, and most informative way for the physician to assess for past drug and diet compliance and long-term glycemic control?

a. Glucose concentration in venous blood sample
b. Glucose tolerance test (oral)
c. HbA_{1c}
d. Plasma levels of the antidiabetic drug
e. Urine ketone levels (in a sample donated at the time of clinic visit)
f. Urine glucose levels

379. Most therapeutic insulins nowadays are modifications of native human insulin, done by substituting some amino acids in the native protein using recombinant DNA technology. For all these genetically modified insulins, what is the one common result of such changes?

a. Changes the onsets, durations of action
b. Enables administration by either subcutaneous or intravenous routes
c. Prevents cellular K^+ uptake as glucose enters cells
d. Reactivates endogenous (pancreatic) insulin synthesis
e. Selectively affects glucose metabolism, little/no effects on lipids

380. You have prescribed an oral agent to help control a patient's blood glucose levels. He has Type 2 diabetes. In explaining how the drug works, you describe it as inhibiting the intestinal uptake of complex carbohydrates in the diet. You advise also that flatus or some cramping or "grumbling sounds" in the belly may develop. Which of the following drugs fits this description?

a. Acarbose
b. Any thiazolidinedione ("glitazone")
c. Glipizide
d. Metformin
e. Tolbutamide

381. A patient with Type 1 diabetes is being treated with insulin glargine. What clinically important property sets this particular insulin apart, or otherwise differentiates it, from nearly all the other insulin formulations that might be used instead?

a. Blood levels, hypoglycemic effects, following insulin glargine injection are more accurately described as a plateau rather as a definite "spike" or peak.
b. Disulfiram-like reactions (acetaldehyde accumulation from inhibited EtOH metabolism) are more common, severe, with insulin glargine.
c. Has an extremely fast onset, useful for immediate postprandial control of plasma glucose elevations.
d. Poses little or no risk of hypoglycemia if the patient skips several meals in a row.
e. Sensitizes parenchymal cells to insulin (eg, the administered insulin itself), not simply providing or replacing insulin, thereby enhancing glycemic control.

382. A patient presents in the emergency department with a massive overdose of a drug. The most worrisome signs and symptoms include excessive cardiac stimulation (severe tachycardia, palpitations, angina, etc). The ED physician orders IV administration a β-adrenergic blocker, saying (correctly) it is the only drug likely to normalize cardiac function quickly and save the patient's life. What was the most likely drug the patient overdosed on?

a. A second-generation sulfonylurea (eg, glipizide, glyburide)
b. Insulin
c. Levothyroxine
d. Prednisone (oral glucocorticoid)
e. Propylthiouracil

383. This week finds you accompanying an attending in her outpatient endocrinology clinic. One patient, a 56-year-old woman, is taking exenatide, which is classified as an incretin mimetic. Which of the following phrases best describes exenatide's actions or main clinical use?

a. Antagonizes testosterone effects, useful for treating hirsutism in men or women
b. Is a new adjunct to metformin and/or sulfonylurea therapy of hyperthyroidism
c. Often used as an add-on to a bisphosphonate for prophylaxis of postmenopausal osteoporosis
d. Preferred stimulant of cortisol production for treating Addison disease
e. Useful adjunct for some patients with poorly controlled Type 2 diabetes mellitus

384. A patient with hypothyroidism following thyroidectomy will require lifelong hormone replacement therapy. What drug or formulation generally would be most suitable?

a. Levothyroxine (T_4)
b. Liothyronine
c. Liotrix
d. Protirelin
e. Thyroid, desiccated

385. A patient develops marked skeletal muscle tetany soon after a recent thyroidectomy. The attending confirms the diagnosis, in part, by lightly tapping the patient's cheek in front of the ear. Stimulating the facial nerves in this manner leads to spasms of the local (oris) muscle (Chvostek sign). Which of the following drugs is most likely to be chosen to manage this adverse response to surgery?

a. Calcitonin
b. Calcium gluconate
c. Plicamycin (mithramycin)
d. PTH (parathyroid hormone)
e. Vitamin D

386. A 40-year-old man with a symmetrically enlarged thyroid gland associated with elevated levels of T_3 and T_4 is treated with propylthiouracil (PTU). Which of the following phrases best summarizes the principal mechanism of action of PTU?

a. Blocks iodide transport into the thyroid
b. Increases hepatic metabolic inactivation of circulating T_4 and T_3
c. Inhibits proteolysis of thyroglobulin
d. Inhibits thyroidal peroxidase
e. Releases T_3 and T_4 into the blood

387. The attending in the endocrine/metabolic diseases clinic prescribes colesevelam as add-on therapy for a 58-year-old man with Type 2 diabetes who is not getting adequate glycemic control (based on high levels of HbA_{1c} measured twice in the last 12 months) from his current medications: metformin and glyburide. The man has been a pack-a-day cigarette smoker for 40 years and says he "can't seem to quit." In addition to the diabetes and nicotine addiction he has several other comorbidities that are not optimally managed with his current medications for each, or recommended lifestyle modifications (he largely ignores them). The attending states that the colesevelam might just help one of those comorbidities in addition to possibly lowering HbA_{1c} levels after a few months on the drug. Which of the following is the "other condition" that is most likely to be favorably and rather directly influenced by the colesevelam?

a. Chronic bronchitis (or emphysema)
b. Hyperlipidemias
c. Hyperuricemia, gout
d. Nicotine addiction
e. Prostatism (ie, benign prostatic hypertrophy)

388. Your patient, who is taking an oral contraceptive, has heard about and asks about the risk of thromboembolism as a result of taking these drugs. To reduce the risk of this potentially severe adverse hematologic response, but still provide reasonably effective contraception, what would you prescribe?

a. A combination product with a higher estrogen dose
b. A combination product with a higher progestin dose
c. A combination product with a lower estrogen dose
d. A combination product with a lower progestin dose
e. An OC that contains only estrogen

389. A woman goes into premature labor, and the physician orders slow intravenous infusion of terbutaline. Uterine contractions are suppressed in a desirable way, but her pulse rate rises. What is the main mechanism of action by which this drug slows or suppresses uterine contractions, and increases cardiac rate too?

a. Blocks prostaglandin synthesis
b. Blocks uterine oxytocin receptors
c. Inhibits oxytocin release from the posterior pituitary
d. Inhibits oxytocin synthesis in the hypothalamus
e. Stimulates α-adrenergic receptors
f. Stimulates β-adrenergic receptors

390. A 27-year-old woman is diagnosed with hypercortism. To determine whether cortisol production is independent of pituitary gland control, you decide to suppress ACTH production by giving a high-potency glucocorticoid. Which of the following drugs would be the best choice for this purpose?

a. Dexamethasone
b. Hydrocortisone
c. Methylprednisolone
d. Prednisone
e. Triamcinolone

391. A patient with Cushing disease is being treated by X-irradiation of the pituitary. It may take several months of this therapy for adequate symptomatic and metabolic improvement. Until that time, which of the following drugs would be administered to suppress adrenal cortical glucocorticoid synthesis?

a. Cimetidine
b. Cortisol (high pharmacologic doses)
c. Fludrocortisone
d. Ketoconazole
e. Spironolactone

392. A woman who has been taking an oral contraceptive (estrogen plus progestin) for several years is diagnosed with epilepsy and started on phenytoin. What is the most likely consequence of adding the phenytoin?

a. Agranulocytosis or aplastic anemia, requiring stopping both drugs immediately
b. Breakthrough seizures from increased phenytoin clearance
c. Phenytoin toxicity, significant and of fast onset
d. Reduced contraceptive efficacy
e. Thromboembolism from the estrogen component of the contraceptive

393. A woman wants a prescription for an oral contraceptive, and your choice is between an estrogen-progestin combination and a "minipill" (progestin only). Compared with a hormone combination product, which of the following is the main difference that would occur if a progestin-only approach were used?

a. Better contraceptive efficacy
b. Direct spermicidal effects
c. Higher risk of thromboembolism
d. More menstrual irregularities (irregular cycle length, amenorrhea, spotting, etc)
e. Poorer compliance due to taking the drug on an irregular cycle, rather than daily

394. A woman is taking an estrogen-progestin combination oral contraceptive. She experiences a multitude of side effects. Which of the following side effects is most likely due to what can be described as an "estrogen excess," and not likely due to the progestin component of the medication?

a. Fatigue
b. Hypertension
c. Hypomenorrhea
d. Increased appetite
e. Weight gain

395. A comatose patient with an endocrine disorder undergoes a computed tomography (CT) diagnostic procedure that involves contrast media that has a tendency to induce lactic acidosis. He is also taking a drug that, in its own right, may cause lactic acidosis. Normally the drug would be stopped, at least temporarily, two days before the CT, but due to the patient's acute and serious illness that could not be done. Lactic acidosis indeed develops and the patient nearly dies. Which of the following drugs is the most likely cause of this severe and potentially fatal metabolic derangement?

a. Insulin glargine, prescribed for Type 1 diabetes mellitus
b. Levothyroxine, prescribed to maintain euthyroid status following thyroidectomy
c. Metformin, prescribed for Type 2 diabetes mellitus
d. Propylthiouracil, prescribed for hyperthyroidism
e. Spironolactone, prescribed for an adrenal cortical tumor

396. A patient with Type 2 diabetes mellitus begins gaining weight after several months of therapy with an oral antidiabetic agent. A complete workup indicates edema and other signs and symptoms of heart failure. Which antidiabetic drug or group was the most likely cause?

a. Acarbose
b. Biguanides
c. Glitazones (thiazolidinediones, such as rosiglitazone)
d. Metformin
e. Sulfonylureas, both first- and second-generation agents (eg, tolbutamide, chlorpropamide, glyburide, glipizide)

397. A woman goes into premature labor early enough that there are great concerns about inadequate fetal lung development and the risk of fetal respiratory distress syndrome. Terbutaline therapy is started to slow labor, but parturition seems imminent. Which other adjunct should be administered prepartum, specifically for the purpose of reducing the risks and complications of the newborn's immature respiratory system development?

a. Albuterol
b. Betamethasone
c. Ergonovine (or methylergonovine)
d. Indomethacin
e. Magnesium sulfate

398. We prescribe etidronate for a postmenopausal woman who is at great risk for developing osteoporosis. Which of the following side effects or adverse responses to this drug is the patient most likely to experience?

a. Cholelithiasis
b. Esophagitis
c. Fluid/electrolyte loss from profuse diarrhea
d. Hepatic necrosis
e. Renal damage from calcium stone formation
f. Tetany

399. A 75-year-old man had surgery for prostate carcinoma, and local metastases were found intraoperatively. Which of the following is the most appropriate follow-up drug aimed at treating the metastases?

a. Aminoglutethimide
b. Fludrocortisone
c. Leuprolide
d. Mifepristone
e. Spironolactone

400. A 53-year-old woman with Type 2 diabetes mellitus is started on glyburide. Diet, exercise, and usually effective doses of metformin have not provided adequate glycemic control based on periodic measurements of HbA_{1c}. What is the primary mechanism by which the glyburide is likely to provide better glycemic control?

a. Decrease insulin resistance by lowering body weight.
b. Enhance renal excretion of glucose.
c. Increase insulin synthesis.
d. Promote glucose uptake by muscle, liver, and adipose tissue via an insulin-independent process.
e. Release insulin from the pancreas.

401. A 75-year-old woman with Type 2 diabetes is taking an oral antidiabetic drug. One day she goes without eating for 18 hours, but takes her drug nonetheless. She is transported to the emergency department after passing out. Her plasma glucose concentration is 48 mg/dL (hypoglycemic) upon arrival at the ED, and she is in very serious condition. Which of the following drugs did she most likely take?

a. Acarbose
b. Glyburide
c. Metformin
d. Pioglitazone
e. Rosiglitazone

402. A man with Type 2 diabetes is receiving a combination of oral drugs to maintain glycemic control. He becomes hypoglycemic one afternoon and ingests some orange juice and two chocolate bars—all containing abundant amounts of sugars. Nonetheless his blood glucose levels remain low, his symptoms persist. Which of the following antidiabetic drugs that he was taking accounted for the failure of oral sugars to restore his plasma glucose?

a. Acarbose
b. Glyburide
c. Metformin
d. Repaglinide
e. Rosiglitazone

403. A 35-year-old woman has Graves disease, a small goiter, and symptoms that are deemed "mild-to-moderate." Propylthiouracil is prescribed. What is the most serious adverse response to this drug, for which close monitoring is required?

a. Agranulocytosis
b. Cholestatic jaundice
c. Gout
d. Renal tubular necrosis
e. Rhabdomyolysis
f. Thyroid cancer

404. A 60-year-old man with Type 2 diabetes mellitus is treated with pioglitazone (in addition to a proper diet and exercise). Which of the following phrases summarizes best this drug's main mechanism of action?

a. Blocks intestinal carbohydrate absorption
b. Causes glycosuria (increased renal glucose excretion)
c. Increases hepatic gluconeogenesis
d. Increases release of endogenous insulin
e. Increases target tissue sensitivity to insulin

405. A 27-year-old woman with endometriosis is treated with danazol. What is the most likely drug-induced side effect or adverse response associated with this drug, and for which you should be monitoring closely?

a. Anemia from excessive vaginal bleeding
b. Abnormal liver function tests
c. Psychosis
d. Thrombocytopenia
e. Weight loss

406. A patient with a history of Type 2 diabetes mellitus presents in the emergency department. His complaints include nonspecific gastrointestinal symptoms, including nausea and vomiting. He states he is bloated and has abdominal pain. His appetite has been suppressed for several days. He has malaise and difficulty breathing. His liver is enlarged and tender; liver function tests indicate hepatic damage. Plasma bicarbonate is low and lactate levels are high. Kidney function is falling rapidly.

The diagnosis is lactic acidosis, and the suspicion is that it was caused by an antidiabetic drug. Which of the following drugs is this patient most likely taking?

a. Acarbose
b. Glipizide
c. Glyburide
d. Metformin
e. Rosiglitazone

407. A patient is transported to the emergency department shortly after taking a massive overdose of her levothyroxine in an apparent suicide attempt. Which of the following drugs should we administer for prompt control of the hormone-related effects that are most likely to lead to her death if not correctly managed?

a. Iodine/iodide
b. Liothyronine
c. Propranolol
d. Propylthiouracil
e. Radioiodine (^{131}I)

408. There are two main formulations of oral contraceptives: those that are estrogen-progestin combinations, and those that contain only progestin ("minipill"). What is the main mechanism by which these drugs exert their desired contraceptive effects?

a. Acidify the cervical mucus, thereby making the mucus spermicidal.
b. Displace/detach a fertilized egg from the endometrium.
c. Inhibit nidation (implantation of a fertilized ovum).
d. Inhibit ovulation.
e. Reduce uterine blood flow such that the fertilized ovum becomes hypoxic and dies.

409. A 55-year-old postmenopausal woman develops weakness, polyuria, polydipsia, and significant increases of plasma creatinine concentration. A computed tomogram (CT scan) indicates nephrocalcinosis. A drug is considered to be the cause. Which of the following drugs is most likely responsible?

a. Estrogens
b. Etidronate
c. Glipizide
d. Prednisone
e. Vitamin D

410. A patient has severe Cushing disease. Surgery cannot be scheduled for several months, so the physician plans to treat the patient in the interim with a drug that she describes as a "potent inhibitor of corticosteroid synthesis." Which of the following drugs best fits that description?

a. Dexamethasone
b. Hydrocortisone
c. Ketoconazole
d. Prednisone
e. Spironolactone

411. We prescribe bromocriptine for a woman with primary amenorrhea. Normal menstruation returns about a month after starting therapy. Which of the following statements best describes the mechanism by which bromocriptine caused its desired effects?

a. Blocked estrogen receptors, enhanced gonadotropin release
b. Increased follicle-stimulating hormone (FSH) synthesis
c. Inhibited prolactin release
d. Stimulated ovarian estrogen and progestin synthesis
e. Stimulated gonadotropin-releasing hormone (GnRH) release

412. A patient has had his parathyroid glands excised during a total thyroidectomy. In addition to requiring supplemental thyroid hormone, interventions aimed at correcting hypoparathyroidism will be necessary. What is the main physiologic action or role of parathyroid hormone—one that necessitates suitable therapy?

a. Decreases active absorption of Ca from the small intestine
b. Decreases excretion of phosphate
c. Decreases renal tubular reabsorption of calcium
d. Decreases resorption of phosphate from bone
e. Increases mobilization of calcium from bone

413. A 55-year-old male patient with a 20-year history of Type 2 diabetes mellitus comes to your clinic for his regular checkup. He looks good, feels well. However, over the last year his HbA_{1c} levels hovered around 9.5% (equivalent to an average plasma glucose of around 225 mg/dL). Current diabetes medications are metformin and glyburide. The patient says he is doing "the best he can" with recommended diet and exercise plans. He has other personal and familial risk factors for coronary heart disease. He takes a statin to control his lipids, but his LDL and triglyceride levels are far too high. He is taking verapamil for Stage 1 hypertension, but his pressure is still higher than you'd like it to be. Two years ago, he had one episode of angina from atherosclerotic coronary disease and underwent angioplasty and placement of a stent. He has had no ischemic episodes since.

You're thinking about adding niacin to get further control of triglyceride levels, adding another antihypertensive drug, and adjusting his diabetes treatment by adding another hypoglycemic drug (perhaps insulin). Which comorbidity or other factor would weigh against your selection of an angiotensin-converting enzyme (ACE) inhibitor or angiotensin receptor blocker (ARB) as the add-on antihypertensive drug for this diabetic patient?

a. Bilateral renal artery stenosis and albuminuria
b. Bradycardia
c. Had two episodes of hyperosmolar hyperglycemic nonketotic syndrome in past 2 years
d. Has heart failure
e. Niacin will indeed be prescribed

Endocrine Pharmacology, Uterine Stimulants and Relaxants

Answers

363. The answer is c. *(Brunton, pp 1627, 1638-1641. Katzung, pp 471-472, 741-742.)* Polycystic ovarian syndrome (PCOS) is the most common endocrine disorder in young postpubertal women, and is characterized by not only the signs and symptoms noted in the question, but also others that are accompanied or caused by relative androgen excess (thus eliminating testosterone, e, as an answer). Just as metformin is often helpful in Type 2 diabetes, through its insulin-sensitizing effects on parenchymal cells (adipocytes, muscle), so it is in PCOS; an added benefit, indirectly, is a reduction of circulating androgen levels. (Glitazones, eg, rosiglitazone, also seem to be effective.)

Higher dosages of estrogen (a) might help the signs and symptoms of PCOS, but obviously that approach would not preserve or improve fertility as long as the drug is being taken. Ketoconazole (b), a powerful inhibitor of steroidogenesis, is too nonselective in terms of its inhibitory effects, affecting synthesis of not only cortisol but also many other steroid hormones—and the metabolism of many drugs. Prednisone (d) or another glucocorticoid would be irrational, if for no other reason than the fact that these drugs will further raise blood glucose levels—a particularly unwanted effect considering the parenchymal cell insulin resistance that is a component of PCOS. Testosterone (e) is obviously inappropriate given the relative androgen excess already present in PCOS.

364. The answer is d. *(Brunton, pp 290, 1530. Katzung, p 677.)* In thyrotoxicosis/thyroid storm, essentially the only effect of administering a β-adrenergic blocker—and it is an important effect, to be sure—is to provide prompt relief of both relatively innocuous manifestations of thyroid hormone excess, such as tremor, and those that are much more dangerous, including significant and potentially life-threatening increases in cardiac rate, contractility, and automaticity. Circulating thyroid hormone levels modulate the responsiveness of β-adrenergic receptors to their agonists (eg, epinephrine, norepinephrine). When thyroid hormone levels are excessive, so is adrenergic receptor responsiveness. Therefore, we can reduce the adrenergic consequences of the hormone excess using a β-blocker. There are no effects on thyroid hormone levels or thyroid gland function or control.

None of the β-adrenergic blockers block the agonist effects of thyroid hormones on their receptors (a), nor do they inhibit thyroid hormone release (b) or synthesis (c). They do not alter TSH levels (e) directly or indirectly.

365. The answer is b. *(Brunton, pp 1636-1637. Katzung, pp 738-740.)* A side effect common to the newer sulfonylureas (glyburide, glipizide, glimepiride) is hypoglycemia, and the relative incidence is higher than with any of the other drugs listed.

Normally insulin release peaks in response to a meal. That occurs even when there is a relative insulin deficiency (Type 2 diabetes mellitus). Our hypothetical meal-skipping patient essentially fasts all day. His blood glucose levels will tend to fall as the meal-free interval progresses, and during this time physiologic insulin release would be relatively low. However, the newer sulfonylureas—glyburide, glipizide, glimepiride—act by causing insulin release, whether one has eaten or fasted. Thus, the hypoglycemic effect of the drug will enhance the tendency for hypoglycemia that accompanies fasting or that occurs with increased physical activity. This is likely to apply even in the presence of insulin resistance, which is common.

Acarbose (a) is an α-glucosidase inhibitor administered to some patients with Type 2 diabetes mellitus. Its main effect is a reduced rate of carbohydrate absorption from the gut. This blunts the insulin response to rising blood glucose levels. Because acarbose's effects center on inhibiting dietary carbohydrate absorption, the drug's effects will not occur in the absence of those foodstuffs. Indeed, effects are better when the drug is taken with or right before meals, and it seems to be more efficacious as the amount of carbohydrate in the meal increases.

Metformin (c) does not directly increase or decrease insulin secretion. In contrast with the sulfonylureas, which are correctly classified as hypoglycemic drugs (ie, they drive blood glucose levels down), the biguanides are antihyperglycemic, tending to keep blood glucose levels from going up rather than driving them down.

Pioglitazone (a thiazolidinedione, or "glitazone" for short) sensitizes parenchymal cells (mainly adipocytes) to insulin and so reduces insulin resistance. (The glitazones apparently activate a nuclear peroxisomal proliferator-activated receptor, PPAR-γ, that participates in the cellular response to insulin.)

Because of the insulin-dependency of their actions, the intensity of the effects of a glitazone increase when insulin levels are high (eg, postprandial) and diminish markedly as insulin levels fall (eg, fasting, which this patient does). Regardless, and unless a glitazone is prescribed with insulin or a sulfonylurea (common), the incidence of drug-induced hypoglycemia is low.

Repaglinide, a meglitinide, seems to trigger pancreatic insulin release in the presence of sufficient (and high) blood glucose levels. However, when blood glucose levels are sufficiently low (as can occur during fasting or meal-skipping), the insulin-releasing effect wanes and so the drug is not likely to cause or worsen hypoglycemia.

366. The answer is a. *(Brunton, pp 1636, 1638-1640. Katzung, pp 471-472, 741-742.)* Antidiabetic drugs, particularly the oral agents, are sometimes described as being weight-neutral, -positive, or -negative. This is based to a great degree on whether, how well, or how often, they increase or decrease appetite. Metformin is often weight-negative. It tends to suppress appetite—good for patients who overeat or otherwise eat improperly and can benefit from even a slight anorexigenic effect. We certainly do not use metformin as an anorexigenic drug, in the presence or absence of diabetes (or such other disorders as polycystic ovarian syndrome), but the effect occurs, quite commonly, nonetheless. Note that in the context of our "meal-skipping" patient further suppression of appetite is not necessarily desirable (except, perhaps, to suppress his excessive evening food intake), but it does happen.

There is no reason to suspect metformin will cause or worsen hypertension (b). In fact, improvement of glycemic control can actually be beneficial to some hypertensive patients, provided other lifestyle modifications and proper antihypertensive drugs are used. Lactic acidosis (c) is a major—if not the most worrisome and severe—adverse response to metformin. However, it's important to stress that this serious condition is unique to metformin, compared with all other antidiabetic drugs, but it occurs rarely. (You still need to be aware of this, however, because should lactic acidosis develop, the mortality rate is quite high.) Metformin is not likely to cause or worsen heart failure (d). Among the oral antidiabetic drugs, that's rather uniquely associated with the glitazones (pioglitazone, rosiglitazone). And you might want to recall that the sulfonylureas—particularly the older ones (eg, tolbutamide, chlorpropamide)—have been associated with sudden cardiac death. Less likely with newer agents such as glipizide and glyburide, but the warning (eg, in the package insert) is there for them too. Metformin has no direct or significant effects on plasma lipid profiles. Here again, controlling diabetes has secondary benefits on dyslipidemias, but no antidiabetic drug is used specifically for that purpose.

367. The answer is e. *(Brunton, pp 1666-1668. Katzung, pp 759, 762.)* Whether used for osteoporosis (prevention or management, men or women, idiopathic or drug-induced) or Paget disease of the bone, bisphosphonates exert their effects on osteoclasts and osteoblasts. The drug is incorporated into bone. When drug-containing bone is resorbed by the osteoclasts, osteoclast function (and, so, subsequent bone resorption) is inhibited. The bisphosphonates also recruit osteoblasts, which then produce a substance that further inhibits osteoclast activity.

Bisphosphonates in general or alendronate in particular, do not activate vitamin D (a); form hydroxyapatite crystals in bone (b); or provide supplemental calcium (c) or phosphate (d).

368. The answer is d. *(Brunton, p 1668. Katzung, pp 754-755, 759, 762.)* You should be able to deduce hyperparathyroidism as the answer by recalling that the bisphosphonates ultimately affect bone Ca^{2+} metabolism, and the parathyroid gland is the main regulator of plasma Ca^{2+} levels. When a bisphosphonate is given to a patient with Paget disease of the bone, after about a week the dramatic inhibition of bone resorption markedly lowers plasma Ca^{2+} levels (because an important portion of plasma Ca^{2+} arises from bone that is being resorbed). When plasma Ca^{2+} falls considerably, parathyroid hyperfunction can develop. The easiest way to prevent this is to administer dietary calcium supplements along with the bisphosphonate.

Bisphosphonate administration is not associated with or a cause of Cushing disease (a), diabetes insipidus (b) or mellitus (c), or hyperthyroidism (e).

369. The answer is d. *(Brunton, pp 1610-1611. Katzung, pp 693-694.)* Metyrapone, because it decreases plasma levels of cortisol by inhibiting the 11β-hydroxylation of steroids in the adrenal, can be used to assess function of the pituitary-adrenal cortical axis. When metyrapone is given to normal persons, the adenohypophysis secretes more ACTH. This causes a normal adrenal cortex to synthesize increased amounts of 17-hydroxylated steroids, which can be measured in the urine. However, patients who have disease of the hypothalamic-pituitary axis do not produce ACTH in response to metyrapone. As a result, we find no increased levels of the steroids in the urine. Before administering metyrapone we need to test responsiveness of the adrenal cortex to respond to administration of ACTH.

Metyrapone has no significant effects on α cells of the pancreas (glucagon-secreting, a) or the β cells (b); on Leydig cells of the testes (testosterone-secreting, c); or on direct responses of the thyroid gland to TSH (e).

370. The answer is e. *(Brunton, pp 1603-1604. Katzung, pp 347-348, 351-352, 635.)* These findings are characteristic of what one would expect with long-term (and/or high-dose) systemic glucocorticoid therapy (ie, prednisone and many others, but not beclomethasone, a, which is given by oral inhalation and is not absorbed appreciably). Psychoses, peptic ulceration with hemorrhage (coffee-grounds stool, indicative of gastric bleeding) or without (possibly causing guaiac-positive stools), increased susceptibility to infection, edema, osteoporosis, myopathy, and hypokalemic alkalosis can occur. Other adverse reactions include cataracts, hyperglycemia, slowed lineal growth in children, and iatrogenic Cushing syndrome.

Hydrochlorothiazide (b; and other thiazide and thiazide-like diuretics, such as chlorthalidone or metolazone) can increase blood glucose levels. However, they typically lower blood pressure (as evidenced by their widespread use as antihypertensives) and tend to raise, not lower, plasma calcium levels (which would be inconsistent with the decreased bone density described in this man). Metformin (c) or pamidronate (d) would not cause responses described in the question.

371. The answer is e. *(Brunton, pp 920-921, 1527, 1532t. Katzung, pp 236-237, 240-241, 596t, 678.)* Amiodarone, an iodine-rich drug, has several actions that can lead to clinical hypothyroidism—or, more often and mainly in persons with iodine-deficient diets, hyperthyroidism. How can these seemingly opposite outcomes occur? Before we get to that, let's summarize the other adverse responses associated with amiodarone therapy: the potential for pulmonary fibrosis (may become serious); abnormal pigmentation of the skin (is photosensitive, too); corneal deposits (often described as "halo vision"); neuropathies; and hepatotoxicity. Now, the thyroid issue:

Amiodarone inhibits a deiodinase that removes iodine on both the 5 and 5′ positions and that converts thyroxine to triiodothyronine (T_3), mainly in the liver. This process is the main contributor to the production of endogenous (circulating) T_3 that is used by most target tissues in the body. Inhibit this enzyme and the peripheral tissues have less T_3 to utilize, and signs and symptoms of hypothyroidism can ensue.

The excess iodine derived from metabolism of amiodarone may also contribute to the hypothyroidism. The mechanism is analogous to the way in which administering large doses of iodide are clinically useful for suppressing thyroid function in hyperthyroid individuals: iodide limits its own transport into follicular cells, and, acutely at least, high circulating levels of iodide inhibit thyroid hormone synthesis.

And how might amiodarone cause hyperthyroidism? The iodine cleaved from the drug during its metabolism can be incorporated, along with dietary iodine, into thyroid hormone synthetic pathways.

Although amiodarone can cause clinically significant effects on thyroid status, it does not affect the metabolism or responses to other hormones, including cortisol (a, b), insulin (d, f), and ADH (c).

372. The answer is b. *(Brunton, pp 665, 1561-1562. Katzung, pp 694-695, 715-717.)* Mifepristone is a synthetic drug used as an abortifacient. (In some other countries, but not in the United States, it is used as a postcoital contraceptive.) Although the drug blocks glucocorticoid receptors, that effect does not account for its use or effects in the context described here. Here the actions arise from blocking uterine progesterone receptors. They include detachment of the conceptus from the uterine wall, softening and dilation of the cervix, and increased myometrial contraction that expels the conceptus. (The latter arises from both a drug-induced increase of local prostaglandin synthesis and greater myometrial responsiveness to them.) If mifepristone fails to induce expulsion of the fetus, misoprostol is usually given to increase uterine contractions further. (Estrogens used alone or in combination with progestins have also proven effective in postcoital contraception.)

Ergonovine and methylergonovine (a) are ergot compounds that cause uterine contraction, and are used postpartum to control bleeding, mainly in the face of postpartum uterine atony, because they cause rather intense and tonic uterine muscle contraction. They are abortifacient drugs, but not used for postcoital contraception. Raloxifene (c) and tamoxifen (d) are estrogen receptor agonists or antagonists (which effect occurs depends on the tissue) that are used to treat certain estrogen-dependent breast cancers.

Terbutaline (e) is a β_2-adrenergic agonist used to slow uterine contractions and reduce overall uterine tone in premature labor. An older related drug used as a tocolytic drug, and no longer available in the United States, is ritodrine.

373. The answer is e. *(Brunton, pp 1533-1535. Katzung, pp 673, 676-677.)* Hypothyroidism is the most common adverse outcome of using ^{131}I to treat hyperthyroidism. No matter how accurately the dose is calculated, according to some studies about 8 of 10 treated patients develop symptomatic hypothyroidism (that needs to be treated) by 10 or more years after treatment. It results, of course, from excessive thyroid cell destruction.

Substantive symptom relief from ^{131}I takes from several weeks to a couple of months to develop (although blood chemistries change somewhat faster). Thus, answer b is incorrect. Until a euthyroid state develops, drugs such as β-adrenergic blockers or oral antithyroid drugs may be needed (not contraindicated, a) for symptom control. (The patient described here seems not to be experiencing thyrotoxicosis, so a β-adrenergic blocker might not be needed.) Oral antithyroid drugs can be given before ^{131}I treatment, but they should be stopped for a couple of days before (not administered up to and including the day of administration, answer d) radiotherapy so as not to prevent radioiodine uptake into the gland. Thyroid and other cancers, metastatic or not, are rare after ^{131}I therapy (c, therefore, is incorrect).

374. The answer is b. *(Brunton, pp 865, 1643-1644. Katzung, pp 180, 746.)* Oral diazoxide is indicated for the very situation described in the question. It is, chemically, a benzothiadiazide (like hydrochlorothiazide, many other diuretic/antihypertensives), but it is more efficacious in terms of reducing parenchymal cell (skeletal muscle, adipocytes) responsiveness or sensitivity to insulin, thereby helping to raise blood glucose levels. (Recall that thiazides tend to cause hyperglycemia as a side effect. That is due to their insulin-desensitizing effects.) Neither diazoxide nor a thiazide diuretic has any significant effects to inhibit insulin synthesis, release, or blood levels. Indeed, they tend to cause hyperinsulinism in response to hyperglycemia.

Atenolol, metoprolol (a), and all other drugs that block β-adrenergic receptors, tend to suppress insulin release, lower blood glucose levels, delay recovery from hypoglycemic episodes by inhibiting hepatic glycogenolysis and suppressing insulin release, and block tachycardia (a tip-off to some diabetic patients that their blood glucose levels are getting quite low) that tends to occur in response to hypoglycemia. (The degree or extent to which β-adrenergic blockers exert their effects on glucose depends on the overall profile of the individual agents—nonselective [propranolol, others]; atenolol or metoprolol [largely β_1 selective]; labetalol or carvedilol (nonselective β- plus α blockade); pindolol [nonselective β-blockade with intrinsic sympathomimetic activity].)

Glucagon (c) is used to manage hypoglycemia, but it is an injectable drug used only as an adjunct to IV glucose for short-term, severe, and symptomatic hypoglycemia. Octreotide (d), identified as a somatostatin analog, is used to inhibit growth hormone (GH) release and the effects of GH on insulin-like growth factor (IGF-1) in such cases as acromegaly and carcinoid syndrome, and is also used to control bleeding from esophageal varices. It is about 40% to 50% more potent than somatostatin in terms of suppressing GH release, but relatively weak in terms of suppressing insulin secretion. It would not be a reasonable choice here, given the alternatives. Oxytocin (e), a posterior pituitary hormone used mainly as a uterine stimulant (that's where we got the terms oxytocic drug or oxytocic effect) has no clinically useful effects on glycemic control or the responses of target tissues to insulin or glucose deficiency or excess.

375. The answer is a. *(Brunton, pp 1384, 1555-1557. Katzung, pp 716-717, 958-959.)* Tamoxifen is often referred to as a selective estrogen receptor modifier (SERM). It blocks estrogen receptors in some tissues and stimulates them in some others. The drug can be used to prevent or treat estrogen-dependent breast cancers, and it works as an estrogen receptor antagonist there. A receptor-agonist action also accounts for one of the drug's more distressing and common side effects, hot flashes. In contrast, the drug activates (not blocks; b) estrogen receptors in the uterus, increasing the risk of endometrial cancers. Other estrogen-activating (estrogen-like) consequences include a reduced risk of osteoporosis (not increased; c), desirable (not unwanted; d) changes in plasma cholesterol profiles (reduced LDL and total cholesterol; increased HDL), and an increased (not decreased; e) risk of thromboembolic events. The related drug, raloxifene, is largely tamoxifen-like with one main exception: it does not activate uterine estrogen receptors, and so does not increase the risk of endometrial cancers.

376. The answer is c. *(Brunton, pp 1638-1639. Katzung, pp 741-742.)* Metformin, classified as a biguanide, "sensitizes" peripheral cells (skeletal muscle, adipocytes) to insulin, thereby facilitating glucose uptake and metabolic use, and suppresses release of glucose from the liver and into the blood. It is ineffective in the absence of insulin and so is approved only for Type 2 diabetes (used alone or in conjunction with such other drugs as a sulfonylurea or insulin). Like other oral agents (and some parenteral drugs such as exenatide), metformin has no beneficial effect in patients with Type 1 diabetes (d).

Weight loss during metformin therapy is much more common than weight gain (e). This is probably due to an appetite-suppressing effect (leading to reduced caloric intake), rather than because of a specific drug-related effect on some metabolic reaction(s) or anorexia secondary to GI side effects.

Why does metformin seldom—if not rarely—cause hypoglycemia? Rather than actively driving down blood glucose levels (as, say, insulin does), the drug acts as if it "puts a lid" on physiologic rises of blood glucose concentrations. (Thus, it has been described as being an antihyperglycemic drug, rather than a hypoglycemic agent.)

Metformin is not metabolized by the liver, but liver dysfunction is one contraindication. That's mainly because of the risks of the drug's most important adverse effect, lactic acidosis, which is rare but often fatal (not common and seldom serious, answer b) when it does occur. Impaired liver function impairs lactate elimination and favors its accumulation to toxic levels (and so answer a is not correct).

However the main primary cause of the lactic acidosis is renal insufficiency (plasma creatinine >1.5 mg/dL in men, 1.4 mg/dL in women), whether caused by renal disease or by renal hypoperfusion (ischemia, as might occur with heart failure and/or hypotension).

377. The answer is c. *(Brunton, pp 268, 272, 1582-1583. Katzung, pp 723, 1063.)* Finasteride competitively inhibits steroid 5-reductase, the enzyme necessary for synthesis of the active form of testosterone (dihydrotestosterone) in the prostate. Testosterone synthesis (d) and circulating testosterone levels (e) do not fall in response to the drug. PSA titers will, however, fall although the prognostic value of PSA measurements apropos prostate cancer is being called into question anyway.

Recall that α_1-adrenergic blockers (eg, prazosin as the overall prototype and, particularly tamsulosin in terms of use for BPH) provide symptomatic relief in some men with enlarged prostates by relaxing smooth muscle in the urethra, bladder neck, and prostate capsule; moreover, they do so without any effects on testosterone or its cellular actions. Finasteride, however, has no α-adrenergic receptor blocking activity (a).

378. The answer is c. *(Brunton, pp 1622-1624.)* Blood-borne glucose reacts nonenzymatically with hemoglobin to form glycated hemoglobin products (eg, HbA_{1c}). The rate of HbA_{1c} formation is related to ambient glucose levels, and the amount of HbA_{1c} measured in any given blood sample reflects the average blood glucose levels over the last 2 to 3 months. Thus, although the patient's plasma glucose levels may be acceptable after a couple of days' fast, HbA_{1c} measurements give the big picture about how good glycemic control was on a longer-term (and more important) timeline. Note that although measuring HbA_{1c} gives important information about the long-term timeline, it does not provide any information about day-to-day fluctuations in glucose levels or what's happening "right now," and such information is important to optimal control of diabetes and its symptoms. Nonetheless, regular, periodic checks of HbA_{1c} should be part of the monitoring for every patient with diabetes (Type 1 or 2), not so much as a way to assess for noncompliance as to make sure that the current treatment plan with which the patient is complying is working. It is a common and relatively inexpensive assay.

Having the clinical lab measure glucose in a venous blood sample (a) won't give any additional or meaningful information: hand-held glucometers, used properly, are remarkably accurate. Glucose tolerance tests, even those done with oral glucose (b), will provide little historic information, and they are expensive. Few clinical labs are set up to measure plasma concentrations of most oral antidiabetic drugs. The cost would be quite expensive, and in the patient described here the results would be of little or no value if the goal is assessing past drug and diet compliance and long-term glycemic control (d). Measuring urine ketone levels (e) are of no benefit for our purposes. All that they might suggest is that our patient has fasted for several days, and even that period without food may not elevate ketones much. And remember that diabetic ketoacidosis is far more prevalent in patients with Type 1 diabetes mellitus than those with Type 2 (who are much more prone to developing hyperglycemic hyperosmolar nonketotic syndrome). Urine glucose monitoring (f) is not very enlightening either. Recall that glucose appears in the urine only when plasma glucose concentrations exceed a renal threshold for reabsorption (around 180 mg/dL or so). A glucose-free urine sample, then, would only indicate that plasma glucose levels are below the threshold: they still could be unacceptably high, or normal, or low, and you would never know just by urine testing.

379. The answer is a. *(Brunton, pp 1624-1630. Katzung, pp 731-734.)* Insulin modifications, whether by rDNA technology to substitute amino acids, or by physical means (eg, in the case of NPH insulin), alter onsets and durations of action. (Recall that regular insulin, given by SC injection, has an onset of about 30 min, peaks in about 3 h, and has a duration of about 7 to 8 h. Lispro and aspart insulins work faster, peak earlier, and have the shortest durations [rapid/short]; NPH insulins [intermediate-acting] have onsets, times to peak, and durations longer than regular insulins; and insulin glargine have the slowest onsets [4 to 6 h], with durations that are on par with NPH.)

Many of the genetically-engineered insulins must not be administered intravenously (b). Like endogenous insulin, all the pharmaceutical formulations facilitate, not prevent (c) cellular potassium uptake along with glucose. They have no ability to reactivate or stimulate pancreatic insulin synthesis (d). Finally, while glucose is the metabolite that is directly affected by insulin, insulin deficiencies that characterize diabetes mellitus (whether Type 1, Type 2, gestational diabetes, etc), have negative impact on the metabolism of fats and proteins, which contribute to many diagnostic signs and symptoms. Thus, it is not correct to say that any insulin "selectively" affects glucose metabolism (to the exclusion of ultimate effects on fat and protein; answer e).

Note: Insulins that can be given intravenously are insulin lispro, insulin aspart, and insulin glulisine (all short duration, rapid acting); and regular insulin (short duration but with a slower onset of action that lispro, aspart, and glulisine).

380. The answer is a. *(Brunton, p 1640. Katzung, pp 743-744.)* Acarbose, and the related drug miglitol, act in intestinal brush border cells to inhibit monosaccharide formation from complex carbohydrates and oligosaccharides, and in so doing inhibit/slow the absorption of monosaccharides (eg, glucose) from the gut. The enzymatic targets are alpha glucosidases in the brush border of intestinal cells. The main consequence in terms of glycemic control is a blunting of usual postprandial rises of blood glucose. The most common side effects of acarbose affect the GI tract, as described in the question. Used alone, hypoglycemia due to acarbose is rare; however, the drug is often used as an adjunct to a sulfonylurea, and their propensity for causing hypoglycemia is not at all reduced by acarbose. It is important to note that the usual patient-centered approach to managing an episode of hypoglycemia, as might occur when certain oral antidiabetic drugs are used (eg, sulfonylureas, glitazones), is to ingest table sugar (sucrose) or some beverage or food that contains it. If the hypoglycemic patient is taking acarbose, this approach will not correct blood glucose levels adequately or promptly.

The mechanism of action described for acarbose is not at all like the mechanisms of glitazones (b), sulfonylureas such as glipizide (c) or tolbutamide (e), or metformin (d).

381. The answer is a. *(Brunton, pp 1624-1630. Katzung, pp 731-734.)* Insulin glargine is a genetically engineered insulin that is poorly (but adequately) soluble at physiologic pH values. The drug dissolves and enters the bloodstream slowly and in such a way that there is more of a stable plateau in terms of blood levels and hypoglycemic effects. It does not cause a well-defined peak in blood levels and effects (a). The plateau is rather "flat" over much of the typical 24-hour period following a subcutaneous injection. Thus, the drug is better able than most other insulins to maintain steady round-the-clock glycemic control, but less able to suppress the postprandial elevation of glucose that is necessary for some patients. Insulin glargine's onset and duration of action are comparable to such preparations as NPH insulin. It is what happens in between, temporally, that distinguishes this formulation from the rest.

Insulin glargine—indeed all the insulin formulations—has no disulfiram-like effects (b). As with all the insulins, insulin glargine poses a risk of hypoglycemia (and so answer d is incorrect). Finally, the drug has no parenchymal cell insulin-sensitizing effects (e), and like all insulins it is given solely as hormone replacement therapy.

382. The answer is c. *(Brunton, pp 1521-1524. Katzung, pp 677-678.)* Tachycardia, palpitations, tachyarrhythmias, and the possibility of acute myocardial ischemia, are among the hallmarks of thyrotoxicosis or somewhat lesser thyroid hormone supplement overdoses. Thyroid hormone levels regulate the "responsiveness" of β-adrenergic receptors to epinephrine and norepinephrine (or exogenous β agonists), and this probably contributes to the cardiovascular problems. Although excesses of thyroid hormone are the cause of the problems, management is symptomatic and aimed at suppressing β-mediated responses. Hence the use of propranolol or some other suitable β-adrenergic blocker for immediate and quite possibly lifesaving symptom controls.

Sulfonylureas (a; first or second generation) would not cause the signs or symptoms noted above, and β-blocker therapy for overdoses of one of those drugs would do more harm than good. The same applies to insulin (b); β-blockers might control increases of cardiac rate, but they are more likely to further lower blood glucose levels and slow or otherwise attenuate rises of blood glucose levels when appropriate therapy to render the patient euglycemic is started. Overdoses of prednisone (d) or propylthiouracil (e) are not likely to present as described, and they are not properly managed with a β-blocker.

383. The answer is e. *(Brunton, pp 1641-1642. Katzung, pp 744-745.)* Exenatide is the first in a new class of antidiabetic agents, the incretin mimetics. It is administered by subcutaneous injection and used adjunctively to improve glucose control in Type 2 diabetes patients already taking metformin, a sulfonylurea, or both. It is not indicated for Type 1 diabetes.

Exenatide is a synthetic analog of glucagon-like peptide-1 (GLP-1), a hormone in the incretin family. Under physiologic conditions, GLP-1 and other incretins are released from cells of the GI tract after a meal. Exenatide binds to receptors for GLP-1. In doing so it slows gastric emptying, stimulates glucose-dependent insulin release, inhibits postprandial release of glucagon, and suppresses appetite.

Dose-related hypoglycemia is common when exenatide is combined with a sulfonylurea (but not when used with only metformin, which seldom causes hypoglycemia). Nausea, vomiting, and diarrhea are the most common side effects. The drug is also apparently linked to the development of pancreatitis, and so monitoring for it is essential.

Some patients taking exenatide develop antibodies directed against the drug. Antigen-antibody reactions to exenatide do not cause adverse effects (eg, allergic or anaphylactoid reactions), but can reduce the intensity of exenatide's effects. At this time, the drug is classified in FDA pregnancy risk category C. Given the years of experience with using insulin for diabetes during pregnancy, and the benefits and safety it provides, there's little justification in using exenatide.

Incretin and incretin mimetics have no effects on testosterone (whether antagonism or intensification; answer a). Metformin and sulfonylureas are, of course, antidiabetic drugs and are not indicated for thyroid disorders (b). Exenatide has no effects on calcium metabolism or osteoporosis management (c); and no direct effects on corticosteroid metabolism (d), whether in hyposecretory (Addisonian) or hypersecretory (Cushingoid) states.

384. The answer is a. *(Brunton, pp 1524-1525. Katzung, pp 667-670, 673-676.)* Levothyroxine is usually considered the first choice for long-term maintenance therapy of hypothyroidism, such as that which occurs after thyroidectomy or radiation therapy of the thyroid. Once absorbed, we get the slow-onset and rather steady, long-lasting effects of the T_4. In addition, some of the administered T_4 is deiodinated in the tissues to T_3, "automatically" providing usually adequate levels and effects of this more rapidly and shorter-acting hormone without the need to administer T_3 (liothyronine) separately.

If the patient develops profound hypothyroidism (eg, myxedema), some clinicians may still prefer T_3 for its prompt effects. However, in this instance too, T_4 is generally regarded as the preferred way to replace both hormones and reestablish a euthyroid state (administered with corticosteroids for myxedema coma).

Liothyronine (b) is synthetic T_3; liotrix (c) is a mixture of synthetic T_3 and T_4; protirelin (d) is a synthetic tripeptide, chemically identical to thyrotropin-releasing hormone (TRH), that is used to diagnose some thyroid disorders; desiccated thyroid products (e) are outmoded for managing hypothyroidism, given the availability of synthetic hormone preparations.

385. The answer is b. *(Brunton, p 1663. Katzung, pp 754-758, 763.)* We're dealing with hypocalcemia in this patient with tetany postthyroidectomy, because the parathyroid gland was damaged or removed during the surgery. Administration of intravenous calcium gluconate would immediately correct the tetany. Parathyroid hormone (d) could be considered appropriate for long-term management of hypocalcemia, but it has a slower onset of action that would not be of much help in a tetanic state. We would then probably use vitamin D (e) and dietary modifications for long-term control of plasma calcium levels.

Calcitonin (a) is a hypocalcemic antagonist of parathyroid hormone. (Note that calcitonin or calcitriol will raise plasma calcium levels faster than vitamin D, but in this emergent situation they will not work fast enough, which is why we need direct administration of ionic calcium.) Plicamycin (c; mithramycin) is used to treat Paget disease and hypercalcemia.

The dose employed is about one-tenth the amount used for plicamycin's cytotoxic action when it is used as a chemotherapeutic drug.

386. The answer is d. *(Brunton, pp 1526-1529. Katzung, pp 671-673, 676, 1034.)* Propylthiouracil, a thioamide used to manage many patients with hyperthyroidism, has three main actions. It inhibits a peroxidase, and in doing so inhibits oxidation of inorganic iodide to iodine, and the iodination of tyrosine. It also blocks coupling of iodotyrosines and inhibits deiodination of T_4 to T_3 in the periphery. Propylthiouracil and the thioamides in general, do not: block thyroid uptake of iodide (a); affect metabolic inactivation of T_3 and T_4 (b); inhibit thyroglobulin's proteolysis (c); or directly release thyroid hormones into the circulation (e).

Note: Most texts and other publications refer to this group of drugs as I have: thioamides. However, occasionally you will find an alternative term used: thionamide, thioamine, and even thionamine.

387. The answer is b. *(Brunton, pp 953-955, 996. Katzung, pp 615, 1081.)* Colesevelam's original approved indication, and its most common use, is for managing hypercholesterolemia. It is classified as a bile acid sequestrant: it binds the cholesterol-rich bile acids in the gut, preventing their enterohepatic recirculation. The main outcome is lowered LDL levels. In early 2008 it was approved as an adjunct for some patients with Type 2 diabetes, such as the gentleman described here. Its antihyperglycemic mechanism of action is not fully understood. There are other bile acid sequestrants (cholestyramine, colestipol), but they are not indicated for nor apparently effective as an adjunct to therapy of Type 2 diabetes. There is at least one probable advantage of colesevelam over the alternative bile acid sequestrants. Cholestyramine and colestipol bind to and inhibit the absorption (rate, extent, or both) of many other oral drugs that are in the GI tract at the same time. That is, they participate in many drug-drug interactions. They also tend to bind to and inhibit absorption of fat-soluble vitamins (A, D, E, K), whether from dietary or vitamin supplement sources. Colesevelam does not significantly inhibit the absorption of other oral medications or fat-soluble vitamins.

Based on what is known about colesevelam's mechanism of action there is nothing to suggest that it has any beneficial effects on the pathophysiology or clinical course of COPD (a) , hyperuricemia (c), nicotine (or any other) addiction/dependency (d), or prostate disease (benign or not).

See Question 256 in the Chapter on Cardiovascular Pharmacology for more information about colesevelam.

388. The answer is c. *(Brunton, pp 1565-1567. Katzung, pp 701-704.)* Thromboembolism associated with OC administration is attributed to the estrogen component. If thromboembolism is a concern, then one approach to reducing the risk would be selecting a product with a lower—not higher (a)—estrogen dose. (Using estrogen alone [e] would be irrational, then; that partially explains why there are no estrogen-only oral contraceptives.) Even reducing the estrogen dose in a combination contraceptive may not be sufficient, long-term, to provide a suitable reduction in thromboembolic risk. Progestins seem to have little impact on the development of thromboembolic disorders during OC therapy, and so increasing (b) or decreasing (d) progestin content will do little more than nothing for most patients.

Smoking is a major risk factor for thromboembolism, especially for women taking an oral contraceptive, so it's essential to encourage the patient to quit (or not start) smoking. As noted above there are no OCs that contain estrogen only—unlike the availability of progestin-only OCs—the so-called minipills (see Question 393).

389. The answer is f. *(Brunton, pp 240t, 253. Katzung, pp 140, 144.)* Terbutaline is a predominantly β_2-selective adrenergic agonist, much like the prototype albuterol. These drugs have no α-adrenergic receptor agonist or antagonist activity (e), nor is there any drug-related effect on prostaglandins (a) or on oxytocin (b, c, d).

In addition to causing bronchodilation—arguably the main overall use for drugs in this class—β_2 agonists slow uterine contractions. And that use, applied to suppression of preterm labor (a tocolytic effect), is the main clinical use of this "bronchodilator" drug.

The sequence of events following binding of terbutaline to its receptor includes increased myometrial cAMP formation, activation of cAMP-dependent protein kinase, and extrusion of Ca^{2+} from smooth muscle cells such that contractile force is reduced. Terbutaline's effects are not at all like those of ergot compounds (eg, methylergonovine), which induce uterine contraction by a mechanism that involves α-adrenergic receptor activation.

Be sure to understand that despite the classification of terbutaline as a "β_2-selective adrenergic agonist," or as a uterine relaxant, the drug can activate all β-adrenergic receptors and cause a host of unwanted side effects or adverse responses that include tachycardia (direct and reflexly, in response to reduced blood pressure), pulmonary edema, and myocardial ischemia. This very effective drug is contraindicated in eclampsia or severe preeclampsia. In these situations the goal is to deliver the fetus (the definitive cure for eclampsia), not prolong labor.

390. The answer is a. *(Brunton, pp 1603, 1610. Katzung, pp 686-692.)* Of the drugs listed, dexamethasone is by far the most potent in terms of glucocorticoid effects relative to other glucocorticoids, and far lower mineralocorticoid (aldosterone) activity. The dexamethasone suppression test has several uses: it allows not only complete suppression of pituitary ACTH production, but also accurate measurement of endogenous corticosteroids, such as 17-ketosteroids, in the urine. The small amount of dexamethasone present contributes minimally to this measurement.

None of the other drugs listed would be suitable for this test, all are less potent than dexamethasone, and they tend to have relatively more (albeit still slight) mineralocorticoid activity: hydrocortisone, b; methylprednisolone, c; prednisone, d; and triamcinolone, e.

391. The answer is d. *(Brunton, pp 1582, 1610-1611. Katzung, pp 693, 723, 839-840.)* Ketoconazole, long used as an antifungal agent (see Chapter 10), is one of the most efficacious inhibitors of corticosteroid synthesis. It is not a primary therapy for pituitary tumors/Cushing disease, but is a useful adjunct. The main problem associated with this drug is the risk of hepatotoxicity and the potential for interactions with some other drugs. An alternative to ketoconazole is aminoglutethimide, which also interferes with synthesis of all the adrenal steroids.

Cimetidine (a), the H_2-histamine blocker that is well known as an inhibitor of P450-mediated metabolism of many drugs, would be of no benefit. Massive doses of cortisol (b), although theoretically "reasonable" (feedback suppression of pituitary function), would be of little help in terms of regulating the pituitary's activity and clearly would aggravate signs and symptoms of adrenal corticosteroid excess that we already have. Fludrocortisone (c) has intense mineralocorticoid activity and is the only drug indicated for replacement therapy in chronic mineralocorticoid deficiencies. Spironolactone (e) blocks aldosterone receptors; it would counteract only the aldosterone-related responses to corticosteroid excess and would not have any effects on adrenal corticosteroid synthesis.

392. The answer is d. *(Brunton, pp 121, 509-510, 523-524. Katzung, pp 64t, 403-405, 1029t, 1147t-1148t.)* Phenytoin is one of several agents that can enhance the hepatic metabolism of oral contraceptives (especially the estrogen component), leading to reduced contraceptive levels and unintended pregnancy (contraceptive failure). It is also one that interacts by inducing synthesis of hormone-binding globulins: more hormone molecules are bound to the protein, and so less free (active) drug is in the circulation. Several other common anticonvulsants interact with the same potential outcome, especially barbiturates (including phenobarbital, mephobarbital, and primidone), carbamazepine, and oxcarbazepine. Be sure to recall that rifampin (and rifabutin) and protease inhibitors (ritonavir, others) are also important interactants with OCs via a metabolism-inducing mechanism. Finally, some antibiotics (eg, tetracyclines) interact with OCs, but here the mechanism differs: the antibiotics suppress gut flora that participate in enterohepatic recycling of the OCs. When the bacteria are suppressed, OCs that are secreted into the gut are lost in the feces, rather than being reabsorbed.

Adding phenytoin to an oral contraceptive regimen is not likely to increase the risk of blood dyscrasias (a), and if dosages are adjusted properly there is little or no risk of breakthrough seizures (b), which would be consistent with subtherapeutic anticonvulsant levels. Conversely, the combination is not likely to cause phenytoin levels to rise to a toxic level (c), even though slight increases in phenytoin doses may cause significant rises of the anticonvulsant's plasma concentration (see Question 115 in the Chapter on Central Nervous System Pharmacology). Adding phenytoin would not increase the risk of estrogen-related thromboembolic disease (e).

393. The answer is d. *(Brunton, p 1564. Katzung, pp 706-709, 715.)* Progestin-only oral contraceptives (minipills) are associated with a higher risk of menstrual irregularities than the more common estrogen-progestin preparations. That is largely due to the lack of estrogen. However, the absence of estrogen also lowers the risk (not increases; c) of thromboembolic disorders—a major advantage, especially, for women who smoke. Progestin-only formulations are, overall, less effective in terms of preventing pregnancy than combination products (and so answer a is incorrect); like combination products they lack definitive spermicidal effects (b) but they thicken cervical mucus, retard sperm motility in that way, and reduce the likelihood of nidation, and their administration schedule is continuous—every day (not answer e), rather than the cyclic schedule used for combination products.

394. The answer is b. *(Brunton, pp 1564-1566. Katzung, pp 701-704.)* Hypertension, which may occur (and usually transiently) in response to OCs, is mainly due to estrogen excess. Fatigue (a), weight gain (e; usually triggered by increased appetite; d), and infrequent or missed menses (c) are mainly associated with progestin excess. Hypomenorrhea (c) may also be due to inadequate estrogen levels in the combination product. Unusually frequent menses—hypermenorrhea—tends to be related to too little progestin in the product.

395. The answer is c. *(Brunton, pp 1638-1639. Katzung, pp 741-742.)* Metformin, a common drug for managing many patients with Type 2 diabetes mellitus, is a very well tolerated and effective drug. This biguanide not only lowers circulating glucose levels, but suppresses appetite, thereby lowering dietary caloric intake. One of the main problems associated with metformin is the development of lactic acidosis—admittedly rare but potentially fatal adverse response to this drug, and associated with none of the other drugs listed as answer choices (insulin glargine or other insulins (a); thyroid hormones (b); sulfonylureas (d), older or newer; or spironolactone or the related drug eplerenone (e).

396. The answer is c. *(Brunton, pp 1639-1640. Katzung, pp 738-739.)* Tolbutamide and the older sulfonylureas (e) have been associated with an increased risk of sudden death. The glitazones, however, have been associated with an increased risk of heart failure, which is why patients taking these drugs should be monitored for weight gain, edema, and other expected signs and symptoms of heart failure. Acarbose (a), an inhibitor of gastrointestinal carbohydrate uptake, is relatively free of any serious toxicities. Biguanides (b), of which metformin (d) is an example, are widely used antidiabetic drugs. The major toxicity or adverse response is a risk of lactic acidosis.

397. The answer is b. *(Brunton, p 1609. Katzung, pp 687t, 689.)* We would give betamethasone to enhance fetal surfactant synthesis and suppress airway inflammation, thereby lessening the chance or severity of fetal respiratory distress syndrome at birth. (The action probably involves stimulating synthesis of fibroblast pneumocyte factor, which then stimulates surfactant synthesis by pneumocytes in the fetus. Recall that surfactant lowers alveolar surface tension, thereby reducing the likelihood of alveolar collapse and its consequences on gas exchange.)

Note: Other corticosteroids, especially dexamethasone, could be used. However, betamethasone is preferred because it binds less to plasma proteins than cortisol and most other glucocorticoids, allowing more steroid to cross the placenta.

Even though albuterol (a) is used as a bronchodilator (eg, for asthma or COPD), it is classified, pharmacologically, precisely as we classify terbutaline, a relatively selective β_2 agonist. With the terbutaline being given already, administering albuterol would be pointless. In obstetrics, ergonovine or methylergonovine (c) are given postpartum; their strong uterine contracting effects are used to reduce postpartum bleeding. Aside from being contraindicated before delivery, they have no pulmonary effects of the sort we want. Indomethacin (d) is sometimes used to slow premature labor. It works by blocking synthesis of prostaglandins that have oxytocic activity, but prostaglandin synthesis inhibition also causes closure of the ductus arteriosus (which, in this setting, would be unwanted). Magnesium sulfate (e) would not cause the desired pulmonary effects; it is used in obstetrics to prevent seizures in preeclampsia/eclampsia. The drug has tocolytic activity, but the jury is out on just how effective and safe the drug is when used to suppress uterine contractions.

Note: Three pharmaceutical preparations of surfactant are now available: calfactant, beractant, and poractant alfa. They are given to neonates with respiratory distress syndrome by direct intratracheal instillation.

398. The answer is b. *(Brunton, p 1668. Katzung, pp 759, 762.)* Esophagitis, sometimes with esophageal ulcers, is the most worrisome adverse response to bisphosphonates such as etidronate. It is not due to any specific metabolic alteration causes by the drug, but rather by direct, prolonged contact of the drug with the esophagus if the oral dose lodges there without passing quickly enough to the stomach. This is why the drug should not be administered to patients with esophageal disease, difficulty swallowing, or an inability to sit or stand up for at least 30 minutes (to help gravity bring the tablet to the stomach) after taking the drug. There is also some concern that long-term therapy with bisphosphonates may cause osteonecrosis of the jaw. Nonetheless, overall the bisphosphonates cause remarkably few side effects in the vast majority of patients.

399. The answer is c. *(Brunton, pp 1387-1388. Katzung, pp 653-655, 661t, 959.)* Leuprolide is a peptide that is related to GnRH or luteinizing hormone-releasing hormone (LHRH), and it is used to treat metastatic prostate carcinoma. By inhibiting gonadotropin release it induces a hypogonadal state; testosterone levels in the body fall significantly, and this appears to be the mechanism for suppression of the cancer.

Aminoglutethimide (a) is an aromatase inhibitor mainly used to treat Cushing disease or syndrome (it inhibits synthesis of adrenal corticosteroids), and some patients with metastatic breast carcinoma. Fludrocortisone (b) is a mineralocorticoid used for chronic adrenal insufficiency (along with glucocorticoids) or congenital adrenal hypoplasia. Mifepristone (d) is an abortifacient/oxytocic drug. Spironolactone (e) is an aldosterone receptor blocker that is used mainly as for patients with primary or secondary hyperaldosteronism, and as an adjunct to the management of severe heart failure. It is also classified as a potassium-sparing diuretic.

400. The answer is e. *(Brunton, pp 1634-1637. Katzung, pp 738-740.)* Gyburide is one of several sulfonylurea antidiabetic drugs. Recall that the sulfonylureas simplistically fall into two main classes, based largely on how long they have been used: the so-called first-generation agents, such as tolbutamide and chlorpropamide, and the newer second-generation drugs, glipizide, glyburide, and glimepiride. Whether older or newer, these drugs mainly lower blood glucose levels by enhancing insulin release from the β cells of the pancreas. The mechanism involves binding to and blocking an ATP-sensitive K^+ channel on β-cell membranes. This depolarizes the membrane, and resulting Ca^{2+} influx triggers insulin release. The mechanistic dependence on insulin release, of course, explains why these drugs are ineffective in Type 1 diabetes.

Other probable actions of the sulfonylureas include reduced plasma glucagon levels and increased binding of insulin to parenchymal tissue cells. These drugs have no direct effects on renal handling of glucose (b) or insulin synthesis (c). Unlike some other oral antidiabetic drugs, such as the glitazones (thiazolidinediones), they do not increase parenchymal cell responsiveness to insulin (d) or do so in any other ways that might be described as "insulin sensitizing." They do not decrease "insulin resistance" (a), which is a common problem for many patients with Type 2 diabetes mellitus, whether by lowering body weight or appetite or by other mechanisms.

401. The answer is b. *(Brunton, pp 1634-1637. Katzung, pp 738-740.)* Of the main groups or chemical classes of oral antidiabetic agents, sulfonylureas are the ones typically associated with causing hypoglycemia, whether from overdose or as a rather expected response in some patients, particularly before meals. As noted in the previous question, sulfonylureas release insulin from the pancreas even if blood glucose levels already are low. Even in a fast-induced hypoglycemic state a sulfonylurea will release insulin and drive blood glucose down even further, with a likely outcome being hypoglycemia.

The elderly are particularly susceptible to sulfonylurea-induced hypoglycemia. Part of this may relate to diet. However, expected age-related falls of renal and/or hepatic function can reduce elimination of these drugs, thereby increasing their plasma levels and their effects unless dosages are reduced accordingly.

This propensity for preprandial hypoglycemia is shared by the meglitinides—repaglinide and nateglinide—because they, too, increase pancreatic insulin release. However, they are not prescribed nearly as often as a sulfonylurea (or metformin) when oral therapy is indicated.

The thiazolidinediones (glitazones; d, e) seldom cause symptomatic hypoglycemia because they do not release insulin. The same applies to metformin (c), the biguanide; and acarbose (a; an α-glucosidase inhibitor, as is miglitol). Because of a longer half-life, compared with glipizide, a sulfonylurea is more likely to cause preprandial hypoglycemia. Glipizide is contraindicated in patients with liver disease because it is metabolized in the liver.

402. The answer is a. *(Brunton, p 1640. Katzung, pp 743-744.)* Acarbose, classified as an α-glucosidase inhibitor, slows the rate and extent of complex carbohydrate absorption from the intestines. The consequence of this for the hypoglycemic patient is that attempts to restore blood glucose levels by consuming sugar or sucrose-containing foods or beverages (eg, orange juice is a popular choice, as are products such as the one our patient took) will be less effective, if effective at all—and certainly slower in terms of symptom relief. If the patient who is taking acarbose becomes hypoglycemic, but not to the extent that it becomes severe or serious, oral glucose must be used. Several glucose-containing products are on the market and are made for such patients.

None of the other oral diabetes drugs have this mechanism of action and so will not hinder attempts to restore euglycemia when sugar is consumed: glyburide (b), a sulfonylurea; metformin (c), a biguanide; repaglinide (d), a meglitinide; or rosiglitazone (e).

403. The answer is a. *(Brunton, p 1528. Katzung, pp 671-673.)* The incidence of agranulocytosis due to propylthiouracil, or the related thio(n)amide, methimazole, is not rare. In addition, it may develop within the first few weeks of starting therapy, and so a "routine" blood test scheduled for several months or more after starting the drug may not catch it. However, if it is detected early (eg, the patient promptly reports a sore throat or other flu-like symptoms) and the drug is stopped, it is usually spontaneously reversible. The most common side effect with the thioamides is urticaria. It may abate spontaneously or require symptomatic management with an antihistamine (either first or second generation) or with a corticosteroid.

None of the other responses listed are recognized as being commonly associated with or caused by thioamides: cholestatic jaundice (b); hyperuricemia or clinical gout (c); renal tubular necrosis (d); rhabdomyolysis (e); or thyroid cancer (f).

404. The answer is e. *(Brunton, pp 1639-1640. Katzung, pp 742-743.)* Pioglitazone and the related drug rosiglitazone (classified as thiazolidinediones, or glitazones for short) work by increasing parenchymal cell responsiveness to insulin. The mechanism seems to involve activation of peroxisome proliferator-activated receptors (PPARs). This apparently increases transcription of insulin—responsive genes that control glucose (and lipid) metabolism and cellular glucose uptake via glucose transporters. The net effects include not only lowered plasma levels of glucose, but also fatty acids and (indirectly) of insulin. Given the necessary involvement of insulin in the drug's effects, it will not work (alone) for patients with Type 1 diabetes. When used for patients who have Type 2 diabetes, and who nonetheless require insulin, a thiazolidinedione can be a valuable adjunct that helps lower daily insulin requirements.

Acarbose would be a good example of an antidiabetic drug that blocks intestinal absorption of complex carbohydrates (a). None of the antidiabetic drugs, whether used for Type 1 or 2 diabetes mellitus, increase renal glucose elimination (b). Metformin is an antidiabetic drug that increases hepatic glucose production (c). Sulfonylureas (d; older agents such as tolbutamide or newer ones such as glyburide) are the ones that mainly trigger pancreatic insulin release, and after a time they may increase target cell sensitivity to insulin (e), as do the glitazones.

405. The answer is b. *(Brunton, pp 1578f, 1581. Katzung, pp 717-718.)* Danazol is a testosterone derivative used to treat endometriosis, and some of the side effects and adverse responses are those you would expect from testosterone itself: liver dysfunction, virilism (acne, hirsutism, oily skin, reduced breast size), and reductions in HDL cholesterol levels. Other reported adverse reactions include amenorrhea, weight gain, sweating, vasomotor flushing, and edema.

Nonetheless, danazol appears to be just as effective as an estrogen-progesterone combination for managing endometriosis, and relatively few patients have stopped (or have had to stop) danazol treatment because of side effects or adverse reactions.

Anemias (a), psychosis (c), reduced platelet counts (d), and weight loss (e) are not common accompaniments of danazol therapy.

406. The answer is d. *(Brunton, pp 1638-1639. Katzung, p 742.)* Metformin (a biguanide) poses the greatest risk, of all the antidiabetic drugs, of causing lactic acidosis. Although the overall risk of lactic acidosis from this drug is low, should it occur, mortality is quite common. Alcohol consumption or renal or hepatic disease increase the risk of lactic acidosis associated with metformin.

Acarbose (a), an α-glucosidase inhibitor (blocks polysaccharide uptake from the gut), the sulfonylureas (older ones such as tolbutamide or newer ones such as glipizide and glyburide; b and c), and rosiglitazone (e; and other glitazones, eg, pioglitazone) are not associated with lactic acidosis (unless they are coadministered with metformin).

407. The answer is c. *(Brunton, pp 1521-1524. Katzung, pp 677-678.)* Cardiovascular and related hemodynamic changes, mostly arising from or related to tachycardia, increased ventricular contractility, and potentially leading to acute myocardial ischemia, are among the hallmarks of thyroid hormone excess, whether drug-induced or idiopathic (eg, thyrotoxicosis of other causes). Increased thyroid hormone levels "up-regulate" the β-adrenergic receptors, leading to heightened and potentially lethal responses that involve overactivation of those receptors. β-Blockade provides important and prompt symptom relief, and may be lifesaving in situations such as this. Other interventions aimed at lowering thyroid hormone synthesis or release (iodine/iodides, a; a thioamide such as propylthiouracil, d) ultimately may be important, but saving the patient's life with administration of propranolol or a suitable alternative is the most important first step.

Liothyronine (b) would be a wholly irrational choice for acute thyroid hormone overdoses. Radioiodine (e) is also irrational for acute and infrequent episodes of hyperthyroidism such as those that occur with thyroid hormone overdoses. It is, of course, one option for managing hyperthyroidism due to a thyroid gland cancer in some patients.

408. The answer is d. *(Brunton, pp 1563-1564. Katzung, pp 710-716.)* There are two main mechanisms by which OCs exert their main effects. Arguably the most important is inhibition of ovulation. This prevents (or reduces the risk of) fertilization, a process that must come before such others as impairing nidation (c). The other is thickening of cervical mucus. That important effect, mainly caused by the progestin component, provides a physical barrier that slows or stops sperm motility. There are changes of cervical mucus pH (a), but that does not cause a spermicidal effect per se, nor is it the major mechanism by which the contraceptive acts. Detaching a fertilized ovum (b) or reducing uterine or endometrial blood flow (e), are not elements of the mechanisms of action.

409. The answer is e. *(Brunton, pp 1660-1661, 1666. Katzung, pp 755-758.)* Overmedication with vitamin D may lead to a toxic syndrome called hypervitaminosis D. The initial symptoms can include weakness, nausea, weight loss, anemia, and mild acidosis. As the excessive doses are continued, signs of nephrotoxicity can develop, such as polyuria, polydipsia, azotemia, and eventually nephrocalcinosis. In adults, osteoporosis can occur. Also, there is CNS impairment, which can result in mental retardation and seizures.

The signs and symptoms described in the question are not associated with estrogens (a) or progestins; etidronate (b) or other bisphosphonates; glipizide (c) or any other sulfonylureas; or prednisone (d) or other glucocorticoids.

410. The answer is c. *(Brunton, pp 1610-1611. Katzung, pp 65t, 693, 723.)* Ketoconazole is typically remembered as an azole antifungal drug, and a common cause of drug interactions due to its powerful cytochrome P450 inhibitory effects. At doses higher than those used when the drug is prescribed as an antifungal, it inhibits corticosteroid synthesis and is one of the preeminent drugs for nonoperable Cushing disease. Alternatives are metyrapone and aminoglutethimide, not listed here. Dexamethasone (a) is a synthetic corticosteroid with powerful glucocorticoid effects and little or no mineralocorticoid activity. Hydrocortisone (b) is cortisol; an efficacious glucocorticoid with useful (but slight) mineralocorticoid activity. The same applies to prednisone (d), predominately a glucocorticoid used as an oral anti-inflammatory drug for asthma, some arthritides, and other steroid-responsive conditions. Spironolactone (e) is an aldosterone receptor antagonist, used mainly for primary or secondary hyperaldosteronism, for heart failure, and for its potassium-sparing diuretic effects.

411. The answer is c. *(Brunton, pp 309t, 1500. Katzung, pp 644-645, 655-657.)* Primary amenorrhea is associated with hyperprolactinemia. Women who are amenorrheic from hyperprolactinemia also often present with galactorrhea and infertility. Bromocriptine, a dopamine receptor agonist, inhibits prolactin release. The site of action is the pituitary, and it involves the same site and ultimate mechanism by which dopamine, released from the hypothalamus, normally suppresses prolactin release. Some causes of hyperprolactinemia, in both men and women, include pituitary cancer, hypothalamic dysfunction, and some drugs (eg, antipsychotics, estrogens). Recall that bromocriptine, by virtue of its central dopaminergic activity, is sometimes used to help correct the dopamine-ACh imbalance that underlies Parkinson disease.

Effects on estrogens or progestin (a, d), gonadotropins (a), FSH (b), or GnRH (e) are not responsible for the therapeutic actions of bromocriptine in the context of managing primary amenorrhea.

412. The answer is e. *(Brunton, pp 1649-1658. Katzung, pp 754-758.)* Parathyroid hormone's main role is to maintain normal plasma Ca^{2+} levels. When plasma Ca^{2+} concentrations become sufficiently low, parathyroid hormone synthesis and release increase, and it helps restore a normocalcemic state by promoting (in concert with vitamin D) Ca^{2+} absorption from the intestines (therefore a is incorrect), promotes renal tubular Ca^{2+} reabsorption and phosphate excretion (the opposite of answers b and c), and increases mobilization of Ca^{2+} and phosphate from bone (the opposite of answer d).

413. The answer is a. *(Brunton, pp 808-809. Katzung, p 187.)* Persistently high plasma glucose and cholesterol levels obviously have many untoward consequences, one of which is renovascular disease that may lead to eventual renal failure and death. The patient already has microalbuminuria, so some renal damage is likely present. When the arterial supply to both kidneys is reduced because of stenosis (or other factors), that weighs against using an ACE inhibitor or an ARB. Angiotensin II has a critical role in maintaining glomerular filtration by increasing efferent arteriolar pressure. Blocking A-II synthesis, or its receptor-mediated vasoconstrictor effects, can significantly reduce renal perfusion and GFR and, eventually and sometimes precipitously, lead to renal failure.

ACE inhibitors or ARBs do not cause bradycardia (b), whether directly or via baroreceptor-related reflex mechanisms. Prior episodes of hyperosmolar hyperglycemic nonketotic syndrome (HHNKA, c) reflect periods of severe, symptomatic hyperglycemia (and poor glycemic control). In the absence of bilateral renal disease or other renal pathologies (or if the patient is not a woman who is pregnant or of child-bearing potential), an ACE inhibitor or ARB would be a logical choice for controlling hypertension; heart failure does not contraindicate (d) the use of these medications. Neither hypercholesterolemia or hypertriglyceridemia (or both), nor the use of niacin or other drugs for dyslipidemias (e), has any impact on the decision to use an ACE inhibitor or ARB in the absence of other contraindications.

Antimicrobial and Antiviral Pharmacology

Antibacterials
Antimycobacterials
Antifungals
Antivirals
Antiprotozoals

Questions

414. You are a physician and epidemiologist employed by the U.S. Centers for Disease Control and Prevention, working in Atlanta. You get an urgent phone call stating that an envelope with no return address was opened in the mail room of a large corporation that received federal bail-out money and has top executives getting salaries and bonuses in "seven figures." Some sort of white powder fell out and was blown around the room, exposing dozens of workers. The suspicion is anthrax. Which of the following drugs would be best, most properly indicated, for prophylaxis if the substance tests positive for *Bacillus anthracis*?

a. Azithromycin
b. Clarithromycin
c. Doxycycline
d. Hydroxychloroquine
e. Metronidazole

415. You are caring for a patient with HIV infection and will start drug therapy initially with the nucleoside analog zidovudine (formerly called azidothymidine, or AZT). Which of the following statements most correctly describes zidovudine or the dideoxynucleoside class to which it belongs?

a. Levels of active metabolite in cerebrospinal fluid usually are not detectable (ie, zero) because it cannot cross the blood-brain barrier.
b. Resistance to these antivirals develops rapidly after monotherapy starts, involves decreased incorporation of active metabolite into viral DNA.
c. The dideoxynucleoside stops viral nucleic acid synthesis.
d. The active metabolite is an equally effective substrate for viral reverse transcriptase and mammalian DNA polymerase, which explains the high incidence of host toxicity.
e. Zidovudine is phosphorylated to form the active metabolite, which is incorporated into viral nucleic acid via HIV reverse transcriptase.

416. A patient on antimicrobial therapy develops the following signs and symptoms that ultimately are found to be drug-induced: cough, dyspnea, and pulmonary infiltrates; neutropenia and bleeding tendencies; and paresthesias. Which of the following is the most likely cause of this patient's symptoms?

a. Amoxicillin
b. Azithromycin
c. Ciprofloxacin
d. Isoniazid
e. Nitrofurantoin

417. A patient with an opportunistic infection with *Pneumocystis jurovecii* is receiving a combination of sulfamethoxazole (SMZ) and trimethoprim (TMP). Which of the following statements describes best the mechanism by which this combination exerts its desired effects—and does so better than if just one of the drugs was administered?

a. The combination exerts significant antiviral activity, thereby reducing the risk of opportunistic *P jurovecii* infections during antiviral therapy with other medications.
b. The SMZ makes bacterial cell walls more permeable, allowing better penetration of the TMP.
c. They inhibit sequential steps in bacterial synthesis of tetrahydrofolic acid.
d. TMP inhibits production of resistance factors (R-factors) directed against SMZ.
e. TMP kills gut flora that otherwise would reduce oral bioavailability of the SMZ.

418. A 39-year-old man with aortic insufficiency and a history of multiple antibiotic resistances is given a prophylactic intravenous dose of antibiotic before surgery to insert a prosthetic heart valve. As the antibiotic is being infused, the patient becomes flushed over most of his body. Which antibiotic most likely caused this cutaneous response?

a. Erythromycin
b. Gentamicin
c. Penicillin G
d. Tetracycline
e. Vancomycin

419. A patient presents with severe, unrelenting diarrhea, and the fluid and electrolyte imbalances one would expect from that. She had been started on an antibiotic recently, and the likely diagnosis is antibiotic-associated pseudomembranous colitis (AAPMC). What drug is the most likely cause?

a. Amoxicillin
b. Azithromycin
c. Clindamycin
d. Metronidazole
e. Trimethoprim plus sulfamethoxazole (TMP-SMZ)

420. A 35-year-old woman complains of itching in the vulval area. Hanging-drop examination of the urine reveals trichomonads. What is the preferred treatment for the trichomoniasis?

a. Doxycycline
b. Emetine
c. Metronidazole
d. Pentamidine
e. Pyrazinamide

421. A 59-year-old woman is diagnosed with tuberculosis (TB). Before prescribing a multidrug regimen, you take a careful medication history because one of the drugs commonly used to treat TB induces some of the microsomal cytochrome P450 enzymes in the liver, and is a common cause of drug-drug interactions. Which of the following is the most likely drug?

a. Ethambutol
b. Isoniazid
c. Pyrazinamide
d. Rifampin
e. Vitamin B_6

422. A patient will be started on primaquine to treat active *Plasmodium vivax* malaria, specifically to target the hepatic forms of the parasite. Before you administer the drug you should screen the patient to assess their relative risk of developing a relatively common and severe adverse response to the drug. Which of the following is that primaquine-associated risk?

a. Cardiac conduction disturbances
b. Hemolytic disease
c. Nephrotoxicity
d. Retinopathy
e. Seizures, convulsions

423. You are on morning rounds in the hospital and encounter a patient being treated with linezolid, the first approved member of the oxazolidine class of antimicrobials. Which of the following most correctly describes a characteristic of this drug?

a. Exerts strong bactericidal effects
b. Mainly used for relatively minor infections with gram-negative organisms
c. Preferred alternative to amoxicillin for children with otitis media
d. Preferred alternative to ciprofloxacin for *B anthracis* infections
e. Suitable for vancomycin-resistant enterococci

424. A patient with HIV infection is receiving a combination of protease inhibitors as part of overall antiviral therapy. What is, ordinarily, the most likely/most common side effect(s) of the protease inhibitors?

a. Anemia and neutropenia
b. Hyperglycemia and hyperlipidemia
c. Lactic acidosis
d. Neuropathy
e. Pancreatitis

425. A 27-year-old woman has just returned from a trip to Southeast Asia. Over the past 24 hours she has developed shaking, chills, and a temperature of 104°F. A blood smear reveals *P vivax*. Which of the following drugs would you prescribe to eradicate the extraerythrocytic phase of the organism?

a. Chloroguanide
b. Chloroquine
c. Primaquine
d. Pyrimethamine
e. Quinacrine

426. A jaundiced 1-day-old premature infant with an elevated free bilirubin is seen in the premature baby nursery. The mother had received an antibiotic combination for a urinary tract infection (UTI) 1 week before delivery. Which of the following antibiotic drugs or classes was the most likely cause of the baby's kernicterus?

a. Aminopenicillin (eg, amoxicillin)
b. Azithromycin
c. Erythromycin
d. Fourth-generation cephalosporin
e. Sulfamethoxazole plus trimethoprim

427. A sputum culture of a 65-year-old man with pneumonia is positive for β-lactamase-positive staphylococci. Which of the following is the best choice for penicillin therapy in this patient?

a. Ampicillin
b. Carbenicillin
c. Oxacillin
d. Penicillin G
e. Ticarcillin

428. A patient has a severe bacterial infection that normally would respond to an oral penicillin or a cephalosporin. However, his chart documents anaphylactoid reactions to both drugs. Given the history, what drug would be preferred for treating the infection, and also poses the least risk of cross-reactivity and an allergic response?

a. Clotrimazole
b. Gentamicin
c. Metronidazole
d. Tetracycline
e. Vancomycin

429. A 40-year-old man is HIV-positive with a cluster-of-differentiation-4 (CD4) count of 200/mm^3. Within 2 months he develops a peripheral white blood cell count of 1000/mm^3 and a hemoglobin of 9.0 mg/dL. Which of the following drugs most likely caused the hematologic abnormalities?

a. Acyclovir
b. Dideoxycytidine
c. Foscarnet
d. Rimantadine
e. Zidovudine

430. An 86-year-old man complains of cough and blood in his sputum for the past 2 days. On admission, his temperature is 103°F. Physical examination reveals rales in his right lung, and x-ray examination shows increased density in the right middle lobe. A sputum smear shows many gram-positive cocci, confirmed by sputum culture as penicillinase-producing *Staphylococcus aureus*. Which of the following antibiotics would be best to administer?

a. Ampicillin
b. Carbenicillin
c. Mezlocillin
d. Oxacillin
e. Ticarcillin

431. When considering all the main antibacterial drugs that work by inhibiting protein synthesis in one way or another, virtually every one exerts bacteriostatic actions. Which of the following drugs differs from all the rest because the usual consequence of therapeutic plasma levels is bactericidal, rather than mere inhibition of bacterial growth and replication?

a. Aminoglycosides
b. Clindamycin
c. Erythromycins
d. Linezolid
e. Tetracyclines

432. A patient with HIV infection and clinical AIDS is treated with a combination of agents, one of which is zidovudine. Which enzyme or replicative process is the main target of this antiviral drug?

a. Nonnucleoside reverse transcriptase
b. Nucleoside reverse transcriptase
c. RNA synthesis
d. Viral particle assembly or fusion
e. Viral proteases

433. A 39-year-old woman with a history of recurrent urinary tract infections develops a new infection. Culture of a urine sample indicated that the offending organism is *Escherichia coli*. She receives therapeutic doses of ciprofloxacin. Symptoms disappear as the offending bacteria are destroyed. What is the main bacterial process or enzyme that was inhibited by the fluoroquinolone?

a. Cell-wall synthesis
b. Folic acid synthesis
c. Protein synthesis
d. RNA polymerase
e. Topoisomerase II (DNA gyrase)

434. A patient with HIV/AIDS, being treated with multiple antiviral and immunosuppressive drugs, develops an opportunistic infection caused by *P jurovecii* (*P carinii*). Which of the following drugs would be best to use to treat the pulmonary infection caused by this protozoan?

a. Carbenicillin
b. Metronidazole
c. Nifurtimox
d. Penicillin G
e. Pentamidine

435. A 25-year-old woman with an upper respiratory tract infection caused by *Haemophilus influenzae* is treated with trimethoprim-sulfamethoxazole. She responds well in a matter of days after starting the TMP-SMZ. Which bacterial process is inhibited by this combination, and accounts for the antibacterial effects?

a. Cell-wall synthesis
b. Folic acid synthesis
c. Protein synthesis
d. RNA polymerase
e. Topoisomerase II (DNA gyrase)

436. A man who has been at the local tavern, drinking alcohol heavily, is assaulted. He is transported to the hospital. Among various findings is an infection for which prompt antibiotic therapy is indicated. Given his high blood alcohol level, which antibiotic should be avoided because of a high potential of causing a serious disulfiram-like reaction that might provoke ventilatory or cardiovascular failure?

a. Amoxicillin
b. Cefoperazone (or cefotetan)
c. Erythromycin ethylsuccinate
d. Linezolid
e. Penicillin G

437. A 43-year-old woman is recovering from major surgery, following discharge from the hospital, in an assisted-care facility. She develops fever, rales, dyspnea, cough, and purulent sputum. Results of a chest radiograph indicate bilateral pulmonary infiltrates. We send blood and sputum cultures to the clinical pathology lab for culturing, but now must turn our attention to what we believe is community-acquired pneumonia caused by antibiotic-resistant pneumococci. We want to start empiric antibiotic therapy until culture results are available. Which drug would be best for this initial therapy?

a. Amoxicillin
b. Cefazolin
c. Erythromycin
d. Levofloxacin
e. Penicillin G
f. Vancomycin

438. Blood and sputum cultures taken in a critically ill 26-year-old woman indicate the presence of MRSA—methicillin-resistant *S aureus*. Which drug is most likely to be effective in treating this infection?

a. Amoxicillin plus clavulanic acid
b. Clindamycin
c. Erythromycin
d. Trimethoprim-sulfamethoxazole (TMP-SMZ)
e. Vancomycin

439. Compared with most other cephalosporins, the administration of cefmetazole, cefoperazone, or cefotetan is associated with a higher incidence of an adverse response that is particularly dangerous for some patients. What is that rather unique adverse response?

a. Acute heart failure
b. Acute renal failure
c. Bleeding tendencies in patients taking warfarin
d. Hypertension
e. Ototoxicity

440. A patient develops muscle aches and pains during the course of antibiotic therapy. A muscle biopsy would clearly show myopathy. Which drug most likely (and rather uniquely) caused this adverse effect on skeletal muscle?

a. Daptomycin
b. Erythromycin
c. Gentamicin
d. Linezolid
e. Vancomycin

441. A patient with an infectious disease routinely takes their antimicrobial medication with milk or other dairy products in an attempt to reduce stomach upset from the drug. The antibiotic fails to work adequately because calcium in the dairy products chelates the drug and reduces its oral bioavailability. Which antimicrobial drug or drug class was the patient most likely taking?

a. Aminoglycoside
b. Antimycobacterial drug, specifically isoniazid
c. Cephalosporin, first-generation
d. Cephalosporin, third-generation
e. Penicillin
f. Tetracycline

442. A patient develops profuse, watery diarrhea, fever, abdominal pain, and leukocytosis in response to antibiotic therapy. *Clostridium difficile* infection in the gut is confirmed. What is the preferred agent for therapy of this antibiotic-associated pseudomembranous colitis (AAPMC)?

a. Amphotericin B
b. Clindamycin
c. Gentamicin
d. Metronidazole
e. Trimethoprim plus sulfamethoxazole (TMP-SMZ)

443. A patient has been taking warfarin for several months and their INR (International Normalized Ratio) and PT (prothrombin time) have been kept within the desired therapeutic range consistently. They develop an infection and are started on antibiotic therapy. Shortly thereafter their INR rises to 8 (very high) and they develop epistaxis and other indicators of excessive bleeding. Which antibiotic most likely interacted with the warfarin, increasing its blood levels and effects, by inhibiting warfarin's metabolism by the hepatic P450 system?

a. Azithromycin
b. Erythromycin
c. Gentamicin
d. Penicillin G
e. Rifampin

444. Ampicillin and amoxicillin are in the same group of penicillins (broad spectrum, or aminopenicillins). However, there is one clinically important difference. Which of the following phrases best states how amoxicillin differs from ampicillin?

a. Has better oral bioavailability, particularly when taken with meals
b. Is effective against penicillinase-producing organisms
c. Is a broad-spectrum penicillin
d. Does not cause hypersensitivity reactions
e. Has great antipseudomonal activity

445. A patient's history notes a documented severe (anaphylactoid) reaction to a penicillin. What other antibiotic or class is likely to cross-react and so should be avoided in this patient?

a. Aminoglycosides
b. Azithromycin
c. Cephalosporins
d. Erythromycin
e. Linezolid
f. Tetracyclines

446. A 30-year-old woman develops a severe *Pseudomonas aeruginosa* infection. The physician chooses to treat it with amikacin, not with gentamicin. Which of the following phrases best describes how amikacin differs from gentamicin?

a. Does not require monitoring of blood levels during therapy
b. Exerts significant bactericidal effects against anaerobes too
c. Has broader spectrum against gram-negative bacilli
d. Lacks ototoxic potential
e. Protects against typical aminoglycoside nephrotoxicity

447. A 19-year-old being treated for leukemia develops a fever. You give several agents that will cover bacterial, viral, and fungal infections. Two days later, he develops acute renal failure. Which of the following drugs is most likely responsible?

a. Acyclovir
b. Amphotericin B
c. Ceftazidime
d. Penicillin G
e. Vancomycin

448. Penicillins, cephalosporins, and amphotericin B are quite different structurally, and the antimicrobial spectrum of amphotericin B is decidedly different from those of the other agents. Nonetheless, they all share a common property or action. Which of the following statements identifies what that is?

a. Act, though various mechanisms, on cell walls or membranes of susceptible organisms.
b. Contraindicated in immunocompromised patients.
c. Interact with many drugs by inducing their hepatic metabolism.
d. Leukopenia (decreased white cell counts) is a common side effect.
e. Nephrotoxicity is common.

449. Given the recent and widespread worldwide outbreaks of "swine flu" (particularly influenza A virus subtype H1N1) there has been a great need for prophylactic measures in certain at-risk populations who may be susceptible. Which of the following drugs is generally recommended by the U.S. Centers for Disease Control and Prevention for this purpose?

a. Acyclovir
b. Amantadine
c. Lopinavir
d. Oseltamivir
e. Ritonavir

450. A patient with a *P aeruginosa* infection is receiving intravenous gentamicin. The aminoglycoside blood levels are well above the minimum inhibitory concentration (MIC), but the clinical response is not satisfactory. A new medication order calls for adding a penicillin, administered in separate IV lines to avoid a physical incompatibility. If this order is carried out, what is most likely to occur?

a. The aminoglycoside will inactivate the penicillin.
b. The aminoglycoside will chemically neutralize and abolish the effects of the penicillin.
c. The patient is likely to develop *C difficile* colitis (superinfection).
d. The penicillin will act synergistically with the aminoglycoside.
e. The penicillin will increase the risk of aminoglycoside nephrotoxicity.
f. The risk of inducing resistance to both drugs increases dramatically.

451. Narrow spectrum penicillins, both penicillinase-sensitive and -resistant, have relatively poor activity against gram-negative bacteria. What is the main property or characteristic that explains why these microorganisms do not respond well to the penicillins?

a. Actively transport any absorbed penicillin back to the extracellular space
b. Have an outer membrane that serves as a physical barrier to the penicillins
c. Lack a surface enzyme necessary to metabolically activate the penicillins
d. Lack penicillin-binding proteins
e. Metabolically inactivate these penicillins by mechanisms not involving β-lactamase

452. We have a patient with an intraabdominal infection, and *Bacteroides fragilis* is the main organism found upon culture. Which cephalosporin has the greatest activity against anaerobes such *B fragilis*?

a. Cefaclor
b. Cefoxitin
c. Cefuroxime
d. Cephalexin
e. Cephalothin

453. You are taking an initial health history from a 22-year-old woman who just moved to your town. She is remarkably fit and healthy, but is wearing two hearing aids for binaural (bilateral) high-frequency hearing loss. You inquire about the possible reason(s) for this. She says she lost most of her hearing after receiving an antibiotic for a severe infection when she was 19, but cannot recall the specific drug. Which drug or drug class was most likely responsible for the ototoxicity?

a. Aminoglycoside (eg, gentamicin)
b. Cephalosporin, first-generation
c. Cephalosporin, third-generation
d. Fluoroquinolone (eg, ciprofloxacin)
e. Penicillin

454. A 26-year-old woman with acquired immunodeficiency syndrome (AIDS) develops cryptococcal meningitis. She refuses intravenous medication. Which antifungal agent is the best choice for oral therapy of the meningitis?

a. Amphotericin B
b. Fluconazole
c. Ketoconazole
d. Metronidazole
e. Nystatin

455. An adult patient is being treated with a parenteral aminoglycoside for a serious *P aeruginosa* infection. He requires immediate surgery. He is premedicated with midazolam, followed by administration of propofol for induction. A dose of succinylcholine is given for intubation, with skeletal muscle paralysis maintained during surgery with pancuronium. Balanced anesthesia is provided with nitrous oxide, isoflurane, and oxygen. What is the most likely outcome of having the aminoglycoside "on board" in the perioperative setting along with all these other drugs?

a. Acute hepatotoxicity from an aminoglycoside-isoflurane interaction
b. Antagonism of midazolam's amnestic and sedative effects
c. Enhanced aminoglycoside toxicity to host cells
d. Increased or prolonged response to neuromuscular blockers
e. Reduced risk of catecholamine-induced cardiac arrhythmias

456. A patient with tuberculosis is started on isoniazid (INH) as part of a multidrug regimen. The physician also starts therapy with vitamin B_6 at the same time. What is the main reason for giving the vitamin B_6 prophylactically?

a. Facilitates INH renal excretion, thereby protecting against nephrotoxicity
b. Inhibits metabolism of INH, thereby increasing INH blood levels
c. Is a cofactor required for activation of the INH to its antimycobacterial metabolite
d. Potentiates the antitubercular activity of the INH
e. Prevents some adverse effects of INH therapy

457. One antibiotic is considered very effective in treatment of *Rickettsia*, *Mycoplasma*, and *Chlamydia* infections? It is also used to manage some patients with acne vulgaris lesions. To which drug does this description apply?

a. Bacitracin
b. Gentamicin
c. Penicillin G
d. Tetracycline
e. Vancomycin

458. We are starting therapy for an established HIV infection in a 28-year-old man. The drugs are ritonavir, lopinavir, zidovudine, and didanosine. We are obviously using two protease inhibitors and two nucleoside reverse transcriptase inhibitors (NRTIs). What is the main purpose of using the ritonavir?

a. Helps maintain adequate saquinavir levels by inhibiting its metabolism
b. Induces the metabolic activation of the NRTIs, which are prodrugs
c. Prevents the likely development of hypoglycemia
d. Reduces, or hopefully eliminates, lopinavir-mediated host toxicity
e. Serves as the main, most active, inhibitor of viral protease in this combination

459. As part of a multidrug attack on a patient's infection with *Mycobacterium tuberculosis*, a physician plans to use an aminoglycoside antibiotic. Which drug is most active against the tubercle bacillus and seems to be associated with the fewest problems with resistance or typical aminoglycoside-induced adverse effects?

a. Amikacin
b. Kanamycin
c. Neomycin
d. Streptomycin
e. Tobramycin

460. Such agents as clavulanic acid, sulbactam, or tazobactam are often added to some proprietary (manufactured) penicillin combination products. What is the main reason for including them, or describes their action best?

a. Add antibiotic activity against *Pseudomonas* and many *Enterobacter* species
b. Facilitate antibiotic penetration into the central nervous system and cerebrospinal fluid
c. Inhibit cell wall transpeptidases
d. Inhibit inactivation of penicillin by β-lactamase-producing bacteria
e. Inhibit the normally significant hepatic metabolism of the penicillin
f. Reduce the risk and/or severity of allergic reactions in susceptible patients

461. A patient with active tuberculosis is being treated with isoniazid (INH) and ethambutol as part of the overall regimen. Which of the following is the main effect expected of the ethambutol?

a. Facilitated entry of the INH into the mycobacteria
b. Facilitated penetration of the blood-brain barrier
c. Retarded absorption after intramuscular injection
d. Retarded development of organism resistance
e. Slowed renal excretion of INH to help maintain effective blood levels

462. A patient has a severe infection caused by anaerobic bacteria. The first-year house officer writes an order for gentamicin. This approach is doomed to fail because aminoglycosides have no activity against anaerobes. Which of the following best explains why anaerobes will be resistant?

a. Cannot metabolize the aminoglycosides, which are all prodrugs, to their bactericidal-free radical forms
b. Cannot oxidatively metabolize aminoglycosides to moieties that are nontoxic to host cells
c. Lack molecular oxygen that is a prerequisite for drug binding to the 50S subunit of bacterial ribosomes
d. Lack the ability to transport aminoglycosides from the extracellular milieu in the absence of oxygen
e. Synthesize more and more active resistance factors than do aerobic bacteria

463. In patients with hepatic coma or portal-systemic encephalopathy decreasing the production and absorption of ammonia from the gastrointestinal (GI) tract will be beneficial. What is the antibiotic of choice in this situation and for this specific purpose?

a. Cephalothin
b. Chloramphenicol
c. Neomycin
d. Penicillin G
e. Tetracycline

464. A 19-year-old women who previously was healthy develops bacterial meningitis. It seems inevitable that with the malignancy of the condition and the degree of distal tissue death she will need to have both arms and legs amputated. Nonetheless, of course, antibiotic therapy is essential. Which of the following would be the drug of choice for this situation?

a. Ceftriaxone
b. Erythromycin
c. Penicillin G
d. Penicillin V
e. Procaine penicillin

465. A patient is being treated with an antibiotic for a vancomycin-resistant enterococcal (VRE) infection. She consumes an over-the-counter medication containing ephedrine and develops a significant spike of blood pressure that leads to a pounding headache. She is transported to the hospital. As part of the workup, blood tests indicate some bone marrow suppression. Which antibiotic is most likely associated with this clinical picture?

a. Azithromycin
b. Ciprofloxacin
c. Erythromycin estolate
d. Gentamicin
e. Linezolid

Antimicrobial and Antiviral Pharmacology

Answers

414. The answer is c. *(Brunton, pp 1122, 1137, 1177. Katzung, pp 819-820, 888t-890t.) Bacillus anthracis* is a gram-positive anaerobe, and of the drugs listed only doxycycline is indicated and apt to be effective. (The equally effective and more often turned-to alternative is ciprofloxacin.) Azithromycin (a) or clarithromycin (b) are first choice drugs for *Mycobacterium avium* complex, used in conjunction with ethambutol (with or without rifabutin too). They are also used widely (particularly azithromycin) for a variety of responsive infections of the respiratory tract; uncomplicated skin infections, otitis media, etc. Azithromycin is the drug of choice for treating *C trachomatis* infections. Clarithromycin is also commonly used, as part of multidrug therapy, as an alternative to penicillin G in penicillin-allergic patients, for *Helicobacter pylori* eradication in patients with severe or recurrent GI tract ulcers. Hydroxychloroquine (d) is an antimalarial drug, wholly inappropriate for anthrax. Metronidazole (e) is primarily used for and effective first-line therapy with gram-positive bacilli (eg, *C difficile*, and *Clostridium tetani*), *Bacteroides* (gram-negative enteric bacteria), and *Gardnerella vaginalis* (gram-negative bacillus). It, too, is one common and effective ingredient in multidrug eradicative therapy of *H pylori* infections.

415. The answer is e. *(Brunton, pp 1249, 1251, 1255, 1276t, 1280-1285. Katzung, pp 856t, 860-861.)* Resistance develops rapidly when only zidovudine or another nucleoside analog is used to treat HIV. It most likely involves decreased incorporation of the active metabolite into viral DNA, or increased excision of it from viral DNA. Zidovudine and other nucleoside analogs must be phosphorylated to form the active metabolite, the dideoxynucleo*tide* triphosphate. It occurs via the actions of several kinases in host cells. That levels of active metabolite in CSF are undetectable (a) is false. In most cases CSF concentrations of active drug reach about 60% of those measured in the plasma at the same time. The ultimate effect of these drugs is, indeed, to stop viral nucleic acid synthesis (c), but that occurs only after the administered drug, the dideoxynucleoside, is phosphorylated. The active metabolite is a good substrate for HIV reverse transcriptase, but a very poor one for DNA polymerases in host cells (and so d is incorrect).

And the main adverse responses to or side effects associated with zidovudine? They include bone marrow toxicity, leukopenia/granulocytopenia, and anemia; potentially severe or persistent insomnia and headache, nausea, and vomiting. The side effects profiles differ somewhat among the other dideoxynucleosides.

416. The answer is e. *(Brunton, pp 1123-1124. Katzung, p 878.)* Although several of the antimicrobial agents listed can cause one (or perhaps two) of the adverse responses noted here, nitrofurantoin is the most likely cause. GI side effects (anorexia, nausea, vomiting) are the most common side effects caused by this drug, which is still widely used for managing acute lower urinary tract infections (eg, from many strains of *E coli*, staphylococci, streptococci, *Neisseria, Bacteroides*). However, the drug can also cause acute or subacute pulmonary reactions such as those described, various hematologic reactions (in particular, leukopenia and thrombocytopenia), and peripheral sensory and motor neuropathies.

Amoxicillin (a)—and most other penicillins—may cause central neurotoxicity if present at extraordinarily high plasma levels. Beyond that, allergic reactions are the most important adverse responses. Pulmonary, hematologic, and peripheral neuropathic adverse responses are not associated with these drugs.

Azithromycin's (b) profile of adverse effects is quite similar to that of erythromycin and other macrolides, and that profile does not include the signs and symptoms noted here. GI upset, mild to severe, are the most common complaints, and azithromycin may be ototoxic.

Ciprofloxacin (c; or other fluoroquinolones) is not likely to cause any of the adverse responses noted. They are quite well tolerated and cause a variety of side effects that, in general, are mild. If one were to recall one "unique" toxicity, it would be alterations of collagen metabolism that may lead to tendon rupture. There is also evidence that the drug can prolong the QT interval, leading to arrhythmias, particularly in patients with long QT syndrome.

Isoniazid (d) can cause peripheral neuropathy (mainly from a drug-induced pyridoxine deficiency) and hepatotoxicity. Pulmonary and bleeding problems are not at all common in terms of drug-induced problems.

417. The answer is c. *(Brunton, pp 1104, 1111-1115. Katzung, pp 816-819, 888-891, 1252f.)* SMZ and TMP act on sequential steps in the synthesis of tetrahydrofolic acid in susceptible bacteria. Sulfamethoxazole (and sulfonamides in general) inhibit incorporation of para-aminobenzoic acid (PABA) into folic acid. Trimethoprim then inhibits dihydrofolate reductase, the enzyme that (in the presence of NADPH) converts dihydrofolate into tetrahydrofolate. This leads to the bacteriostatic effect in susceptible organisms, and a clinical response that is better than with either drug used alone.

Note that this mechanism accounts for the selectively toxic effect on microbes, as opposed to host cells, because mammalian cell dihydrofolate reductases are largely insensitive to the effects of TMP, and host cell viability is not dependent on tetrahydrofolate synthesis (they use "preformed" folic acid, folate from the diet) and so they are unaffected by the sulfonamide.

Neither SMZ nor TMP, alone or in combination, exerts antiviral activity (a). Sulfamethoxazole does not permeabilize bacterial cell walls (b); trimethoprim does not inhibit R-factors (d) or affect the bioavailability of SMZ by any mechanism (e).

418. The answer is e. *(Brunton, pp 632, 1196. Katzung, pp 786-787.)* This "red man" syndrome is characteristically associated with vancomycin, and is not a manifestation of drug allergy. The flushing (redness) of the skin, often most prominent on the chest, neck, and face, is thought to be caused by histamine release. The risk or severity can be reduced dramatically by infusing the drug more slowly, and by pretreatment with antihistamines (H_1-receptor blockers, eg, diphenhydramine).

Macrolides such as erythromycin (a) and tetracycline (d) do not cause a similar response. Nor do the aminoglycosides (eg, gentamicin, b) or penicillins (c; at least in patients who are not allergic to these drugs).

419. The answer is c. *(Brunton, pp 1188-1190. Katzung, pp 801-802, 889t.)* More than any other antibiotic, clindamycin is associated with the highest risk of AAPMC (*C difficile* superinfection). Thus, it is mainly reserved for certain anaerobic infections located outside the CNS (susceptible anaerobes include *B fragilis*, *Fusobacterium*, and *Clostridium perfringens*, plus anaerobic streptococci). Tetracycline use is also associated with AAPMC. The phenomenon is not typically attributed to treatment with amoxicillin (a), azithromycin (b), or the trimethoprim-sulfamethoxazole combination (e). Metronidazole (d) or vancomycin (not listed) are considered preferred treatments for AAPMC—and the offending drug should be stopped as soon as AAPMC is suspected.

420. The answer is c. *(Brunton, pp 1050, 1058-1060. Katzung, pp 596t, 877, 889t, 913-914.)* Metronidazole is distributed to all body fluids and tissues. Its spectrum of activity is limited largely to anaerobic bacteria—including *B fragilis*—and certain protozoa. It is considered to be the drug of choice for trichomoniasis in females and carrier states in males, as well as for intestinal infections with *Giardia lamblia*.

Doxycycline (a), emetine (b; an antiprotozoal), pentamidine (d; used for treatment of *P jirovecii; [P carnii]* pneumonia, or prophylactically for that condition in high-risk HIV-positive patients), and pyrazinamide (e; a bactericidal agent used for *M tuberculosis* infections) would not be appropriate for the patient described in the question.

421. The answer is d. *(Brunton, pp 121, 1209. Katzung, pp 825-826, 1149t.)* Rifampin induces cytochrome P450 enzymes, which causes a significant increase in elimination rates of many interacting drugs, such as oral contraceptives, warfarin, ketoconazole, cyclosporine, and chloramphenicol. It also promotes urinary excretion of methadone, which may precipitate withdrawal.

Ethambutol (a), isoniazid (b), pyrazinamide (c), and vitamin B_6 (e) are not P450 inducers, although the metabolism of some of these drugs can be induced by rifampin.

422. The answer is b. *(Brunton, pp 101-102, 1040-1045. Katzung, pp 907-908.)* Hemolysis is the most common and serious adverse response to primaquine. The risk is clearly highest in patients who have red cell deficiencies in glucose-6-phosphate dehydrogenase, a heritable trait and one that can be screened for before giving the drug. (This G6PD deficiency is more common in blacks, and whites with darker skin [eg, some from certain regions of the Middle East or the Mediterranean countries].) Regardless of the results of pretreatment screening, periodic blood counts should be done, and the urine checked for unusual darkening (indicating the presence of hemoglobin from lysed red cells), during treatment.

Cardiac conduction disturbances (a), nephrotoxicity (c), and seizures (e) are not typically associated with primaquine. If you selected answer d, "retinopathy," you were probably thinking about chloroquine, which may cause that response.

423. The answer is e. *(Brunton, pp 432, 1098, 1136, 1192-1193, 1203-1204, 1212, 1690. Katzung, pp 804, 824t, 829.)* Linezolid is a bacteriostatic (not cidal, so answer a is wrong) inhibitor of protein synthesis. Its unique mechanism of action, binding to the 23S portion of the 50s ribosomal subunit, ultimately blocks formation of the initiator complex that is necessary for bacterial replication. This unique mechanism means linezolid is not susceptible to cross-resistance that may have developed to other antibiotics, but the more the drug is used the greater the likelihood that resistance to it will develop.

Linezolid is, indeed, the preferred drug for vancomycin-resistant enterococci, and vancomycin is often used as a "drug of last resort" for serious infections that cannot be treated with first-line alternatives. Another major use is for methicillin-resistant *S aureus*, for which linezolid and vancomycin seem to be equally efficacious. (There are other approved uses for linezolid, but since few bacteria are resistant to it—so far—it should be used sparingly, only when absolutely needed.) It is not at all indicated for relatively minor infections, especially those with gram-negative causes (b). It is not a preferred alternative to amoxicillin for otitis media (c). Doxycycline, not linezolid, is the preferred alternative to ciprofloxacin for anthrax prophylaxis or treatment (d).

The most serious adverse effect associated with linezolid is reversible myelosuppression. Complete blood counts need to be done at least once a week if this drug is being administered to myelosuppressed patients (including those taking other myelosuppressive drugs) or if linezolid therapy lasts more than about 14 days.

424. The answer is b. *(Brunton, pp 122, 1209, 1217, 1276t, 1295t, 1302-1303. Katzung, pp 862-867.)* Protease inhibitors, as a class, tend to cause hyperglycemia (probably involves insulin resistance in parenchymal cells) and hyperlipidemia (precise mechanism not known).

The other adverse responses listed are more typical of those caused by nucleoside reverse transcriptase inhibitors (NRTIs; zidovudine, others), and it is worthwhile commenting on that here. Anemias and neutropenia (myelosuppression, a) are fairly common with NRTIs. The risk of NRTI-induced lactic acidosis is rare, but the risks go up significantly if the patient receives more than one NRTI. Lactic acidosis tends to develop along with hepatomegaly and fatty liver degeneration (steatosis). Peripheral neuropathies (d) tend to be associated with didanosine and stavudine but not with other members of the NRTI class including the prototype, zidovudine. Pancreatitis (e) is also mainly associated with NRTIs (and among the class, mainly didanosine and stavudine), not with protease inhibitors.

425. The answer is c. *(Brunton, pp 1025t, 1040-1045. Katzung, pp 907-908.)* Primaquine is effective against the extraerythrocytic forms of *P vivax* and *P ovale*. It is used to eradicate plasmodia from the liver, and in doing so it not only provides a cure but also helps prevent relapse.

Chloroguanide (a) is a very old antimalarial drug but is seldom used instead of primaquine. Chloroquine (b) would not be used because it is effective only in the erythrocytic phase of the malarial parasites' life span: it will not work against the exoerythrocytic forms of malaria parasites, nor can it serve as primary prevention. This 4-aminoquinoline derivative is a weak base that selectively concentrates in infected red blood cells. There it probably interferes with the ability of plasmodia to convert heme—a toxin to the parasite—to nontoxic metabolites.

Pyrimethamine (d) and quinacrine (e) are not suitable agents for treating the patient described in the question.

426. The answer is e. *(Brunton, pp 1102, 1116. Katzung, pp 815-819.)* Sulfonamides cross the placenta and enter the fetus in concentrations sufficient to produce toxic effects. They compete with and displace bilirubin from plasma protein binding sites, raising free bilirubin levels and causing the jaundice and other manifestations of kernicterus. For the same reason, sulfonamides should also not be given to neonates, especially premature infants. This woman should not have been given the sulfonamide, whether alone or in combination with trimethoprim. Nitrofurantoin usually would be preferred for uncomplicated urinary tract infections in pregnant women. None of the other drugs are associated with this neonatal hyperbilirubinemia: amoxicillin or other aminopenicillins, a; azithromycin, b; erythromycin, c; or cephalosporins, fourth-generation or other, d.

427. The answer is c. *(Brunton, pp 1129t, 1333-1343. Katzung, pp 774-780, 790t, 888-890.)* Oxacillin is classified as a penicillinase-resistant penicillin that is relatively acid-stable and, therefore, is useful for oral administration. Major adverse reactions include penicillin hypersensitivity and interstitial nephritis. With the exception of methicillin, which is no longer used, all penicillinase-resistant penicillins are highly bound to plasma proteins. Oxacillin has a very narrow spectrum and is used primarily as an antistaphylococcal agent.

428. The answer is e. *(Brunton, pp 1194-1196. Katzung, pp 41t, 728f, 786-787, 888-890.)* Vancomycin has an antimicrobial spectrum closest to those of penicillins and cephalosporins, and it does not cross-react in patients with a history of hypersensitivity or allergic reactions to the penicillins. As is true with penicillins and cephalosporins, there is a growing risk of resistance to vancomycin (particularly in hospital settings, where the drug is mainly used), but it nonetheless is considered the best (if not the last resort) drug for these patients. Clotrimazole (a) is an antifungal drug, mainly for infections involving *Candida*. Metronidazole (c) is also used mainly for systemic or urinary tract fungal infections, although it does have some broader antibacterial activity. Gentamicin (b) would be inappropriate, in part because its spectrum of activity is not likely to include organisms killed or inhibited by penicillins, cephalosporins, or vancomycin. The same applies to tetracyclines (d).

429. The answer is e. *(Brunton, pp 1280, 1284-1285, 1440. Katzung, pp 856t, 859-861.)* One of zidovudine's major adverse effects is bone marrow depression that appears to be dose- and length-of-treatment-dependent. The severity of the disease and a low CD4 count contribute to the bone marrow depression.

430. The answer is d. *(Brunton, pp 1129-1133. Katzung, pp 774-780, 790t, 888-890.)* Unlike the other listed drugs, oxacillin is resistant to penicillinase. The other four agents are broad-spectrum penicillins, whereas oxacillin is generally specific for gram-positive microorganisms. Use of penicillinase-resistant penicillins should be reserved for infections caused by penicillinase-producing staphylococci.

431. The answer is a. *(Brunton, pp 1156-1158, 1159t. Katzung, pp 807-810.)* Of all the protein synthesis inhibitors, only the aminoglycosides are routinely bactericidal. Clindamycin (b), the erythromycins (c), linezolid (d), and the tetracyclines (e), are bacteriostatic with usual therapeutic doses and plasma concentrations.

432. The answer is b. *(Brunton, pp 1283-1284, 1290. Katzung, pp 810, 860-861.)* Zidovudine competitively inhibits HIV-1 nucleoside reverse transcriptase. It is also incorporated in the growing viral DNA chain to cause termination. Each action requires activation via phosphorylation of cellular enzymes. Zidovudine decreases the rate of clinical disease progression and prolongs survival in HIV-infected patients.

Efavirenz is an example of a nonnucleoside reverse transcriptase inhibitor (a), and it is considered to be the only member of its group that is considered a preferred agent for treating HIV infections. Interferon alfa preparations, such as those used for hepatitis (c), interfere with viral mRNA and protein synthesis (b), and also block viral entry into and eventual release from host cells. Enfuvirtide inhibits viral particle fusion (d), and so far is the only antiviral drug that works that way. Indinavir, ritonavir, and saquinavir are among the antivirals classified as protease inhibitors (e).

433. The answer is e. *(Brunton, pp 1119-1121. Katzung, pp 819-821.)* Bacterial DNA gyrase (topoisomerase II) is composed of four strand-cutting subunits to which ciprofloxacin, levofloxacin, and other quinolones bind. In doing so they inhibit bacterial growth and replication. (The original member of this group was nalidixic acid.) These antibiotics have a broad spectrum of antibiotic activity and are relatively free from common or serious side effects (some members associated with significant toxicities were withdrawn from the market), and tend not to be associated with rapidly developing antibiotic tolerance to their actions.

Penicillins, carbapenems (eg, imipenem), cephalosporins, and vancomycin, are examples of cell wall synthesis inhibitors (a). Aminoglycosides also inhibit bacterial protein synthesis, but they are bactericidal. Sulfonamides and trimethoprim, often used together, are bacteriostatic drugs that work by inhibiting folic acid synthesis (b). Tetracyclines, erythromycin and other macrolides, and such other drugs as clindamycin and linezolid, are examples of bacteriostatic protein synthesis inhibitors (c). Rifampin, which is active against most gram-positive bacteria and many gram-negative ones and is noteworthy because it exerts bactericidal effects against *M tuberculosis* and *Mycobacterium leprae*—inhibits bacterial DNA-dependent RNA polymerase (d).

434. The answer is e. *(Brunton, pp 1064-1066. Katzung, pp 817-819, 915-917.)* Both trimethoprim-sulfamethoxazole (not listed) and pentamidine are effective in pneumonia caused by *P jurovecii*. This protozoal disease usually occurs in immunodeficient patients, such as those with AIDS. Nifurtimox (c) is effective in trypanosomiasis and metronidazole (b) in amebiasis and leishmaniasis, as well as in anaerobic bacterial infections. Penicillins (d) are not considered drugs of choice for this particular disease.

435. The answer is b. *(Brunton, pp 1104, 1111-1115. Katzung, pp 815-818.)* Trimethoprim inhibits dihydrofolic acid reductase. Sulfamethoxazole inhibits p-aminobenzoic acid (PABA) incorporation into folic acid by folate, but by giving the combination we inhibit two essential and sequential steps in the formation of folate-dependent metabolites that are necessary for bacterial viability and replication. See the answer and explanation for Question 433 for a short summary of key drugs that exert antimicrobial effects by other mechanisms.

436. The answer is b. *(Brunton, pp 1145t, 1149. Katzung, pp 781-784.)* Cefoperazone (third-generation cephalosporin) or cefotetan (second-generation) inhibit aldehyde dehydrogenase and cause accumulation of acetaldehyde (as does disulfiram), and so can cause all the typical and potentially serious consequences of a disulfiram-like reaction. Cefmetazole, a second-generation cephalosporin, and metronidazole, also cause a similar adverse interaction with alcohol. (Note that these three cephalosporins are also the ones that are associated with vitamin K–related bleeding problems, as addressed in Question 439.)

Erythromycin (c; whether administered as the base or one of the common salts, eg, ethylsuccinate, estolate, or stearate) can inhibit the hepatic P450 system sufficient to cause adverse interactions with (excessive effects of) such drugs as warfarin, carbamazepine, and theophylline. However, based on current evidence there is no specific inhibition of aldehyde dehydrogenase, nor resulting accumulation of acetaldehyde, that would correctly qualify as a disulfiram-like interaction.

Amoxicillin (a), penicillin G (e), and other penicillins do not participate in disulfiram-like reactions. Linezolid (d) inhibits monoamine oxidase (MAO), albeit weakly, and so can trigger potentially significant adverse interactions in persons receiving such sympathomimetics as cocaine, ephedrine, or pseudoephedrine; or those consuming tyramine-rich foods or beverages. However, the drug does not inhibit alcohol metabolism or cause the adverse responses noted in this question.

437. The answer is d. *(Brunton, pp 1119-1121, 1146. Katzung, pp 819-821.)* Levofloxacin or another quinolone would be a good choice, not only because of their antibiotic spectrum of activity, but also because our working hypothesis is that we're dealing with a community-acquired respiratory infection caused by resistant bacteria. The resistance is likely to render penicillins (a, e), cephalosporins (b), and even erythromycin or other macrolides (c) ineffective. Resistance to fluoroquinolones has not become that much of a problem yet. Note that cefazolin (b), a first-generation cephalosporin, is ineffective against pneumococci, and is mainly suitable only for infections with *S aureus* or streptococci that are not resistant to penicillins. Vancomycin (f) might ultimately be needed, but since it must be given parenterally (and I never mentioned that the patient was unable to take oral medications) it would be premature to use this otherwise "last resort" antibiotic.

438. The answer is e. *(Brunton, pp 1096, 1098, 1131-1132, 1146-1147, 1194-1196. Katzung, pp 786-787.)* The only suitable drug listed for this potentially fatal infection is vancomycin. The finding of MRSA is not uncommon, particularly in hospitals, rendering therapy with penicillins (including amoxicillin with clavulanate, the β-lactamase inhibitor; a) ineffective. Macrolides (including clindamycin, b; and erythromycin, c) are also unsuitable, in part because of a growing resistance problem. Resistance to the trimethoprim-sulfamethoxazole (d) combination is also a major problem, regardless of the infections for which this folate reductase inhibitor therapy is prescribed.

439. The answer is c. *(Brunton, pp 1145, 1149. Katzung, pp 780-784.)* Cefmetazole and cefotetan, both second-generation cephalosporins, and cefoperazone (third-generation) can interfere with hepatic vitamin K metabolism, leading to what amounts to a deficiency of vitamin K–dependent clotting factor activity. Because this is the general mechanism by which warfarin exerts its anticoagulant effects, combined use of one of these cephalosporins can cause further (and potentially dangerous) prolongations of the International Normalized Ratio (or prothrombin time); the clinical consequence can be spontaneous, prolonged, or excessive bleeding. One should also be cautious when these cephalosporins are given to patients taking aspirin or other antiplatelet drugs (eg, clopidogrel) or thrombolytics.

Although most cephalosporins are excreted unchanged by the kidneys, renal failure (b, especially severe and acute) seldom occurs with these or other cephalosporins. There is no link between administration of even high doses of these cephalosporins (or others) with the development of acute heart failure (a). Hypertension (d) or other substantial changes of blood pressure are not associated with cephalosporins, nor are these drugs ototoxic (e).

Although a history of severe allergic reactions to penicillins requires caution when considering a cephalosporin (indeed, cephalosporins should be avoided, if possible, in such patients), there is nothing unique about cefmetazole, cefoperazone, or cefotetan in this context. None of the cephalosporins are contraindicated for patients with mild allergic reactions due to penicillins.

440. The answer is a. *(Brunton, pp 1197-1198. Katzung, pp 787-788.)* Daptomycin, classified as a cyclic lipopeptide and rapidly bactericidal against nearly all gram-positive bacteria, is uniquely associated (among antimicrobial agents) with myopathy and its typical signs and symptoms. Daily dosages currently recommended pose a low risk of myositis and myopathy, but nevertheless creatine kinase levels (marker of muscle damage) should be measured periodically during the course of therapy and the patient should be advised to report any relevant symptoms at once.

None of the other drugs listed are associated with myopathy. GI side effects are quite common with usual doses of erythromycin (b) and other macrolides, and sudden cardiac death (from QT prolongation) has been reported when erythromycin blood levels get too high. The estolate salt of erythromycin estolate (salt) may cause cholestatic hepatitis. Gentamicin (c, and most other aminoglycosides) generally cause few minor side effects; their major adverse effects are ototoxicity and nephrotoxicity. The main common side effects associated with linezolid (d) are nausea and diarrhea, and the potential for usually reversible myelosuppression and pancytopenia. Vancomycin (e) tends to cause facial and neck flushing, pruritus, and urticaria (so-called "red man syndrome"), probably secondary to local histamine release. Histamine release may also contribute to the development of tachycardia and hypotension. As with the aminoglycosides, vancomycin is ototoxic at high plasma levels.

441. The answer is f. *(Brunton, pp 121, 1175-1176. Katzung, pp 795-799.)* Tetracyclines interact with many polyvalent metal cations such that their absorption from the gut (ie, bioavailability) is reduced. The extent of this reduction can be clinically significant, that is, leading to inadequate blood levels and effects of the antibiotic.

Calcium is, of course, abundant in dairy products, some OTC antacid products, and in supplements touted for "bone health." Other metals that can interact with tetracyclines by this mechanism include iron, magnesium, aluminum, and zinc. Note that one or several of these interactants are typically found in antacid products, multivitamin/mineral supplements, and even (the trend is growing) in some (mineral-) fortified foods, such as cereals, and citrus juices.

Although foods (in general) and most antacid combination products (usually containing both aluminum and magnesium salts) may interfere with the oral absorption of several other antibiotics (oral aminoglycosides such as neomycin and paromomycin, a; isoniazid (b); cephalosporins, c, d; and penicillins, e), the cation-antibiotic interaction is most important to and amply documented for the tetracyclines.

442. The answer is d. *(Brunton, pp 1058-1060. Katzung, pp 596t, 877, 912.)* Among the indications for metronidazole is management of *C difficile* (and other *clostridia*) infections, including AAPMC. Many other obligate anaerobes, mainly gram-positive bacilli, will respond. So will various types of intestinal or systemic amebiasis infections (the drug is generally used adjunctively with iodoquinol for gut infections—symptomatic amebiasis); and for giardiasis and *Trichomonas vaginalis* infections (generally the drug of choice). An alternative to metronidazole in the setting of AAPMC would be vancomycin.

None of the other drugs listed would be suitable. Amphotericin B (a) is an antifungal agent. Clindamycin (b) is not at all the preferred treatment; indeed, it is the most likely cause of the superinfection. Gentamicin (c) is not effective against anaerobes, *C difficile* of course included. Trimethoprim plus sulfamethoxazole (e) is not indicated for *C difficile* infections. The main uses of this broad spectrum antibiotic combination are most uncomplicated urinary tract infections (especially if chronic or recurrent), and treating pneumonia and other *P carnii* infections (mainly in immunocompromised patients with AIDS, cancer, or organ transplants).

443. The answer is b. *(Brunton, pp 951, 988, 1182-1187. Katzung, pp 799-800.)* Erythromycin (and clindamycin) is macrolide antibiotic that rather powerfully inhibits P450-mediated metabolism of many other drugs, raising blood levels of the interactants. Warfarin is eliminated almost exclusively by P450 metabolism, and so the excessive effects described in the question are quite likely. Although azithromycin (a) is a macrolide, it is not a P450 inhibitor (or inducer). Gentamicin (c) and other aminoglycosides are eliminated solely by renal excretion and have no direct effects on hepatic drug metabolism or any other important aspects of liver function. The same applies to penicillin G (d) and other penicillins, including those classified as penicillinase-resistant, broad-spectrum (aminopenicillins), and extended-spectrum (mainly used against *Pseudomonas* in combination with an aminoglycoside). Rifampin (e) is a P450 inducer, not an inhibitor, and is obviously a cause of many drug-drug interactions as a result of its stimulatory effect on hepatic metabolism.

444. The answer is a. *(Brunton, pp 1139-1140. Katzung, pp 779-780.)* Compared with ampicillin, amoxicillin absorption is affected less by the presence of food, so the bioavailability is better and dosing may be more convenient for many patients. Both drugs are inactivated by β-lactamases, and so neither is effective against penicillinase-producing organisms (b). Both drugs are broad spectrum (c) and share the same antimicrobial spectrum as penicillin G, and additionally are effective, for example, against *E coli*, *H influenzae*, *Salmonella*, and *Shigella*; both also can cross-react in patients with a history of hypersensitivity reactions (d) to other penicillins. Neither amoxicillin nor ampicillin has antipseudomonal activity. The penicillins capable of that are the extended-spectrum penicillins, for example, piperacillin and ticarcillin; note that the extended-spectrum penicillins are susceptible to inactivation by β-lactamase and so are not effective against several strains of organisms, notably *S aureus*.

445. The answer is c. *(Brunton, pp 1143-1150. Katzung, pp 780-784.)* Unless there are no reasonable alternatives, cephalosporins should be avoided for patients with prior severe allergic responses to penicillins because of their cross-reactivity. "Mild" allergic or hypersensitivity reactions to penicillins do not necessarily contraindicate cephalosporin use. None of the other drugs or drug groups listed cross-react in penicillin-sensitive patients: aminoglycosides, a; azithromycin, b; erythromycins, d; linezolid, e; and tetracyclines, f.

446. The answer is c. *(Brunton, pp 1155-1159, 1166-1167. Katzung, pp 808, 812.)* Amikacin stands out among all the aminoglycosides in two main ways: it has the broadest spectrum against gram-negative bacilli, and it is least susceptible to bacterial enzymes that inactivate aminoglycosides and lead to resistance. (Recall that among gram-negative bacteria, genetic information that codes for the production of these inactivating enzymes is transferred via R factors.) It is best to monitor blood levels of either amikacin or gentamicin, mainly to help ensure that concentrations are neither subtherapeutic nor toxic, and so answer a is incorrect. Aminoglycosides are not effective against anaerobes (b). Amikacin and gentamicin are ototoxic (d) and nephrotoxic (e), as are all aminoglycosides.

447. The answer is b. *(Brunton, pp 1228-1229. Katzung, pp 835-838, 1052.)* Amphotericin B, given intravenously, often alters kidney function. The most common and most easily detected manifestation of this is decreased creatinine clearance. If this occurs, the dose must be reduced. Amphotericin B also commonly increases potassium loss, leading to hypokalemia; and can cause anemia and neurologic symptoms. A liposomal preparation of amphotericin B may reduce the incidence of renal and neurologic toxicity (see the note at the end of the explanation for Question 448). Vancomycin (e) may cause renal damage, but the overall incidence is lower, the severity less. Acyclovir (a), ceftazidime (c) and penicillins (d) rarely are causally related to the development of acute renal failure.

448. The answer is a. *(Brunton, pp 1128-1132, 1225-1229. Katzung, pp 773-789, 835-838.)* Penicillins, cephalosporins, and amphotericin B exert their desired clinical effects by altering the structure or function of cell walls of susceptible organisms. Penicillins interfere with bacterial cell wall synthesis: their β-lactam structures bind to and inhibit enzymatic function of transpeptidases that normally provide susceptible bacteria with cell walls that are capable of maintaining an osmotically stable intracellular milieu. Cephalosporins, by virtue of their β-lactam ring, work in essentially the same way. Amphotericin B (a polyene antifungal drug) binds to ergosterol in the fungal cell membrane; the ultimate outcome is increased cell permeability. Nonetheless, the ultimate effect is osmotic instability of the organism, leading to cell death.

Neither penicillins, cephalosporins, or amphotericin B are contraindicated in patients with immunodeficiencies (b). Indeed, they may play a key role in managing opportunistic infections in such patients.

They do not induce the metabolism of other drugs (c), or interact in most of the typical pharmacokinetic ways.

Amphotericin B can cause decreased platelet counts and leukopenia, but this is rare. The most common hematologic adverse response to this drug is a normochromic, normocytic anemia. Penicillins and cephalosporins do not share these properties (and so answer d is incorrect).

Finally, amphotericin B is clearly nephrotoxic (see note). When given intravenously, renal dysfunction is the most serious and most common long-term manifestation of this antifungal drug's toxic spectrum. Penicillins and cyclosporins may cause interstitial nephritis, but compared with amphotericin B the incidence and clinical consequences are quite low.

Note: There are new lipid formulations of amphotericin B—amphotericin B colloidal dispersion, liposomal amphotericin B, and a lipid complex of the drug—and they apparently cause much less nephrotoxicity than conventional amphotericin B formulations. That is probably because these newer formulations alter distribution of the antifungal drug such that renal concentrations, and so the nephrotoxic potential, are lower.

449. The answer is d. *(Brunton, pp 1257t, 1258-1259. Katzung, p 872.)* Oseltamivir is the recommended drug; zanamivir is a recommended alternative. The biochemical mechanism of action is inhibition of viral neuraminidase; that, in turn, inhibits the ability of newly formed viral particles to "bud off" of host cell membranes and spread the virus to other cells. Oseltamivir or zanamivir are also used prophylactically for outbreaks of other influenza A (or B) infections.

Acyclovir (a) is active only against herpesviruses (including herpes simplex, which is most sensitive to acyclovir); varicella-zoster; and cytomegalovirus (but most strains are resistant). Acyclovir must form an active metabolite, acyclo-GTP, which in turn inhibits viral DNA polymerase. Amantadine (b) is an antiviral drug for flu prophylaxis (mainly A strains) and treatment, but its use has declined sharply (as oseltamivir or zanamivir use has grown) because many viral strains quickly develop resistance. In addition, amantadine tends to cause disturbing CNS effects (dizziness, irritability, insomnia, impaired mental concentration in a large number of patients) and cardiovascular depression. Amantadine is also used occasionally as an adjunct to treatment of Parkinson disease. Lopinavir (c) and ritonavir (e) are protease inhibitors/antiretroviral drugs. Those two drugs are used in combination, and with a nucleoside/-tide reverse transcriptase inhibitor (eg, zidovudine) for HIV infections.

Note: Given the number of H1N1 cases, and worries about a pandemic, in 2009 the FDA gave formal authorization to use either of these drugs for flu-related indications for which they were not previously approved, including children younger than the preapproved minimum age.

450. The answer is d. *(Brunton, pp 1104, 1155-1159. Katzung, pp 807-810.)* The rationale behind this combination is that penicillins essentially weaken the cell walls of susceptible bacteria, which in turn facilitates access of the aminoglycoside to its site of action, where bacterial protein synthesis is inhibited. This usually provides better antibiotic response than with either antibiotic used alone, and with the aminoglycoside, plasma levels aren't necessarily so high that they are more likely to cause ototoxicity, nephrotoxicity, or other adverse responses. The combination does not increase the risk of superinfection (c), increase the risk of aminoglycoside nephrotoxicity (e), or increase the risk of resistance (f) compared with the risks of resistance if either drug were used alone.

You should also recall at least two other things: (1) the penicillin in this combination is usually an extended-spectrum penicillin, such as ticarcillin; and (2) as I specifically noted in the question, the administration of these drugs is by separate IV lines. That is because if the two drugs were mixed together in sufficiently high concentrations, the penicillin may chemically inactivate the gentamicin (but the aminoglycosides do not inactivate penicillins, a, b).

451. The answer is b. *(Brunton, pp 1134-1138. Katzung, pp 773-776.)* Both susceptible and resistant gram-negative and gram-positive bacteria have penicillin-binding proteins (PBPs). Resistance to the narrow spectrum penicillins by gram-negative bacteria arises from the presence of an outer membrane with pores that are too small to allow adequate penetration of the drug and access to the PBPs. Thus, we are dealing with what amounts to a physical barrier to the drug.

Gram-negative bacteria do not actively transport the narrow spectrum penicillins out of the organisms (a). A lack of penicillin-binding surface enzymes (c) or other penicillin-binding proteins (d) do not explain the low efficacy of narrow spectrum penicillins, whether penicillin-sensitive or -resistant. Most penicillins (with few exceptions, such as bacampicillin) are active in the form in which they are administered (ie, they are not prodrugs), and so no subsequent metabolic activation is required (making answer e incorrect).

452. The answer is b. *(Brunton, pp 1143-1150. Katzung, pp 781-783.)* Cefoxitin or cefmetazole (not listed) are suitable for treating intra-abdominal infections caused by many aerobic and anaerobic gram-negative bacteria, including and especially *B fragilis*. Cefoxitin alone has been shown to be as effective as the traditional therapy of clindamycin plus gentamicin. The other cephalosporins (cefaclor, a; cefuroxime, c; cephalexin, d; and cephalothin (e) have much lower antibiotic activity against these organisms, and so generally are not appropriate.

453. The answer is a. *(Brunton, pp 1160-1163. Katzung, pp 810-813.)* Aminoglycosides (gentamicin, tobramycin, others) are classic examples of ototoxic drugs, and they can affect both branches of the eighth cranial nerve.

The risks of aminoglycoside-induced ototoxicity (and nephrotoxicity) are among the reasons why it is important to keep an eye on peak and trough drug levels during therapy, adjust dosages accordingly, and avoid concomitant use of other ototoxic drugs. That is because the hearing loss is blood level-dependent (as opposed to being an idiosyncratic or allergic reaction). Aminoglycoside-induced ototoxicity is usually irreversible. The risk and severity of hearing loss from aminoglycosides are increased if they are administered with other ototoxic drugs.

Recall that there are two main forms of drug-induced ototoxicity. Cochlear toxicity includes hearing loss, tinnitus (ringing in the ears), or occasionally both. Hearing loss may also occur with loop diuretics (particularly ethacrynic acid), cis-platinum, and the vinca alkaloids (anticancer drugs). These drugs are intrinsically ototoxic; use one or more of them together or with an aminoglycoside and the risk of ototoxicity increases greatly.

Tinnitus (usually reversible) is typically associated with such drugs as aspirin (and, possibly, some other NSAIDs) and quinidine.

The other main form of ototoxicity is vestibular toxicity, which is typically manifest as balance and gait problems, vertigo, and nausea resulting from vestibular apparatus dysfunction.

Nephrotoxicity may develop during or after the use of an aminoglycoside. It is generally more common in the elderly when there is preexisting renal dysfunction. In most patients, renal function gradually improves after discontinuation of therapy. Aminoglycosides rarely cause neuromuscular blockade that can lead to progressive flaccid paralysis and potential fatal respiratory arrest. Hypersensitivity and dermatologic reactions occasionally occur following use of aminoglycosides.

None of the other antibiotics listed are linked to ototoxicity, whether from excessive blood levels or due to a hypersensitivity or true allergic reaction: cephalosporins (b, c), fluoroquinolones (d); and penicillins (e). Azithromycin (not an answer choice) is, however, another antibiotic for which there is evidence of a link to sudden onset hearing loss. Several case reports have noted permanent, near-complete, and binaural hearing loss after only one dose. The mechanism is unknown, the incidence is neither dose-dependent nor predictable, and no cause-effect relationship has been proved.

454. The answer is b. *(Brunton, pp 1233-1234. Katzung, pp 839-841.)* Fluconazole, an azole antifungal, penetrates into cerebrospinal fluid, where it exerts good antifungal activity against *Cryptococcus neoformans*. When it is given orally, blood levels are almost as high as when it is given parenterally. Amphotericin B (a) is administered intravenously and even when given intrathecally does not appear to be highly effective in fungal meningitis. Ketoconazole (c) is often used as an alternative to amphotericin B for systemic mycotic infections. It is much less toxic than amphotericin B, and somewhat less efficacious. However, it is highly plasma protein bound and does not cross the blood-brain barrier well, making it a poor choice for brain infections. Metronidazole (d) is mainly used for protozoal infections and infections caused by obligate anaerobes. It would not be an appropriate choice for this patient. Nystatin (e), a polyene antibiotic, is used only for candidiasis. It is the drug of choice for intestinal candida infections, and is also used for candida infections of the esophagus, mouth, skin, and vagina. Systemic absorption is nil whether the drug is given orally or topically, and it cannot be given parenterally.

455. The answer is d. *(Brunton, pp 227, 1164. Katzung, pp 807-813.)* Aminoglycosides, at sufficiently high blood levels, can cause skeletal neuromuscular blockade in their own right. This probably arises from a combination of effects: inhibition of neuronal ACh release and perhaps direct blockade of nicotinic receptors on skeletal muscle. This would add to and prolong the effects of both neuromuscular blockers the patient has received. In addition, isoflurane and other halogenated hydrocarbon volatile liquid anesthetics have some neuromuscular-blocking effects in their own right—but not to a degree that is sufficient to obviate the need for succinylcholine and/or nondepolarizing blockers when skeletal muscle paralysis is indicated. So here we have a combination of drugs that affect skeletal muscle activation.

The greatest concern, of course, would be the prolongation of neuromuscular blockade. A "greater degree" of paralysis is largely inconsequential, so long as ventilation is supported. It is the prolonged blockade—and especially the return of skeletal muscle weakening and ventilatory insufficiency after mechanical ventilation has been discontinued and additional doses of aminoglycoside are given—that poses the greatest risk if the patient had already been taken off ventilatory support.

(Note, too, in your studies, that some other antimicrobials seem to have some skeletal neuromuscular-blocking activity, including polymyxin B and clindamycin.)

You should recall that although such agents as isoflurane and other halogenated hydrocarbon volatile liquid anesthetics may potentiate the effects of a neuromuscular blocker, once they are eliminated (that occurs fairly rapidly when administration stops) there is no added risk of prolonged or greater skeletal muscle weakness or paralysis.

I should add that in settings where the overall incidence of aminoglycoside resistance is low (or in the absence of documented resistance to a particular aminoglycoside in a particular patient), tobramycin or gentamicin is usually the aminoglycoside of choice. Amikacin should be reserved for situations where there is proven resistance to the alternatives.

As with other aminoglycosides, periodic monitoring of peak and trough blood levels is essential to help insure optimal antibiotic effects while reducing the risk of ototoxicity and nephrotoxicity—both of which can be caused by any aminoglycoside (although with varying relative risks). No aminoglycoside has "nephroprotective" effects.

There is no known phenomenon involving hepatotoxicity from an aminoglycoside-isoflurane (or any other halogenated hydrocarbon anesthetic) interaction (a); aminoglycosides do not counteract any of the effects of midazolam (b) or other benzodiazepines; typical anesthesia premedications or induction/maintenance drugs do not enhance host toxicity from aminoglycosides (c); and, finally, aminoglycosides have no impact on myocardial sensitivity to catecholamines (e) as might be caused by some anesthetics (notably halothane).

456. The answer is e. *(Brunton, pp 1102, 1206-1207, 1451. Katzung, pp 65t, 824-825.)* Isoniazid (INH) inhibits cell-wall synthesis in mycobacteria. Increasing vitamin B_6 levels prevents some common and potentially significant complications associated with this inhibition, including peripheral neuritis, insomnia, restlessness, muscle twitching, urinary retention, convulsions, and psychosis, without affecting the antimycobacterial activity of INH.

Vitamin B_6 has no influence on INH excretion (a) or metabolism (b); it is not a cofactor for activating INH to an active drug (c; metabolism, specifically acetylation, is responsible for INH inactivation, not the formation of an active moiety), nor does the vitamin potentiate the actions of INH on mycobacteria (d).

457. The answer is d. *(Brunton, pp 1173-1174, 1178, 1690. Katzung, pp 796-798.)* Tetracyclines are drugs of choice in the treatment of *Rickettsia*, *Mycoplasma*, and *Chlamydia* infections. The antibiotics that act by inhibiting cell-wall synthesis have no effect on *Mycoplasma* because the organism does not possess a cell wall; penicillin G (c), vancomycin (e), and bacitracin (a) will be ineffective. Gentamicin (b) also has little or no antimicrobial activity against these organisms.

458. The answer is a. *(Brunton, pp 1297, 1301-1302. Katzung, pp 855t, 859t, 865.)* Ritonavir is a powerful inhibitor of the liver's P450 system. Ritonavir is used in combination with lopinavir solely to inhibit lopinavir's metabolism and enhance its ability to inhibit the final step in HIV maturation. Thus, the ritonavir helps keep lopinavir's plasma concentration in a therapeutic range longer. Ritonavir does have protease inhibitory activation but it is weak (especially at the dosages used in combination with other protease inhibitors: in this combination the ritonavir dose would be subtherapeutic if it were the only protease inhibitor used). In this combination it is the lopinavir, not the ritonavir (e) that is causing the main therapeutic effect. The protease inhibitors do not cause hypoglycemia (c), nor does ritonavir reduce the ability of lopinavir to alter plasma glucose levels. In fact, whether used alone or in combination, protease inhibitors typically cause hyperglycemia (and may cause clinical diabetes mellitus, and quite often raise cholesterol and triglycerides levels too).

The NRTIs (zidovudine, didanosine) are, indeed, prodrugs that must be metabolically activated to the triphosphate form in order to serve as a substrate for reverse transcriptase. However, neither lopinavir nor ritonavir facilitate that metabolism (b).

459. The answer is d. *(Brunton, pp 1158-1159, 1164-1165, 1211. Katzung, p 811.)* Streptomycin is bactericidal for the tubercle bacillus organism.

Other aminoglycosides (eg, amikacin [a], gentamicin, kanamycin [b], neomycin [c], tobramycin [e]) have activity against this organism but are seldom used clinically because of toxicity or development of resistance. Streptomycin is arguably the most ototoxic aminoglycoside.

460. The answer is d. *(Brunton, pp 1132-1133, 1151-1152. Katzung, p 785.)* These agents are inhibitors of penicillinase (β-lactamase) and are used in conjunction with β-lactamase-sensitive penicillins to potentiate their activity. These drugs are found in several brand-name fixed-dose penicillin combination products (amoxicillin and clavulanic acid; sulbactam with ampicillin; tazobactam with piperacillin). Clavulanic acid is an irreversible inhibitor. These agents do not, per se, add activity against *Pseudomonas* or Enterobacter (a; an activity already possessed by piperacillin but not by ampicillin or amoxicillin). Likewise, they have no intrinsic effect on transpeptidases (c) or facilitate entry into the CNS or CSF (b). They do not inhibit hepatic metabolism of the penicillins, and you should recall that renal excretion (not metabolism, e) is the main pathway for penicillin elimination. Importantly, the penicillinase inhibitors have no impact on the risks or severities of allergic reactions to penicillins (f).

461. The answer is d. *(Brunton, pp 1203-1204, 1210, 1214-1215. Katzung, pp 823-830.)* An important problem in the chemotherapy of TB is bacterial drug resistance. For this reason, concurrent administration of two or more drugs should be employed to delay the development of resistance. Ethambutol is often given along with INH for this purpose. Streptomycin or rifampin may also be added to the regimen to delay even further the development of drug resistance. Ethambutol does not facilitate mycobacterial entry of INH (a), affect penetration of the blood-brain barrier (b), alter absorption rates (c), or slow renal excretion of INH (e), which is mainly eliminated by metabolism (acetylation).

462. The answer is d. *(Brunton, pp 1097, 1155-1158. Katzung, pp 807-811.)* Aminoglycosides, which are mainly used for parenteral therapy of severe infections from aerobic gram-negative bacilli (eg, *E coli, Serratia, Klebsiella*), require oxygen in order for the drug to be transported across the bacterial cell membrane. Such incorporation is necessary for these drugs to exert their bactericidal effects, which arise from binding to the 30S subunit of susceptible bacteria. Ultimately the aminoglycoside-ribosomal binding leads to premature termination of bacterial protein synthesis and the formation of abnormal bacterial proteins. Such abnormal proteins ultimately insert into the bacterial cell membrane, causing leakiness and cell death.

The aminoglycosides are not prodrugs (a), and so metabolism (whether aerobic or otherwise) is not necessary for activity. Formation of an oxygen-free radical or an aminoglycoside-free radical has nothing to do with their antibiotic effects. Moreover, metabolism by host cells (b) is not an important process in the elimination of aminoglycosides, nor of reducing host cell toxicity (eg, to the kidneys or auditory nerve). Renal excretion is the main route of elimination for these drugs, which explains why renal function is such an important consideration in dosing adjustments.

Clearly, both aerobic and anaerobic bacteria can elaborate resistance factors (or develop resistance in other ways) to a variety of antibiotic classes. From a clinical viewpoint, the presence or absence of molecular oxygen is not a crucial or even relevant issue in this matter, however.

463. The answer is c. *(Brunton, pp 1167-1168. Katzung, p 813.)* Neomycin, an aminoglycoside, is not significantly absorbed from the GI tract. After oral administration, the intestinal flora are suppressed or modified and the drug is excreted in the feces. This effect of neomycin is used in hepatic coma to decrease coliform flora, thus decreasing the production of ammonia and reducing levels of free nitrogen in the bloodstream. Other antimicrobial agents (eg, cephalothin [a]; chloramphenicol [b]; penicillin G [d], and tetracycline [e]) do not have the efficacy or potency of neomycin in causing this effect. Note that chloramphenicol is no longer available in the United States.

464. The answer is a. *(Brunton, p 1150. Katzung, pp 773-780, 781t, 783-784, 888-890.)* Penicillins were used in the treatment of meningitis because of their ability to pass across an inflamed blood-brain barrier. The third-generation cephalosporin, ceftriaxone, is preferred because it is effective against β-lactamase producing strains of *H influenzae* that may cause meningitis in children. Erythromycins (b) or penicillins (c, d, e) would not be drugs of choice.

465. The answer is e. *(Brunton, pp 1992-1993. Katzung, p 804.)* There are several pieces of information you should link together to help arrive at the answer, for which a relatively new drug is the correct answer. (1) Although linezolid has several uses, it is best reserved for vancomycin-resistant enterococci (VRE) and methicillin-resistant *S aureus* (MRSA) infections. (It's seldom a first-line antibiotic because of the risk of resistance.) (2) Linezolid is occasionally linked to bone marrow suppression that is usually reversible upon discontinuation of the drug. (Granted, such other antibiotics as chloramphenicol [no longer used in the United States] pose greater risks of bone marrow suppression, but this property is nonetheless associated with linezolid.) (3) The third piece of evidence is the rise of blood pressure in response to ephedrine, a mixed-acting sympathomimetic (adrenomimetic) that works, in part, by releasing neuronal norepinephrine. Linezolid has monoamine oxidase inhibitory activity (albeit relatively weak compared with traditional MAO inhibitors). Piece these three lines of evidence together and the only reasonable choice is linezolid, and that azithromycin (a), fluoroquinolones (b), erythromycins (c), and aminoglycosides (d) are not correct.

Cancer and Immune System Pharmacology

Cell cycle, cell cycle specificity
Alkylating agents
Anticancer hormones and their antagonists
Antitumor antibiotics
Antimetabolites
Plant alkaloids
Immunomodulators

Questions

466. A 47-year-old woman with choriocarcinoma is treated with very high doses of methotrexate (MTX). You anticipate significant host cell toxicity in response to the high MTX dose. Which of the following drugs would you give to limit toxic effects of the MTX on normal host cells?

a. Deferoxamine
b. Leucovorin
c. *N*-acetylcysteine
d. Penicillamine
e. Vitamin K

467. We administer vincristine, the prototype of the vinca alkaloids, to a patient with a tumor that is likely to be responsive to this drug. Which of the following is the most likely adverse response to this drug?

a. Nephrotoxicity, renal dysfunction or failure
b. Neutropenia
c. Peripheral sensory and motor neuropathy
d. Pulmonary damage
e. Thrombocytopenia, bleeding

468. A cancer patient develops severe, irreversible cardiomyopathy because the maximum lifetime dose of an anticancer drug was exceeded. Which of the following drugs is most likely responsible for this patient's symptoms?

a. Asparaginase
b. Bleomycin
c. Cisplatin
d. Cyclophosphamide
e. Doxorubicin
f. Vincristine

469. A patient with Wilms tumor is receiving a chemotherapeutic agent that is described as working by intercalating into DNA strands, and that is efficacious regardless of which stage of the cell cycle the tumor cells are in. Which of the following drugs best fits this description?

a. Anastrozole
b. Cytarabine
c. Doxorubicin
d. Fluorouracil
e. Tamoxifen

470. A 42-year-old woman is diagnosed with metastatic breast cancer. You consider use of raloxifene, toremifene, or fulvestrant. Which of the following summarizes why fulvestrant might be the best choice, all other factors being equal?

a. Exerts antiplatelet, rather than thrombotic, effects
b. Lacks ability to cause hot flashes or other disturbing side effects
c. Lower risk of causing endometrial cancer
d. Provides clinical cure, rather than palliation, in all patients
e. Significantly improves mineral density in, strength of, long bones

471. The FDA soon will be requiring manufacturers of an anticancer drug to avoid concomitant administration of certain SSRI antidepressants (fluoxetine, paroxetine, and sertraline) to women receiving a particular anticancer drug. The anticancer drug in question is mainly used to treat certain types of breast cancers and is also used to prevent breast cancer recurrence. It commonly causes hot flashes and is associated with a high incidence of nausea and vomiting. The SSRIs listed here are strong inhibitors of CYP2D6 and so they can interfere with the anticancer drug's metabolic activation, which is required for its chemotherapeutic effects. Which one of the following drugs is the most likely target of interactions with these SSRIs?

a. Bleomycin
b. Interferon alpha
c. Mercaptopurine
d. Tamoxifen
e. Vinblastine

472. A patient with chronic myelogenous leukemia (CML) is being treated with imatinib. Which of the following side effects or other situations should you anticipate in response to imatinib therapy?

a. A high rate of therapeutic failure, and the need to switch to interferons α-2a and α-2b
b. Hypotension and hypovolemia due to significant drug-induced diuresis
c. Interactions with other drugs that depend on or affect the cytochrome P450 system
d. Significant toxicity to normal host cells due to profound inhibition of tyrosine kinase
e. Thrombocytosis, with a high risk of intravascular clotting

473. As a rule, large (and older) solid tumors are more difficult to eradicate when chemotherapy is started. Which of the following tumor-based properties explains best the reason for this chemotherapeutic limitation?

a. Growth fraction slows; more cells enter G_0.
b. Higher tumor blood flow washes away anticancer drugs faster.
c. P-glycoprotein activity decreases as tumors get older.
d. Their higher metabolic rate makes them less vulnerable to chemotherapeutic agents.
e. Topoisomerase activity (ability to self-repair DNA strand damage) increases with tumor size.

474. A man has prostate cancer that will be treated with leuprolide. Which of the following drugs are we most likely to use adjunctively when starting chemotherapy?

a. An aromatase inhibitor (eg, anastrozole)
b. Flutamide
c. Prednisone or another potent glucocorticoid
d. Tamoxifen
e. Testosterone

475. A Hodgkin disease patient received mechlorethamine as part of his treatment plan. Which of the following best describes the anticancer mechanism of action of this drug?

a. Alkylates DNA, causing cross-links between parallel DNA strands
b. Blocks microtubular assembly and mitosis during M-phase
c. Inhibits topoisomerase, preventing repair of DNA strand breaks
d. Intercalates in DNA strands, thereby preventing DNA replication by mRNA
e. Stabilizes microtubular arrays, thereby preventing mitosis

476. The oncology team has treated many patients with acute lymphocytic leukemia using a combination of drugs. One drug tends to cause a high incidence of lumbar and abdominal pain, significant increases of plasma amylase and transaminase activity, and other symptoms of hepatic and/or pancreatic dysfunction. Some patients developed serious hypersensitivity reactions upon drug administration, and there have been occasional sudden deaths. Which of the following drugs best fits this description?

a. Asparaginase
b. Azathioprine
c. Doxorubicin
d. Methotrexate
e. Vincristine

477. A 30-year-old woman being treated for ovarian cancer develops high frequency hearing loss and declining renal function in response to anticancer drug therapy. Which of the following drugs is the most likely cause?

a. Bleomycin
b. Cisplatin
c. Doxorubicin
d. 5-Fluorouracil
e. Paclitaxel

478. A 41-year-old woman is admitted to the outpatient area of the hematology-oncology center for her first course of adjuvant chemotherapy for metastatic breast cancer following a left modified radical mastectomy and axillary lymph node dissection for infiltrating ductal carcinoma of the breast. Two biopsies were positive for cancer.

Following premedication with dexamethasone and ondansetron, she will receive combination chemotherapy with doxorubicin, cyclophosphamide, and fluorouracil. Twenty-four hours after the first course of chemotherapy she will start a 10-day regimen with filgrastim. Which of the following is the most likely reason for administering the filgrastim?

a. Control of nausea and emesis
b. Potentiate the anticancer effects of the chemotherapeutic agents
c. Prevent doxorubicin-induced cardiotoxicity
d. Reduce the risk/severity of chemotherapy-induced neutropenia, and related infections
e. Stimulate the gastric mucosa to repair damage caused by the chemotherapy drugs

479. While reviewing charts in a general medicine clinic you see that a patient, 55-year-old and with no history of cancer at all, is taking methotrexate (MTX). What is the most likely condition for which this "anticancer drug" is being given?

a. Asthma or emphysema
b. Hyperthyroidism
c. Hyperuricemia or clinical gout
d. Myasthenia gravis
e. Rheumatoid arthritis or psoriasis

480. A cancer patient receives prophylactic allopurinol before a course of chemotherapy. Which of the following is the main reason for giving the allopurinol?

a. Facilitate host cell detoxification of the chemotherapeutic drug, thereby reducing host cell toxicities
b. Inhibit the potential for DNA repair, by topoisomerases, that otherwise might lead to chemotherapy failure
c. Potentiate the action of a nitrogen mustard or nitrosourea to bind to (cross-link) purine moieties in DNA strands
d. Prevent myelosuppression and related blood dyscrasias
e. Reduce the risk of hyperuricemia and its main consequences (renal damage, gout) that can occur with a massive cell kill

481. Allopurinol is commonly administered before initiating chemotherapy of leukemias and other blood-based cancers to prevent hyperuricemia and its consequences. It is also important in preventing hyperuricemia in response to chemotherapy of some solid tumors. However, it may potentiate the host toxicity of certain anticancer drugs by inhibiting their metabolic inactivation and detoxification. With which of the following drugs should concomitant use of allopurinol be avoided, or be used with extra caution?

a. Bleomycin
b. Cisplatin
c. Cyclophosphamide
d. Doxorubicin
e. Mercaptopurine

482. A 48-year-old patient who was in renal failure received a kidney transplant. We start her on cyclosporine to reduce the risk of graft rejection. Which of the following are the most common and worrisome adverse responses associated with this immunosuppressant?

a. Cardiotoxicity and hepatotoxicity
b. Hepatotoxicity and nephrotoxicity
c. Hypotension and pulmonary fibrosis
d. Nephrotoxicity and infection risk
e. Thrombosis and pulmonary embolism or ischemic stroke

Cancer and Immune System Pharmacology

Answers

466. The answer is b. *(Brunton, pp 1335, 1339, 1694. Katzung, pp 631-632, 944-946, 975, 1090-1091.)* This essential technique to reduce host cell toxicity in response to MTX therapy is known as leucovorin rescue. Methotrexate, a folic acid analog/antimetabolite, can be curative for women with choriocarcinoma and is also useful for non-Hodgkin lymphomas and acute lymphocytic leukemias in children. The drug kills responsive cancer cells by inhibiting dihydrofolate reductase, an enzyme necessary for forming tetrahydrofolic acid (FH_4). The FH_4, in turn, is critical for eventual synthesis of DNA, RNA, and proteins. Inhibition of thymidylate synthesis is probably the single most important consequence in the overall reaction scheme.

Some cancer cells are resistant to MTX because they lack adequate mechanisms for transporting the drug intracellularly. These include some head and neck cancers and osteogenic sarcomas. In such cases we need to give very large doses of MTX to establish a high concentration gradient that essentially "drives" it into the cells. Unfortunately, normal host cells depend on folate metabolism, they take up MTX well, and they will be affected.

To protect normal cells we administer leucovorin (also called citrovorum factor or folinic acid) right after giving the MTX. It is taken up by the normal cells, bypasses the block induced by the MTX, and so spares normal cell metabolism. The leucovorin does not spare cancer cells: just as they cannot take up MTX well, they cannot take up the rescue agent and save themselves from cytotoxicity.

Leucovorin rescue is not done "automatically" in every case when MTX is given. When low MTX doses are used leucovorin may be withheld until and unless blood counts show evidence of MTX-induced bone marrow suppression. However, it is quite usually given along with MTX when MTX doses are very high (as in severe or MTX-resistant cases), and host toxicity is very probable.

There is another important and growing use of MTX: as a disease-modifying or slow-acting antirheumatic drug (DMARD, SAARD, respectively).

Owing to toxicity it had been relegated to second- or third-line therapy of severe and/or refractory rheumatoid arthritis. Now that we have a better appreciation of the drug's toxicity, and how to recognize it earlier and minimize its occurrences, it is being used much more, earlier on in therapy, for rheumatoid arthritis that is "moderate" and likely to progress rapidly.

The main adverse responses to MTX, regardless of the purpose for which it is given, include bone marrow suppression, pulmonary damage (infiltrates, fibrosis), stomatitis, and lesions in the GI tract. High doses can be nephrotoxic (risk reduced by maintaining adequate hydration and alkalinizing the urine). MTX is also teratogenic.

Recall that deferoxamine (a) is used to treat iron poisoning (it is an iron chelator). *N*-acetylcysteine (c) is mainly used either as a mucolytic (mucus-thinning) drug for certain pulmonary disorders (eg, COPD) or as an antidote for acetaminophen poisoning. Penicillamine (d) is mainly a copper chelator, used for copper poisoning or Wilson disease. Vitamin K (e) is used for deficiency states, for combating excessive effects of warfarin, or for managing bleeding disorders in newborns of mothers who have been taking certain drugs (eg, anticonvulsants such as phenytoin) during pregnancy and delivery.

467. The answer is c. *(Brunton, pp 1350-1354. Katzung, pp 949, 950t.)* Vincristine is one of relatively few cytotoxic anticancer drugs that does not cause bone marrow suppression (and all the potential accompanying consequences of that, including neutropenia, b) as its main toxicity. Rather, it causes neuropathies involving both sensory and motor nerves. Paresthesias are a common example of the former (hearing loss can also occur); muscle weakness and obtunded reflexes are examples of the latter.

Important note: Vincristine differs from vinblastine and vinorelbine, which do cause bone marrow suppression (and not neuropathies) as their main dose-limiting toxicity. Nephrotoxicity (a), pulmonary damage (d), and reduced platelet counts or bleeding disorders of other etiologies (e) are not typically associated with vincristine.

468. The answer is e. *(Brunton, pp 1357-1360. Katzung, pp 950-953.)* Doxorubicin, an antitumor antibiotic, is cardiotoxic, and the risk for and severity of cardiomyopathy is dose-related and cumulative: there is a maximum recommended lifetime (cumulative) dose for this drug, and if it is exceeded the risk of cardiac damage rises significantly.

Asparaginase (a), used only for acute lymphocytic leukemia, tends to cause mainly pancreatitis, hepatic dysfunction, and allergic/hypersensitivity reactions. Pulmonary damage that usually presents initially as pneumonitis is the main organ-specific toxicity of bleomycin (b), which is also an antitumor antibiotic. It occurs in about 1 of 10 patients treated with this drug. In some cases the pulmonary damage will progress to pulmonary fibrosis that is, of course, irreversible.

Renal damage is the main dose-limiting toxicity of cisplatin (c). It can be prevented somewhat by ensuring that the patient is adequately hydrated and producing adequate amounts of urine. Diuretics may be used as adjuncts. The goal is to minimize accumulation of the nephrotoxic drug in the renal tubules and urine. (A related drug, oxaliplatin, tends to cause peripheral sensory neuropathies and does so in most patients who receive this drug.)

Cyclophosphamide (d) has no particular organ-specific toxicity. Rather, main manifestations of toxicity affect rapidly growing cells such as those in the bone marrow, intestinal tract mucosae, and hair follicles.

Vincristine's (f) main dose-limiting toxicities involve dysfunction of motor, sensory, and occasionally autonomic nerves. It probably arises in a manner related to the drug's anticancer effect: inhibition of microtubular function—or, in the case of nerves, neurotubules—as a result of drug binding to tubulin.

469. The answer is c. *(Brunton, pp 1356-1357. Katzung, pp 951-953.)* Antrhacycline-type antitumor antibiotics (doxorubicin, daunorubicin, idarubicin, etc) intercalate between and eventually bind to DNA base pairs. This distortion of the DNA chains makes the DNA an unsuitable template for RNA polymerase, and ultimately RNA and protein synthesis is inhibited. Dactinomycin is phase-nonspecific.

Anastrozole (a) is a relatively new aromatase inhibitor. This is an oral agent used for postmenopausal women with early or advanced breast cancer. In postmenopausal women, the major source of estrogen (which supports growth and replication of estrogen-dependent tumors) is adrenal androgens. Those androgens are metabolized by aromatase to estrogens. As a result, anastrozole depletes estrogens and can arrest tumor cell growth.

Cytarabine (b, also called cytosine arabinoside) is a pyrimidine analog (antimetabolite) that is metabolized to the active moiety, ara-CTP. The ara-CTP becomes incorporated into DNA, with the main ultimate effect being suppression of DNA synthesis. It is highly specific for cells in S-phase.

Fluorouracil (d), also an antimetabolite, inhibits thymidylate synthetase through its active metabolite, 5-fluoro-2′-dexoyuridine-5′-monophosphate (FdUMP). It is not phase-specific, but its activity depends on cells not being in the G_0 stage.

Tamoxifen (e) is used for breast cancers. It blocks estrogen receptors on the breast cancer cells (for which the main physiologic agonist is estradiol). Recall that tamoxifen is classified as a selective estrogen receptor modifier (SERM). Although it blocks estrogen receptors on responsive breast cancer cells and is therapeutic for them, it acts as an estrogen receptor agonist in the uterus. Thus, one of the main risks of therapy with tamoxifen is endometrial hyperplasia that may lead to endometrial cancer. Because the drug acts as an estrogen receptor agonist in some tissues and an antagonist in others, risk-benefit ratios must be considered carefully. The beneficial effects in active breast carcinoma may outweigh the risks of inducing endometrial disease. However, the preventative use in the absence of breast cancer has a much lower benefit-to-risk ratio.

470. The answer is c. *(Brunton, pp 1383-1384, 1556-1557. Katzung, p 718.)* Fulvestrant is associated with a much lower risk of causing endometrial pathology, including cancer. It is a "pure" estrogen antagonist. That effect, in breast tissue, is what accounts for the drug's beneficial effects in some patients with metastatic, estrogen-supported, breast cancer. The effects are usually of palliative benefit, not a clinical cure (d), and certainly not in all patients. In contrast, raloxifene and toremifene (and tamoxifen, not mentioned in the question) are classified as selective estrogen receptor modifiers (SERMs). Although SERMs block estrogen receptors in breast tissue (just as fulvestrant does), they also have estrogenic (agonist) activity in some other tissues, notably the uterus. There they can cause endometrial proliferation, hyperplasia, and (apparently) an increased risk of endometrial cancer. (For more information about SERMs, see the answer to Question 375, in Chapter on Endocrine Systems.)

Because fulvestrant lacks estrogen agonist activity, it will not enhance bone mineralization (e) nor favorably modify cholesterol profiles, as the SERMs tend to do. The SERMs slightly increase the risk of thromboembolism. Fulvestrant may too, but it also lacks any ability to prevent platelet aggregation or thromboembolism (a). Hot flashes (b) are fairly common with any of these drugs.

471. The answer is d. *(Brunton, pp 1383-1384, 1555-1557. Katzung, pp 716, 958-959.)* Of all the drugs listed as possible answers, only tamoxifen, a selective estrogen receptor modifier (SERM), fits the description: it requires metabolic activation for anticancer effects (the active metabolite is about 100 times more potent than tamoxifen itself), it is indicated for estrogen-sensitive breast carcinoma (treatment or prophylaxis against recurrence), is associated with a high incidence of severe nausea and vomiting, and tends to cause hot flashes in many women (typically a delayed response occurring late in, or after, treatment with tamoxifen). Data suggest that women taking one of the listed SSRIs with tamoxifen, used for breast cancer prophylaxis, have higher rates of recurrence than those taking other SSRIs, or no antidepressants at all. At this time the same concerns over interactions between SSRIs and the other listed anticancer drugs (bleomycin, a; interferon alpha, b; mercaptopurine, c; and vinblastine, e) have not been raised.

Note: It should not be surprising that many women who have cancer, or are at risk of recurrences, might benefit from an antidepressant, and SSRIs generally are the preferred drugs. Although fluoxetine, paroxetine, and sertraline interact adversely with tamoxifen, due to strong CYP2D6 inhibition, not all SSRIs do. Citalopram, escitalopram, and fluvoxamine are not strong 2D6 inhibitors, and so they are generally preferred when concomitant SSRI therapy is warranted.

472. The answer is c. *(Brunton, pp 1366-1368. Katzung, pp 953-954.)* One of several problems with imatinib therapy is that it is a substrate for, and rather powerful inhibitor of, several cytochromes (CYP3A4, 2C9, and 2D6) that are important for the metabolism of many other drugs—warfarin, theophylline, and many others—whose actions can be increased excessively if dosages are not adjusted accordingly. Conversely, imatinib is a target of interactions by this mechanism. Phenytoin, carbamazepine, barbiturates, and rifampin are examples of drugs that can induce imatinib metabolism and reduce the clinical response to it; and such drugs as azole antifungals and erythromycin can reduce imatinib's metabolic clearance and increase the risk of toxicity.

Because of the issue of drug interactions, a high frequency of adverse responses, limited use, and even cost, imatinib is generally reserved for use after a trial of interferons has proven inadequate. The reverse—using imatinib first—usually isn't done.

Hypotension and hypovolemia (b) are not what one would expect with this drug. Rather, we see a high incidence of fluid retention (and not diuresis, as noted in answer b) that may not only affect blood pressure, but also cause other problems such as ascites, pericardial and pleural effusions, and possibly pulmonary edema. Likewise, thrombocytosis (e) is the opposite of what typically occurs: thrombocytopenia and bleeding problems, plus neutropenia and an increased risk of infection are fairly common.

Recall that chronic myelogenous leukemia cells do synthesize an abnormal constitutively active tyrosine kinase (Bcr-Abl) that is involved in (abnormal) protein phosphorylation. It is that aberrant tyrosine kinase—not ones found in normal host cells—that is affected by the drug and that confers selectivity for the drug's actions. Thus, tyrosine kinase inhibition does not seem to account for the adverse effects of this drug on host cells (d).

473. The answer is a. *(Brunton, pp 1315-1322. Katzung, pp 935-939.)* Gompertzian analysis (a plot of the log of the number of cancer cells in a tumor vs time) shows that after a tumor has reached a certain size, the rate of tumor growth (and "overall metabolic rate") slows: lower growth fraction or, stated differently, the longer it takes for the tumor to double in size. This slowed growth is partially due to more cells entering the G_0 (resting) phase of the cell cycle, where responsiveness to many chemotherapeutic agents is low. One reason for this is the sheer size of the tumor as related to blood flow and the delivery of nutrients that the rapidly dividing cells need. Reduced nutrient and oxygen delivery not only reduces cell replication, but also delivery of the chemotherapeutic agents. Thus, higher tumor blood flow (b) and/or higher tumor cell metabolic rates (d) are not correct explanations. Increased topoisomerase activity (e) is also not correct.

Finally, P-glycoprotein activity does not necessarily decrease with time or tumor size (c). However, even if it did, that would predict increased responsiveness to most anticancer drugs, because it is P-glycoprotein that normally pumps drugs out of the cancer cell. Self-repair mechanisms, as by topoisomerase, is not a factor in explaining reduced vulnerability of very large tumors.

474. The answer is b. *(Brunton, pp 1387-1390. Katzung, p 724.)* Flutamide, one of a small number of androgen receptor blockers used for managing prostate cancer, is used as an adjunct to leuprolide. Leuprolide acts like gonadotropin-releasing hormone (GnRH; or luteinizing hormone-releasing hormone). When leuprolide therapy is started, it stimulates release of interstitial cell–stimulating hormone from the pituitary, thereby increasing testosterone production and supporting tumor growth. It is only with continued exposure to leuprolide that GnRH receptors become desensitized, and the eventual inhibition of testosterone production (and, thereby, support of tumor growth) occurs. Flutamide, by blocking androgen receptors, prevents the potential worsening of the tumor in the early phase of leuprolide therapy when testosterone levels rise. Even when leuprolide's pituitary-desensitizing effects occur, androgens that can support prostate tumor growth will come from the adrenal gland. Their effects, too, are blocked by the flutamide.

Aromatase inhibitors such as anastrozole (a), glucocorticoids (c), tamoxifen (d) and certainly not testosterone (e) would be used adjunctively with leuprolide for prostate or other cancers.

475. The answer is a. *(Brunton, pp 1320, 1322f, 1325, 1327. Katzung p 943.)* Mechlorethamine, like cyclophosphamide (and carmustine and several others), is an alkylating agent. They are called bifunctional alkylating agents because they can covalently bind to DNA in two places (nucleophilic attack), thereby forming cross-links between two adjacent strands or between two bases in one strand. This ultimately disrupts DNA and RNA synthesis or may cause strand breakage. Cyclophosphamide (which can be considered the prototype of the alkylating agents) is actually a prodrug—it requires metabolic activation in order for its effects to occur. Cyclophosphamide (and other alkylating agents) is cell cycle-nonspecific, although its efficacy is greater when cells are not in G_0.

Bleomycin, dactinomycin, and doxorubicin are good examples of drugs that intercalate in DNA strands (d). As a result, the altered DNA no longer serves as an adequately precise template for eventual synthesis of more functional DNA and RNA. They are classified as antitumor antibiotics.

Etoposide and topotecan are examples of drugs that inhibit topoisomerase II (c). The consequence is inhibited ability of affected cells to repair DNA strand breaks. This stops the cell cycle in G_2.

The taxoids (eg, paclitaxel) impair mitosis (b), but by stabilizing assembled microtubules rather than by exerting a vinca alkaloid-like inhibition of microtubular assembly.

476. The answer is a. *(Brunton, pp 1363-1364. Katzung, pp 954-955.)* Asparaginase is an enzyme that catalyzes the hydrolysis of plasma asparagine to aspartic acid and ammonia. Major toxicities from asparaginase are related to antigenicity (it is a foreign protein, and some fatal anaphylactic reactions have occurred), pancreatitis, and a 50% incidence of some hepatic dysfunction based on the presence of elevated transaminases. The drug, which is largely G_1 phase-specific, is not cytotoxic to cells other than leukemic lymphoblasts. Host (and other cells) can synthesize and replace asparagine that has been hydrolyzed by the drug; the lymphoblasts cannot, and so they are killed.

Azathioprine (b) is mainly used as an immunosuppressant and disease-modifying antirheumatic drug (DMARD) for such conditions as severe or refractory rheumatoid arthritis. It is usually used adjunctively with a corticosteroid. The most serious concerns with azathioprine therapy relate to bone marrow suppression. Recall, too, that azathioprine's metabolism (to mercaptopurine) is xanthine oxidase-dependent and so is inhibited by allopurinol or febuxostat, leading to an increased risk or severity of adverse effects.

Doxorubicin (c), whether administered as the standard or the liposomal formulation, tends to cause cardiotoxicity and bone marrow suppression as major toxicities. Methotrexate's (d) main toxicities, whether used for cancer or as a DMARD, tend to cause bone marrow suppression, pulmonary damage (infiltrates, fibrosis), and ulceration of the oral and gastrointestinal mucosae. Neurotoxicity (including dysfunction of the auditory nerves [Question 477]) is the main adverse effect of vinca alkaloids such as vincristine (e).

477. The answer is b. *(Brunton, pp 1326t, 1334. Katzung, pp 953-954.)* Cisplatin, which is sometimes classified along with traditional alkylating agents, is unique among all the common anticancer agents in terms of the relative incidence of hearing loss and nephrotoxicity.

You are correct in associating vincristine with hearing loss, but nephrotoxicity is very rare; in contrast, you may have recalled that methotrexate can cause nephrotoxicity, but it does not cause hearing loss, and it is indicated for a variety of cancers, but not ovarian.

Bleomycin's (a) main targeted toxicity is the lungs (pulmonary infiltrates, fibrosis, etc). Doxorubicin (c), as noted above, is cardiotoxic. The drug is mainly used for testicular carcinomas, squamous cell cancers, and lymphomas. 5-FU (d), a pyrimidine antimetabolite, is used for a variety of solid tumors. However, peripheral neuritis or neuropathy (and, especially, hearing loss) or renal damage are uncommon; rather, we are faced with a relatively high incidence of bone marrow suppression and oral and GI mucosal damage. Paclitaxel (e) is a microtubular stabilizing drug (and plant alkaloid). It is considered first-line for some patients with advanced ovarian cancer or non-small-cell lung cancers, causes dose-dependent bone marrow suppression and peripheral neuropathy, and a fairly high incidence of acute infusion-related hypersensitivity reactions (probably due to the vehicle in which the drug is delivered).

478. The answer is d. *(Brunton, pp 1440-1441. Katzung, p 581.)* Filgrastim, also known as granulocyte colony-stimulating factor (GCSF), enhances neutrophil production. One use, therefore, is to prevent neutropenia and infection associated with bone marrow depression from cancer chemotherapy. (Hint: Look at the generic name, filgrastim: *gra*nulocyte *stim*ulating.) The drug lacks antiemetic effects (a), potentiates the chemotherapeutic actions of no drug (thus b is incorrect), has no effect on doxorubicin-mediated cardiotoxicity (c), and does not stimulate growth or repair of the gastric mucosa (e).

479. The answer is e. *(Brunton, pp 690, 706, 1339-1340. Katzung, pp 631-632, 944-946, 975, 1090-1091.)* The main uses of MTX for conditions other than responsive cancers are management of rheumatoid arthritis (RA) and psoriasis. Doses and dosage schedules differ from those typically used for cancers. It is not used or approved for managing asthma (a), thyroid disorders (b), hyperuricemia or clinical gout (c), or myasthenia gravis (d; even though there is a strong autoimmune component to the etiology of myasthenia gravis).

MTX is one of many disease-modifying antirheumatic drugs (DMARDs), which are also called slow-acting antirheumatic drugs (SAARDs) because their onset of symptom relief is much slower than traditional NSAIDs (salicylates and other first-generation COX-1/-2 inhibitors, or second-generation/COX-2 inhibitors, ie, the "coxibs").

Nonetheless, although the onset is considered slow, meaningful symptom relief usually occurs with as little as 3 to 4 weeks of therapy—faster than the other DMARDs. (Several other DMARDs, including hydroxychloroquine and sulfasalazine, have no cancer-related uses.) All the potential side effects, adverse responses, and contraindications that apply to using MTX for cancer apply to the drug's use for RA or psoriasis.

480. The answer is e. *(Brunton, pp 708-709, 1015-1016, 1414.)* Hyperuricemia is associated with many cancers and is a common outcome of massive cell kills induced by chemotherapeutic drugs. The uric acid is derived from cellular purine degradation, eventually formed from hypoxanthine and xanthine *via* xanthine oxidase, the enzyme that is inhibited by allopurinol and the very new and largely similar alternative, febuxostat. Recall that renal damage (and other damage, such as gout) is due to uric acid's poor solubility in body fluids, especially at low pH.

Allopurinol and febuxostat have no effect on the P450 system or on cellular transitions from one phase of the cell cycle to another. There is no effect on DNA synthesis or repair (b), or any direct cytoprotective effect on myeloid or other tissues (d). Xanthine oxidase inhibitors do not potentiate any actions of nitrogen mustards (c).

Be sure to remember that the metabolic detoxification of azathioprine and its active metabolite 6-mercaptopurine (itself an anticancer drug) depends on xanthine oxidase. Inhibiting that enzyme with allopurinol or febuxostat, therefore, may increase (not decrease, answer a) the risk of toxicity to host cells.

481. The answer is e. *(Brunton, pp 708-709, 1015-1016, 1414. Katzung, pp 945t, 948-949.)* Mercaptopurine is a (thio)purine antimetabolite that is metabolically inactivated (detoxified) by xanthine oxidase. This purine degradation pathway in which xanthine oxidase participates not only leads to formation of uric acid, but also is important to reducing host cell toxicity to the thiopurines. Thus, concomitant use of allopurinol increases the risk of host cell toxicity. The same applies to the newest approved xanthine oxidase inhibitor, febuxostat. Note that azathioprine (an inhibitor of B and T lymphocyte proliferation, typically used as an immunosuppressant) is metabolized to mercaptopurine, which is used as an anticancer drug. As a result, azathioprine's metabolism is also inhibited by a xanthine oxidase inhibitor.

The metabolism of the other drugs listed is not xanthine oxidase–dependent, and so is not affected by allopurinol or febuxostat.

482. The answer is d. *(Brunton, p 1695. Katzung, pp 630-631, 1144t.)* Nephrotoxicity, or at least some clinically significant degree of renal dysfunction, occurs in about 8 of 10 patients receiving cyclosporine. It is typically dose-dependent and, particularly in renal transplant patients, could be due to either the drug (too much) or to rejection. Infection occurs about as often as renal dysfunction. Cyclosporine can cause hepatotoxicity, but the incidence is far lower than that of renal responses or infection. Cardiotoxicity, pulmonary toxicity, and hepatotoxicity also are extremely uncommon in response to cyclosporine, and so answers a, b, and c are incorrect). Blood pressure changes can occur, but with cyclosporine the change usually involves increased pressure (not reduced pressure, as mentioned in answer c), and it is common. Thromboembolism (e) due to cyclosporine is very rare.

Toxicology, Bioterrorism, and Chemical Warfare Agents

Alcohols, ethylene glycol
Antidotes for common drugs
Bioterrorism or chemical warfare agents
Heavy metals
Poisonings of unknown cause
Poisoning syndromes
Toxic gases

Questions

483. A farm worker in California is brought emergently, and dead on arrival, to a local emergency department. He had been exposed to an agricultural toxin. A coworker, who was not poisoned but was nearby right after the time of exposure, said, "He just started shaking bad, collapsed, and immediately stopped breathing. I didn't see anything else happening. He looked perfectly normal one minute, then he was just dead." Gross and microscopic examination of all the major organs at autopsy revealed no pathology. What is the most likely cause of this man's death?

a. Cholinesterase inhibitor insecticide, sprayed by a crop duster airplane
b. Kerosene from a barn heater, ingested
c. Long-term and cumulative cutaneous exposure to arsenic, today's exposure proving rapidly fatal
d. Petroleum distillates used to clean grease off machinery, inhaled
e. Strychnine, ingested

Questions 484 and 485

Here is an excerpt from a newspaper article entitled *Weed Users Chase High All the Way to the Hospital*. Use it to answer the next two questions.

"Teenagers seeking a hallucinogenic high from the seeds of a poisonous weed that now is in bloom are landing in hospitals across the country, police and health officials say… "Lunatic, crazy kids," says Dodge County, Wis., Sheriff Todd Nehls, whose deputies picked up three hallucinating teenagers in October….

"Poison centers last year recorded 975 incidents involving plants such as [the] weed…according to the American Association of Poison Control Centers' annual report.

"[The weed has]…pods that contain seeds that when eaten or brewed in a tea can cause severe hallucinations [delirium] and other reactions, including dry mouth, overheating [fever], agitation, [and] urinary retention… Some cannot urinate and need to have a catheter inserted… [Severe] overdoses can lead to seizures, coma, or death… Most people hospitalized after eating [the] weed have hallucinations that make them so erratic they are a danger to themselves…."

a. Acetylcholine
b. Amphetamine
c. Belladonna alkaloids
d. Bethanechol
e. Cocaine
f. Cyanide
g. Fluoxetine
h. Neostigmine
i. Opium
j. Phencyclidine (PCP)
k. Physostigmine
l. Strychnine

484. Which drug listed above causes signs and symptoms that are most similar to—indeed, virtually identical to—those described in the scenario?

485. Which drug would be most rational and most effective for treating the overdose?

486. Your patient developed acute poisoning as a result of inhaling cyanide gas in an industrial accident. In addition to providing symptomatic, supportive care and other appropriate interventions, administering which one of the following would most likely be effective as an adjunctive drug in treating the cyanide poisoning?

a. Ammonium chloride
b. Deferoxamine
c. Dimercaprol (British anti-Lewisite [BAL])
d. *N*-acetylcysteine
e. Pralidoxime
f. Sodium thiosulfate

487. A patient has taken a potentially lethal dose of acetaminophen. We begin administering repeated doses of oral *N*-acetylcysteine, which can be lifesaving in many such cases. What is the main mechanism by which this antidote exerts its beneficial effects?

a. Alkalinizes the urine to facilitate acetaminophen excretion
b. Causes metabolic acidosis to counteract metabolic alkalosis caused by a toxic acetaminophen metabolite
c. Inhibits P450 enzymes, thereby inhibiting formation of acetaminophen's toxic metabolite
d. Inhibits synthesis of superoxide anion radical and hydrogen peroxide
e. Is rich in sulfhydryl (–SH) groups that react with and inactivate the toxic metabolite

488. A mother calls to report that her 6-year-old child appears to have swallowed a large amount of an over-the-counter sleep aid about an hour ago. The product contained only one active drug, and knowing your drugs you suspect the poisoning is due to diphenhydramine. Assuming your reasoned guess about the cause of poisoning was correct, which of the following signs or symptoms would you expect to find, upon physical examination, to confirm your hunch?

a. Fever; clear lungs; absence of bowel sounds; urinary retention, dry, flushed skin; mydriasis and photophobia; bizarre behavior
b. Bradycardia and profuse diarrhea
c. Miosis with little/no papillary response to bright lights; spontaneous micturition; lack of response to painful stimuli
d. Hypothermia; bounding pulse; hypertension
e. Skeletal muscle weakness or paralysis; profound hypermotility of gut and bladder smooth muscle; bronchospasm

489. A patient presents in the emergency department with a drug overdose. Among other things, the physician correctly orders IV infusion of sodium bicarbonate to alkalinize the urine, which increases the toxin's elimination through pH-dependent inhibition of its tubular reabsorption and helps correct the combined metabolic and respiratory acidosis it caused. Which one of the following drugs most likely caused the toxicity?

a. Amphetamine
b. Aspirin (acetylsalicylic acid)
c. Cocaine
d. Morphine
e. Phencyclidine (PCP)

490. A 3-year-old girl ingests 30 tablets of aspirin, 325 mg each. We've gotten her to the emergency department within 30 minutes of the poisoning. Which one of the following drugs would be the most rational and hopefully effective to administer as part of the initial treatment plan for what otherwise could have a fatal outcome?

a. Activated charcoal
b. Deferoxamine
c. Dimercaprol
d. *N*-acetylcysteine
e. Penicillamine

491. A 50-year-old man has been consuming large amounts of ethanol on an almost daily basis for many years. One day, unable to find any ethanol, he ingests a large amount of methanol (wood alcohol) that he had bought for his camp lantern. Which of the following is the most likely consequence of his methanol poisoning?

a. Atrioventricular conduction defect (block)
b. Blindness
c. Bronchospasm
d. Delirium tremens
e. Metabolic alkalosis

492. A 15-year-old adolescent attempts suicide with a liquid that he found in his parents' greenhouse. His dad used it to get rid of "varmints" around the yard. The toxin causes intense abdominal pain, skeletal muscle cramps, projectile vomiting, and severe diarrhea that lead to fluid and electrolyte imbalances, hypotension, and difficulty swallowing. On examination he is found to be volume-depleted and is showing signs of a reduced level of consciousness. His breath smells "metallic." Which of the following probably accounts for these symptoms?

a. Arsenic
b. Cadmium
c. Iron
d. Lead
e. Zinc

493. A 5-year-old boy consumed a liquid from a container in the family garage. He presents with central nervous system (CNS) depression, obtunded reflexes, and ventilatory depression. A blood sample indicates profound metabolic acidosis and an anion gap. A check of the urine reveals crystals that are presumed to be oxalate. What is the most likely cause of the poisoning?

a. A halogenated hydrocarbon from a can of spray paint
b. An insecticide
c. Ethylene glycol
d. Gasoline
e. Paint thinner

494. A 22-year-old is brought to the emergency department by a friend. They had been at a bar for about an hour, and then the patient suddenly became drowsy but was still conscious. She fell and cut her head, and has little difficulty feeling the pain from the trauma. Her ventilatory rate and depth are depressed, but not to a worrisome degree. Her patellar reflexes are blunted and she is ataxic. She responds slowly to questions but is unable to recall anything that happened after arriving at the bar and sipping her first (and last) adult beverage. Her friend stated that she had only one Cosmopolitan and hadn't been drinking before they went out. With what was this patient's drink most likely "spiked?"

a. A barbiturate
b. A benzodiazepine
c. An opioid
d. Chloral hydrate
e. Cocaine
f. Pure (grain) alcohol

495. Let's assume the profoundly CNS-depressed patient in the previous question indeed was overdosed with a benzodiazepine. Which drug is most likely to be effective, indeed would be a preferred pharmacologic antidote, if that were the case?

a. Amphetamine
b. Flumazenil
c. Methylphenidate
d. Naltrexone
e. Physostigmine

496. Recent occupational health studies in several heavily populated urban areas have revealed an astonishingly large number of homes that have lead-based paint and children living in them. However, a number of environmental poisons that could lead to acute or chronic poisoning have also been found there. Which signs and symptoms would be consistent with chronic exposure to toxic levels of inorganic lead?

a. Anorexia and weight loss; weakness, especially of extensor muscles (eg, wrist drop); recurrent abdominal pain
b. Gingivitis, discolored gums, loosened teeth, or stomatitis; tremor of the extremities; swollen parotid or other salivary glands
c. Hallucinations, insomnia, headache, generalized CNS irritability
d. Hyperventilation in response to metabolic acidosis; hypotension; abdominal pain, diarrhea, brown or bloody vomitus; pallor or cyanosis
e. Severe, watery diarrhea; garlicky or metallic breath; encephalopathy, hypovolemia and hypotension

497. Lab tests conducted by the local health department are positive for chronic lead exposure in a child. Lead levels are significantly elevated, but symptoms fortunately are mild and not at all imminently life-threatening. What is the most appropriate antidote for reducing the child's body load of lead?

a. Ca-Na_2-EDTA
b. Deferoxamine
c. Dimercaprol
d. *N*-acetylcysteine
e. Penicillamine
f. Succimer

498. Not long ago, several patients (and a rather shady health care "provider" who is now incarcerated) seeking "relief" from facial wrinkles nearly died because they received injections of botulinum toxin that was improperly obtained and inadequately diluted. Which is a correct characteristic, finding, or mechanism associated with this toxin?

a. Complete failure of all cholinergic neurotransmission
b. Favorable response to administration of pralidoxime
c. Impairment of parasympathetic, but not sympathetic, nervous system activation
d. Massive overstimulation of all structures having muscarinic cholinergic receptors
e. Selective paralysis of skeletal muscle

499. A terrorist drops a vial of "nerve gas" into a crowded subway at rush hour. The patients are brought to the nearest emergency centers and are given atropine. Which effect of the nerve gas will persist after giving the atropine?

a. Bradycardia
b. Bronchospasm
c. Excessive lacrimal, mucus, sweat, and salivary secretions
d. GI hypermotility, fluid and electrolyte loss from profuse diarrhea
e. Skeletal muscle hyperfunction or paralysis

500. A neighbor calls you for advice and help. She knows you are not a veterinary student, but since you're going to be a physician soon she figures you know everything. Her pet puppy, Pookie, a precocious Pekingese, has eaten a large amount of rodent (rat and mouse) poison. She's panicked and pleads to know if the precious pooch is poisoned. The rodenticide indeed contains a powerful poison intended to kill rats and mice, but it can do the same to any other animals that have ingested it too, including humans. What is the most likely toxic ingredient in these rodenticides, and probably will cause poor Pookie pronounced problems?

a. Amphetamine–cocaine combination
b. Morphine
c. Pancuronium (or a similar curare-like neuromuscular blocker)
d. Succinylcholine
e. Warfarin

Toxicology, Bioterrorism, and Chemical Warfare Agents

Answers

483. The answer is e. *(Brunton, pp 404-405. Katzung, pp 11t, 359t.)* Strychnine is a convulsant, and death from exposure is just as described in the question. The mechanism involves strychnine's ability to antagonize the neuronal-inhibitory effects of glycine, which is an important neurotransmitter, particularly in the spinal cord. These spinal cord receptors are sometimes called strychnine-sensitive receptors. They are coupled to a chloride channel, and in the presence of strychnine the motor neurons become hyperpolarized. The ultimate effect is a disinhibition of (primarily) skeletal motor neurons; that rapidly leads to generalized convulsions (he just started shaking bad) and soon thereafter ventilatory failure and death (stopped breathing, didn't see anything else happening). There is no antidote.

Cholinesterase inhibitors (a), typically used in agriculture as insecticides, ultimately can prove fatal. However, depending on which inhibitor is involved, and depending on the exposure route (oral, cutaneous, pulmonary) the time-course leading to death can be up to several (or many) minutes or hours. Exposure is accompanied, and death is preceded, by all the expected skeletal muscle-stimulating (N_M) and peripheral muscarinic activating effects (heart, gut, airways, exocrine secretions) that are consistent with what amounts to peripheral "ACh excess." Depending on the causative agent, CNS/spinal cord manifestations may occur and be prominent too.

As a generalization, kerosene (b) and other petroleum distillates (d; found in many solvents/cleaners/degreasers, including those for household use) tend to affect multiple organ systems, including: the lungs (pulmonary complications are the most common and include alveolar hemorrhage, alveolar edema and inflammation, and aspiration that contributes further to pneumonitis); heart (cardiomyopathy from chronic exposure, catecholamine-enhanced arrhythmias mainly with acute poisoning); brain (medullary stimulation, then depression; remember that most of these petroleum-based products are highly lipid soluble and enter the CNS readily); gut (typically a painful burning sensation and frequent vomiting if the toxin is ingested); liver (chronic hepatotoxicity with centrolobular necrosis, usually caused by free radical-mediated peroxidation of membrane lipids); and kidneys (renal tubular necrosis and metabolic acidosis). Long-term exposure can also cause aplastic anemia, myelomas, and leukemias (mainly acute myelogenous).

Arsenic toxicity (c) and its management are described in the answer to Question 492. The clinical presentation is much different than the sudden, convulsive death described here. You should also recall that arsenic, too, is widely used as a pesticide and for other pest- and plant-disease control applications.

Note: Before we appreciated the extreme toxicity of strychnine, many decades ago, the drug was used "therapeutically," for humans, as a stimulant, a laxative, and a remedy for a host of other common but ordinarily innocuous GI maladies. Not any more, of course. However, this deadly poison is still readily available in pesticides (mainly those used to kill pesky birds). According to a quick web search, in California alone more than half a ton of strychnine was used agriculturally a mere two to three years ago.

484. The answer is c. *(Brunton, p 195. Katzung, p 122.)* The weed in question is Jimson Weed, also known as stinkweed, locoweed, and a few other names. The signs and symptoms described in the article are among the classic ones associated with severe atropine (or, in general, antimuscarinic drug) poisoning—the original pharmacologic source being alkaloids isolated from various species of *Belladonna*. No other drug listed causes responses that even come close to these in terms of the peripheral autonomic responses described above.

485. The answer is k. *(Brunton, p 195. Katzung, p 122.)* "Atropine poisoning," or the anticholinergic syndrome caused by a host of drugs and by the plants noted in the question, is treated symptomatically and supportively and with administration of physostigmine. Physostigmine is basically the only clinically useful AChE inhibitor that gets into the brain, a major target of atropine/antimuscarinic poisoning. That is because it lacks the quaternary structure that nearly all the other common alternatives possess. And so, since it is not charged, it can cross the blood-brain barrier readily to reverse the CNS consequences of the poisoning—not just those in the periphery, where the quaternary cholinesterase inhibitors work.

Alternatives such as neostigmine, pyridostigmine, and others, will combat peripheral effects of atropine poisoning, just as physostigmine will. Unfortunately, some of the CNS manifestations (eg, severe fever, leading to seizures) contribute greatly to the morbidity and mortality associated with high doses of antimuscarinics, and the quaternary agents simply will not combat them in the CNS.

You won't encounter too many patients overdosed on atropine itself, but you'll see many poisoned with older antihistamines (eg, diphenhydramine); some of the centrally acting antimuscarinics that are used for parkinsonism (eg, benztropine and trihexyphenidyl); scopolamine (used for motion sickness); and most of the phenothiazine antipsychotics (eg, chlorpromazine). Owing to the often strong antimuscarinic side effects of these drugs, treating overdoses of most of them probably will involve managing what amounts to "atropine poisoning"—and many other problems too.

Note: Older antidepressants—for example, the tricyclics such as amitriptyline and imipramine—have strong antimuscarinic actions. Physostigmine can be used adjunctively, as it would be for most cases of antimuscarinic poisoning. However, because of the multiplicity of tricyclic effects (including blockade of neuronal reuptake of norepinephrine and dopamine in the periphery and in the CNS), and a generally complicated clinical picture, cholinesterase inhibitors may not work as well as they would in other situations, and they certainly will not be a panacea for the toxicity.

486. The answer is f. *(Brunton, p 885. Katzung, pp 196, 1022-1023.)* Whether cyanide poisoning occurs from leakage of gas, the combustion of plastics, nitroprusside overdoses, or other causes, management includes many common elements. Cyanide reacts with Fe(III) in mitochondrial cytochrome oxidase, inhibiting oxidative phosphorylation. The shift in metabolism from aerobic metabolism to glycolysis soon leads not only to ATP depletion, but also to severe lactic (anion gap) acidosis as the glycolytic end-product accumulates.

We manage cyanide poisoning first by dealing with the high reactivity of CN^- with Fe(II) in hemoglobin and the subsequent formation of Fe(III) hemoglobin. We do that by administering sodium nitrite (IV) to regenerate active cytochromes and oxidize hemoglobin to the more cyanide-reactive methemoglobin (forming cyanmethemoglobin). (Amyl nitrate can be administered by inhalation until venous access is established and sodium nitrite and sodium thiosulfate can be given.) Once the nitrite is on board we administer sodium thiosulfate IV. Cyanide normally reacts with endogenous thiosulfate, and the hepatic enzyme rhodanese catalyzes the formation of relatively less toxic and more easily excreted thiocyanate. In cyanide poisoning endogenous thiosulfate stores are quickly depleted, so this provides the basis for infusing sodium thiosulfate (f, the correct answer) to lower cyanmethemoglobin levels. In cases of severe methemoglobinemia, we can also give methylene blue intravenously. (Note that large doses of inorganic nitrites can be intrinsically toxic as a result of methemoglobin formation. However, in the context of cyanide poisoning we can capitalize on the reactivity of otherwise toxic inorganic nitrite, in conjunction with thiosulfate administration, to help treat an otherwise fatal toxic scenario.)

Ammonium chloride (a) would be ineffective and may actually make matters worse by exacerbating metabolic acidosis. Deferoxamine (b), an iron chelator, would be of no benefit, nor would dimercaprol (c), a heavy metal (mainly lead) chelator. *N*-acetylcysteine (d), routinely used as an antidote for acetaminophen poisoning, would not alleviate or shorten signs and symptoms in cyanide poisoning. Pralidoxime (e) is a cholinesterase "reactivator" that is used for poisoning with organophosphate insecticides, nerve gases (sarin, soman), or other drugs that cause profound and "irreversible" inactivation of acetylcholinesterase.

487. The answer is e. *(Brunton, pp 82-83, 693-694, 1741. Katzung, p 1020.)* We give *N*-acetylcysteine for acetaminophen poisoning and use it because it is a sulfhydryl-rich drug that, if given soon enough and properly enough, can prevent hepatic necrosis. At safe blood levels, the major pathways of acetaminophen elimination involve glucuronidation and sulfation. When these pathways are overwhelmed, as occurs with acetaminophen poisoning, a cytochrome P450–dependent pathway attempts to handle the metabolic load. The active toxic metabolite, *N*-acetyl-benzoqinoneimine, is formed in levels that exceed the ability of intrinsic sulfhydryl compounds to inactivate it. So long as ample hepatocyte stores of glutathione (a –SH compound) are available, cytotoxicity will not occur. However, severe poisoning depletes –SH stores, and so the hepatotoxic metabolite attacks key cellular macromolecules. That leads to hepatic necrosis.

N-acetylcysteine acts as a substitute for endogenous glutathione to react with the toxic metabolite, thereby sparing –SH groups on key hepatocyte macromolecules.

Alkalinization of the urine is of no benefit with acetaminophen poisoning, as it can be with severe salicylate poisoning (because raising urine pH reduces tubular reabsorption of salicylate and increases its excretion). Moreover, *N*-acetylcysteine does not directly change urine pH. Superoxide anion radical, or hydrogen peroxide, is not directly involved in the cytotoxicity (d).

See the answer to Question 317, for a summary of the "stages" of acetaminophen poisoning.

488. The answer is a. *(Brunton, pp 198, 637-642. Katzung, p 122.)* Most OTC sleep aids contain a first-generation antihistamine (sedating agent, almost always an ethanolamine, either diphenhydramine or the very similar drug, doxylamine). The preponderant signs and symptoms of toxicity arise not from any histamine receptor-blocking activity, but from intense antimuscarinic (atropine-like) effects, plus dose-dependent CNS depression that ultimately (and early on, in children) can lead to seizures. The signs and symptoms of this "anticholinergic syndrome" include many, if not all, that you will see in "atropine poisoning." Aside from symptomatic and supportive care, including the use of traditional drugs for status epilepticus, physostigmine (the nonquaternary, centrally and peripherally acting acetylcholinesterase inhibitor) may be lifesaving. It will certainly help reverse many of the central and peripheral signs and symptoms of the overdose.

489. The answer is b. *(Brunton, pp 686, 691-692, 1749-1750. Katzung, pp 624, 1021.)* Alkalinizing the urine interferes with the renal tubular reabsorption of organic acids (such as aspirin and phenobarbital) by increasing the ionized form of the drug in the urine (per the Henderson-Hasselbach equation). This increases their net renal excretion. Conversely, excretion of organic bases (such as amphetamine, cocaine, phencyclidine, and morphine) would be reduced by alkalinizing the urine.

Note that another consequence of severe aspirin (salicylate) toxicity is a combined metabolic plus respiratory acidosis. So in addition to enhancing urinary excretion of salicylate, the administration of sodium bicarbonate also tends to counteract the fall of blood pH. See the answer explanation for Question 330 for more information on the sequence of events that occur with a potentially lethal overdose of aspirin.

490. The answer is a. *(Brunton, pp 691-692, 1746-1749. Katzung, p 1018.)* Activated charcoal, a fine, black, powder with a high adsorptive capacity, is considered to be a valuable agent in the treatment of many kinds of oral drug poisonings—primarily if administered early on and then removed by gastric lavage. Drugs that are well adsorbed by activated charcoal include primaquine, propoxyphene, dextroamphetamine, chlorpheniramine, phenobarbital, carbamazepine, digoxin, and aspirin. Mineral acids, alkalis, tolbutamide, and other drugs that are insoluble in acidic aqueous solution are not well adsorbed.

Deferoxamine (b), dimercaprol (c; also known as BAL, or British anti-Lewisite), and penicillamine (e) are polyvalent cation chelators (iron, lead, copper) and play no role in managing aspirin (salicylate) poisoning, nor poisoning with any substances other than the metals they chelate. *N*-Acetylcysteine (d) is the preferred antidote for acetaminophen overdoses (Question 334).

Note: The term adsorb—means to bind—is decidedly different from the more common pharmacologic/therapeutic term absorb.

491. The answer is b. *(Brunton, p 600. Katzung, p 1024.)* Methanol is metabolized by the same enzymes that metabolize ethanol, but the products are different: formaldehyde and formic acid in the case of methanol. Headache, vertigo, vomiting, abdominal pain, dyspnea, and blurred vision can occur from accumulation of these metabolic intermediates. However, the most dangerous (or at least permanently disabling) consequence in severe cases is hyperemia of the optic disc, which can lead to blindness. The rationale for administering ethanol to treat methanol poisoning is fairly simple. Ethanol has a high affinity for alcohol and aldehyde dehydrogenases and competes as a substrate for those enzymes, reducing metabolism of methanol to its more toxic products. Important adjunctive treatments include hemodialysis to enhance removal of methanol and its products; and administration of systemic alkalinizing salts (eg, sodium bicarbonate) to counteract metabolic acidosis. Administration of systemic acidifying substances such as ascorbic acid would aggravate the condition.

492. The answer is a. *(Brunton, pp 1763-1766. Katzung, pp 1000t, 1003-1005.)* Arsenic is a constituent of fungicides, herbicides, and pesticides. Symptoms of acute toxicity include tightness in the throat, difficulty in swallowing, and stomach pains. Projectile vomiting and severe diarrhea can lead to hypovolemic shock, significant electrolyte derangements, and death. Chronic poisoning may cause peripheral neuritis, anemia, skin keratosis, and capillary dilation leading to hypotension. Dimercaprol (British anti-Lewisite [BAL]) is the main antidote used for arsenic poisoning.

Note: If dimercaprol is also known as *anti*-Lewisite, what is Lewisite? It is an obsolete organic arsencial (arsenic-containing substance, specifically chlorovinyl dichloroarsine—don't memorize that!) developed as a chemical warfare agent in World War II. Arsenic reacts and forms chelates with sulfhydryl moieties on various substances, including many enzymes involved in essential metabolic reactions. It is a vesicant (causes blistering) that targets many body tissues, but exerts its main toxic effects in the lungs when inhaled. Dimercaprol is a relatively simple molecule with two sulfhydryl groups in its structure. It reacts with the Lewisite, chelating it and thereby reducing attack on and inactivation of cellular –SH-rich enzymes.

493. The answer is c. *(Brunton, p 1749. Katzung, p 1024.)* The tip-off to the correct answer should come from the metabolic acidosis, the anion gap (= $[Na^+] - [HCO_3^- + Cl^-]$), and the oxalate crystals in the urine. Ethylene glycol (ordinary antifreeze) forms, among other metabolites, glycolic, hippuric, and oxalic acids. It is the latter that tends to crystallize in the renal tubules, which may lead to acute renal failure. Ethylene glycol is basically an alcohol, and as with an overdose of ethanol can cause CNS depression and an overall state of inebriation. None of the other agents listed tend to cause a similar poisoning syndrome.

Note: The signs and symptoms of methanol poisoning reflect, in some ways (eg, CNS depression, stupor) those of ethylene glycol or ethanol. However methanol's main toxicity arises from its metabolism to formic acid, the consequences of which can lead to permanent blindness. Whether the poisoning is from ethylene glycol or methanol, treatment includes administration of ethanol; it will be preferentially metabolized by alcohol dehydrogenase, reducing the metabolism of the toxin to its cytotoxic products.

494. The answer is b. *(Brunton, pp 404-412. Katzung, pp 380, 382-383.)* Arguably the most important tip-off in this presentation is the antegrade amnesia, which (among other things) is rather uniquely associated with benzodiazepines. The most likely benzodiazepine used in this scenario was rohypnol (flunitrazepam, better known as "roofies" on the street and by those who use it as a date-rape drug).

Unless this patient were a very atypical responder, it is unlikely that any of the other CNS depressants—a barbiturate, an opioid, chloral hydrate—would cause the same responses. She's had one drink yet still feels pain from her head gash. She apparently hasn't had enough alcohol to be so obtunded that she doesn't feel pain, and a barbiturate is likely to enhance the sensation of pain (hyperalgesic effect). Chloral hydrate is still used medically, mainly as a sedative for children, although its use is declining dramatically. It indeed causes powerful CNS depressants when used in combination with just a little alcohol: chloral hydrate has been known for years as "knock-out drops" and the combination with alcohol has been called a "Mickey Finn." However, chloral hydrate is not nearly as readily available as the illicit benzodiazepines; it does not cause antegrade amnesia (important to the perpetrator, because he or she anticipates no recall of what happened by the victim), but it is not readily available, and it simply doesn't have the "reputation" as a preferred date-rape drug among those who use such drugs.

495. The answer is b. *(Brunton, pp 402-403. Katzung, pp 382-383.)* Flumazenil is the specific benzodiazepine receptor antagonist, and it is both specific and almost always effective for excessive effects of any benzodiazepine. It's tempting to use a CNS stimulant (a, amphetamines; or c, methylphenidate) to overcome the effects of any CNS depressant. It may help, but more likely the outcome of giving a stimulant is excessive effects manifest as seizures and unwanted cardiovascular stimulatory effects. Naltrexone, like naloxone, specifically blocks opioid receptors and will be of no benefit to this poisoned patient. Some benzodiazepines do cause antimuscarinic effects, but weakly. For that reason, and others, physostigmine (or any other AChE inhibitor) would not at all be an effective or problem-free drug to give.

496. The answer is a. *(Brunton, pp 1754-1758. Katzung, pp 999-1003.)* The presentation of chronic lead exposure, as from being exposed to (or even eating) older lead-based paints, differs from the typical presentation of acute organic lead poisoning (answer c). Answer b, with the predominant gingival/head/neck signs and symptoms, is typical of chronic or acute mercury intoxication. Answer d, with the hyperventilation, GI disturbances (including discolored vomitus) and pallor, is what you are likely to encounter in acute iron poisoning (as from a consuming ferrous sulfate supplements in large doses). A characteristic breath (garlicky or metallic), profuse diarrhea, encephalopathy, and hypotension (answer e) are typical of acute inorganic arsenic poisoning. Knowing more about the patient's history and environment will help immensely in sorting out what the "most likely" cause of intoxication is.

497. The answer is f. *(Brunton, pp 1754-1758. Katzung, pp 999-1003, 1008-1009.)* Succimer (a more polar salt of dimercaprol; British anti-Lewisite [BAL]) would be the choice, given the proof of lead poisoning, the lack of acute symptoms, and the fact that our patient is a child. Succimer is easy to give orally and is tolerated far better than the alternatives: Ca-Na_2-EDTA (a), penicillamine (e; traditionally viewed as a copper chelator, but it also chelates lead), or dimercaprol (c) itself. Although the heavy metal chelation profiles for succimer are not drastically different from those of dimercaprol, the fact that succimer is more polar (and, therefore, less likely to enter cells) seems to account for far fewer and milder side effects than those of dimercaprol (especially with respect to risks of tachycardia and hypertension). *N*-acetylcysteine (d), as noted elsewhere, is the drug of choice for acetaminophen poisoning. It has no ability to chelate lead or other cations.

498. The answer is a. *(Brunton, pp 151-152, 171. Katzung, pp 81-82, 465.)* Botulinus (botulinum) toxin prevents release of acetylcholine (from storage vesicles) by virtually all cholinergic nerves. Thus, there is no activation of any cholinergic receptors, whether nicotinic or muscarinic. Noteworthy findings, then, include an inability to activate all postganglionic neurons (sympathetic and parasympathetic), no physiologic release of epinephrine from the adrenal medulla, and flaccid skeletal muscle paralysis due to failure of ACh release from motor nerves. The cause of death is ventilatory failure because the intercostal muscles and diaphragm are nonfunctional.

Pralidoxime is a cholinesterase reactivator, an antidote and adjunct (along with atropine) for poisonings with "irreversible" cholinesterase inhibitors such as soman, sarin, VX ("nerve gases"), and many organophosphorus insecticides. Because no ACh is being released in botulinus poisoning, "reactivation" of the enzyme that normally metabolizes the neurotransmitter is irrelevant (and ineffective).

499. The answer is e. *(Brunton, pp 189-190, 195-197, 209-211. Katzung, p 104.)* Most of the adverse responses to nerve gases (irreversible ACh esterase inhibitors such as soman and sarin) are due to a build-up of ACh at muscarinic receptors (ie, ACh released from postganglionic parasympathetic nerves or sympathetic/cholinergic nerves innervating sweat glands). Those responses will be attenuated by atropine, because it is a highly specific competitive muscarinic antagonist. However, skeletal muscle stimulation (or eventual paralysis) involves nicotinic receptor activation. That will not be affected by atropine, and unless other supportive measures are provided, the patient is likely to die from ventilatory arrest/apnea.

500. The answer is e. *(Brunton, pp 1475-1479. Katzung, pp 594-597.)* No, this is not a frivolous question, nor one intended for veterinarians, your local pest control expert, or even Ace Ventura, Pet Detective. Someday you may be working in an emergency department or a poison center, so you need to know. The critters that eat the rodenticide ultimately bleed to death from a warfarin overdose. When treating such poisonings in humans or poisoned pets, the approach is the same as with therapeutic warfarin: administer vitamin K (orally or parenterally, whichever is indicated), and provide other symptomatic and supportive measures. Amphetamine or cocaine, alone or in combination (a), as well as morphine (b), are controlled substances with high potential for dependence and abuse. Such substances simply wouldn't be permitted in products that virtually anyone could obtain at their local home care or hardware store. What about succinylcholine (d)? It's ineffective when ingested; it has to be injected. The same applies to tubocurarine, pancuronium (c), and all the other "curoniums" or "curines." (You'll remember that some peoples indigenous to the Amazon killed their prey with curare-tipped darts. And they ate that curare-laced meat with absolutely no ill effects from the drug.)

Appendix A

Drug Interactions Involving the P450 System

SELECTED CLINICALLY RELEVANT DRUG-DRUG METABOLISM INTERACTIONS INVOLVING THE CYTOCHROME P450 (CYP) SYSTEM: SUBSTRATES, INDUCERS, AND INHIBITORS		
	CYP1A2	
Substrates	**Inducers**	**Inhibitors**
Acetaminophen, amitriptyline, clomipramine, clozapine, desipramine, fluvoxamine, haloperidol, imipramine, methadone, ropinirole, tacrine, theophylline, warfarin	Carbamazepine, charcoal-broiled foods, phenobarbital, phenytoin, primidone, rifampin, ritonavir, tobacco smoke (smoking), St. John's wort	Cimetidine, ciprofloxacin, clarithromycin, erythromycin, fluvoxamine, isoniazid, nalidixic acid, oral contraceptives (estrogen), troleandomycin, zileuton[a]
	CYP2C9	
Substrates	**Inducers**	**Inhibitors**
Celecoxib, diazepam, losartan, phenytoin, warfarin	Carbamazepine, phenobarbital, phenytoin, primidone, rifampin, ritonavir, St. John's wort	Amiodarone, chloramphenicol,[a] cimetidine, fluconazole, fluoxetine, fluvoxamine, isoniazid, metronidazole, zafirlukast

(*Continued*)

SELECTED CLINICALLY RELEVANT DRUG-DRUG METABOLISM INTERACTIONS INVOLVING THE CYTOCHROME P450 (CYP) SYSTEM: SUBSTRATES, INDUCERS, AND INHIBITORS (CONTINUED)

CYP2C19		
Substrates	**Inducers**	**Inhibitors**
Diazepam, phenytoin, propranolol, thioridazine	Carbamazepine, phenobarbital, phenytoin	Fluconazole, fluoxetine, fluvoxamine, modafinil, omeprazole, topiramate

CYP2D6		
Substrates	**Inducers**	**Inhibitors**
Amitriptyline, clozapine, codeine, desipramine dextromethorphan, donepezil, doxepin, duloxetine, fentanyl, flecainide, haloperidol, hydrocodone, imipramine, meperidine, methadone, nortriptyline, oxycodone, propafenone, propoxyphene, thioridazine, tramadol, trazodone	None with documented clinical relevance	Amiodarone, cimetidine, duloxetine, paroxetine, propranolol, quinidine, ritonavir, sertraline

CYP3A4[b]		
Substrates	**Inducers**	**Inhibitors**
Acetaminophen, alfentanil, alprazolam, amlodipine, atorvastatin, busulfan, carbamazepine, cisapride, clarithromycin, colchicine, cyclosporine, dihydroergotamine, disopyramide,	Carbamazepine, efavirenz, ethosuximide, garlic, macrolide antibiotics, modafinil, nevirapine,	Amiodarone, cimetidine, clarithromycin, cyclosporine, diltiazem, erythromycin, fluconazole,

SELECTED CLINICALLY RELEVANT DRUG-DRUG METABOLISM INTERACTIONS INVOLVING THE CYTOCHROME P450 (CYP) SYSTEM: SUBSTRATES, INDUCERS, AND INHIBITORS (CONTINUED)

CYP3A4[b]		
Substrates	**Inducers**	**Inhibitors**
doxorubicin, dronabinol, eplerenone, ergotamine, erythromycin, estrogens, ethosuximide, etoposide, felodipine, fentanyl, fluticasone, indinavir, isradipine, itraconazole, ketoconazole, lidocaine, lovastatin, methadone, midazolam, nefazodone, nicardipine, nifedipine, nimodipine, nisoldipine, ondansetron, oral contraceptives (estrogen), paclitaxel, pimozide, quinidine, rifabutin, ritonavir, saquinavir, sertraline, sildenafil, simvastatin, sirolimus, tadalafil, tamoxifen, tolterodine, trazodone, triazolam, vardenafil, verapamil, vinca alkaloids, warfarin	oxcarbazepine, phenobarbital, pioglitazone, phenytoin, primidone, rifabutin, rifampin, ritonavir St. John's wort	fluvoxamine, grapefruit, indinavir, isoniazid, itraconazole, ketoconazole, Seville (blood, or bitter) oranges, troleandomycin

[a]No longer available in the United States.
[b]CYP3A5 has substrate, inducer, inhibitor profiles similar to those noted for CYP3A4, but is usually less active in terms of its metabolic roles.
(Modified, with permission, from BG Katzung, SB Masters, AJ Trevor. Basic and Clinical Pharmacology, *11th ed. McGraw-Hill; 2009: Table 4-2, p 58.)*

Appendix B

Common Serum Chemistries (Normal Values)

Albumin	3.5-4.8 g/dL
Bicarbonate [HCO_3^-]	20-30 mEq/L
Blood gases (arterial, whole blood)	
pH	7.35-7.45
p_{O_2}	80-105 mm Hg
p_{CO_2}	34-45 mm Hg
Calcium	
Total	9.0-10.3 mg/dL
Free	4.5-5.0 mg/dL
Carbon dioxide content (bicarbonate)	20-30 mEq/L
Chloride	95-105 mEq/L
Creatinine	
Male	0.8-1.3 mg/dL
Female	0.6-1.1 mg/dL
Glucose (fasting, plasma)	65-110 mg/dL
Magnesium	1.7-2.7 mg/dL (1.4-2.3 mEq/L)
Osmolality	280-290 mOsm/kg water
Phosphorus (inorganic)	2.5-4.5 mg/dL
Potassium	3.5-4.5 mEq/L
Protein (total)	6.5-8.5 g/dL
Sodium	135-145 mEq/L
Urea nitrogen (BUN)	8-25 mg/dL

Appendix C

Web Sites for More Information

Most texts that have been published in the last few years, and many that will be published, have a variety of on-line resources that are well worth a look. These are usually "free," but of course that usually means they're free if you purchased the book on which the web site is based.

However, there are many other sites where you can get good information (and lots more where the information you get is sketchy or of dubious accuracy or objectivity, at best). Access to some sites is free, but others require payment. Here are a selected few that I visit frequently, and believe are worth your time and trust. I've listed them alphabetically.

Drug Facts and Comparisons (http://www.factsandcomparisons.com/). This is usually my go-to web site for all the need-to-know information about drugs and drug products, including drug-drug interactions. The site provides excellent summary tables about all sorts of things pharmacologic and therapeutic, and in a way that will help you glean what's important. Access to the information is not free. However, your school should have a site license for access; if they don't, pester the appropriate administrative person to buy one. After all, look at how much tuition you're paying!

FDA (Food and Drug Administration) (http://www.fda.gov). The FDA has a great (and free!) site for all things medical, not just drugs. Some parts are targeted to the public; others are for health care professionals. You can stay on top of latest drug or device approvals, concerns, warnings, or recalls, and get much more information that ultimately will be of interest and importance to you.

One part of the web site, MedWatch (http://www.fda.gov/medwatch) is a must-see, especially once you hit the wards. The information there will keep you up-to-date on the latest drug safety concerns, recalls, and so on. You can subscribe, for free, to get personal e-mails about the very latest concerns and warnings. That's important to you as a future practitioner and caregiver. (And once you hit the wards it will give you current and important information that you can casually mention to your clinical team—or the attending who gives you your clerkship grade—showing that you're really on top of things.)

The Medical Letter (http://www.medicalletter.com/). This is another excellent web site that will keep you up to date. One important and rather unique facet of The Medical Letter's updates is an unbiased look at, for example, whether a new drug is any better or safer than older alternatives. The publisher frequently provides excellent tables that compare, for example, costs of otherwise similar and alternative drugs; summaries of recommended drugs for a particular condition, and much more.

The Medical Letter also publishes "*Treatment Guidelines from the Medical Letter*," which collects and presents in a concise and unbiased way key information usually derived from prior Medical Letter issues. Access to The Medical Letter requires a subscription (and you can also subscribe to snail-mail updates). Here, too, see if your school has a site license, and if they don't urge them to get one.

Prescriber's Letter (http://www.prescribersletter.com/). This is another web site for which you'll either have to pay, or pester your med ed dean or medical library folks to get a site license. Prescriber's Letter keeps you updated with new and practical information on the latest drugs and drug therapies in just about any area you might find of interest. It is objective and unbiased, and excels (in my opinion) in terms of debunking myths about new drugs or therapies, and giving you a decent "heads up" about drug-related issues that are likely to be important to you. You'll get relevant information much sooner with Prescriber's Letter than with just about any other web site I've visited. With a subscription you can access all sorts of good information about drugs, and be assured that you're not getting anything but current and important information.

RxList (http://www.rxlist.com/). This is another comprehensive site where you can find abundant, current, and objective information about drugs. You can also get interesting (if not important) information about, for example, the "most prescribed drugs," the latest news, and so on. All the information on rxlist.com is free.

Index

N

T

Notes

Notes